MEDICAL
INTELLIGENCE
UNIT

BREAST CANCER SCREENING

Ismail Jatoi, M.D., Ph.D., FACS

Assistant Professor of Surgery
Uniformed Services University of the Health Sciences
Bethesda, Maryland, U.S.A.
and
Brooke Army Medical Center
Fort Sam Houston, Texas, U.S.A.

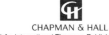

CHAPMAN & HALL
I⊕P An International Thomson Publishing Company

New York • Albany • Bonn • Boston • Cincinnati • Detroit • London • Madrid • Melbourne •
Mexico City • Pacific Grove • Paris • San Francisco • Singapore • Tokyo • Toronto • Washington

AUSTIN, TEXAS
U.S.A.

MEDICAL INTELLIGENCE UNIT
BREAST CANCER SCREENING
LANDES BIOSCIENCE
Austin, Texas, U.S.A.

Please address all inquiries to the Publishers:
Landes Bioscience, 810 South Church Street, Georgetown, Texas, U.S.A. 78626
Phone: 512/ 863 7762; FAX: 512/ 863 0081

North American distributor:

Chapman & Hall, 115 Fifth Avenue, New York, New York, U.S.A. 10003

CHAPMAN & HALL

U.S. and Canada ISBN: 0-412-14161-2

Library of Congress Cataloging-in-Publication Data
CIP applied for, but not received as of publication date.

PUBLISHER'S NOTE

Landes Bioscience produces books in six Intelligence Unit series: *Medical, Molecular Biology, Neuroscience, Tissue Engineering, Biotechnology* and *Environmental*. The authors of our books are acknowledged leaders in their fields. Topics are unique; almost without exception, no similar books exist on these topics.

Our goal is to publish books in important and rapidly changing areas of bioscience for sophisticated researchers and clinicians. To achieve this goal, we have accelerated our publishing program to conform to the fast pace at which information grows in bioscience. Most of our books are published within 90 to 120 days of receipt of the manuscript. We would like to thank our readers for their continuing interest and welcome any comments or suggestions they may have for future books.

Shyamali Ghosh
Publications Director
Landes Bioscience

DEDICATION

This book is dedicated to my parents.

CONTENTS

EDITOR

Ismail Jatoi, M.D., Ph.D., FACS
Assistant Professor of Surgery
Uniformed Services University of the Health Sciences
Bethesda, Maryland, U.S.A.
and
Brooke Army Medical Center
Fort Sam Houston, Texas, U.S.A.
Chapter 3

CONTRIBUTORS

Cornelia J. Baines, M.D., M.Sc.
Associate Professor
Department of Preventive Medicine
  and Biostatistics
Faculty of Medicine
University of Toronto
Toronto, Ontario, Canada
Chapter 6

D. David Dershaw, M.D.
Director, Breast Imaging Section
Department of Radiology
Memorial Sloan-Kettering
  Cancer Center
Professor of Radiology
Cornell University
College of Medicine
New York, New York, U.S.A.
Chapter 4

Sarah A. Fox, Ed.D., M.S.P.H.
Associate Professor, Medicine
University of California, Los Angeles
and Senior Behavioral Scientist
RAND
Santa Monica, California, U.S.A.
Chapter 9

Bart J. Harvey, M.D., Ph.D.,
  FRCP(C)
Assistant Professor
Department of Preventive
  Medicine and Biostatistics
Faculty of Medicine
University of Toronto
Toronto, Ontario, Canada
Chapter 6

Lars Holmberg, M.D., Ph.D.
Associate Professor
Department of Surgery
University Hospital
Uppsala, Sweden
Chapter 1

Daniel B. Kopans, M.D.
Associate Professor of Radiology
Harvard Medical School
Director of Breast Imaging
Massachusetts General Hospital
Boston, Massachusetts, U.S.A.
Chapter 2

Anthony B. Miller, M.B., FRCP
Professor
Department of Preventive
  Medicine and Biostatistics
Faculty of Medicine
University of Toronto
Toronto, Ontario, Canada
Chapter 6

Indraneel Mittra, MBBS,
  Ph.D.(Lond), FRCS
Surgeon and Scientist
Department of Surgery
Tata Memorial Hospital
Mumbai, India
Chapter 7

David Plotkin, M.D.
Director
Memorial Cancer Research
  Foundation of Southern
  California
Los Angeles, California, U.S.A.
Chapter 8

Richard Roetzheim, M.D., M.S.P.H.
Associate Professor,
  Family Medicine
University of South Florida
Tampa, Florida, U.S.A.
Chapter 9

S. Eva Singletary, M.D., FACS
Professor of Surgery
Chief, Surgical Breast Section
Department of Surgical Oncology
The University of Texas
  M.D. Anderson Cancer Center
Houston, Texas, U.S.A.
Chapter 11

Clairice T. Velt, Ph.D.
Senior Research Psychologist
RAND
Santa Monica, California, U.S.A.
Chapter 9

Jeffrey N. Weitzel, M.D.
Director
Department of Clinical Cancer
  Genetics
City of Hope National
  Medical Center
Duarte, California, U.S.A.
Chapter 10

Charles J. Wright, M.B., Ch.B.,
  M.Sc., FRCSC, FRCSE, FRCSEd
Director, Clinical Epidemiology &
  Evaluation
Vancouver Hospital & Health
  Sciences Centre
Vancouver, British Columbia,
  Canada
Chapter 5

PREFACE

Worldwide, breast cancer causes about 400,000 deaths each year. In the United States it is the second leading cause of cancer-related mortality among women, responsible for about 46,000 deaths annually. In order to reduce this mortality, attention has turned to breast cancer screening. Three methods are commonly employed: mammography, self-examination and physical examination by trained personnel. In addition, genetic testing for breast cancer susceptibility has aroused considerable interest and controversy. In this book, various topics pertaining to breast cancer screening are reviewed. We have asked authors with a wide range of views to contribute chapters.

The breast cancer screening trials have given us important insights into the natural history of breast cancer, and Dr. Holmberg reviews this topic in the first chapter. The controversy over mammographic screening for younger women is presented in the subsequent two chapters. Dr. Kopans favors mammographic screening for women below the age of 50, and I present the opposing view. In the following chapter, Dr. Dershaw discusses mammographic screening for women over the age of 50. Dr. Wright then presents his perspective on the relative benefits and harm of mammographic screening. Little is known about the impact of screening by self-examination or physical examination on breast cancer mortality. Drs. Miller, Baines and Harvey review self-examination and Dr. Mittra discusses the evidence for physical examination by trained personnel. In the United States, the failure to diagnose breast cancer in a timely manner is a very common cause for litigation. Dr. Plotkin covers this subject and its relevance to breast cancer screening. In the following chapter, the various socioeconomic, cultural and communication barriers to breast cancer screening and strategies to overcome them are reviewed by Drs. Fox, Roetzheim and Veit. Women at high risk for breast cancer pose a dilemma. Dr. Weitzel reviews genetic testing for breast cancer susceptibility and Dr. Singletary discusses her views on the management of patients at high risk.

Breast cancer screening is an extremely controversial topic, and the contributors strongly disagree on many issues. However, by including authors with many different views, I believe we have provided a balanced perspective on this subject. Despite their differences of opinion, the contributors to this book share a common goal: reducing breast cancer mortality and improving the quality of life for all women.

Ismail Jatoi, M.D., Ph.D.
Fort Sam Houston, Texas

══════ CHAPTER 1 ══════

NATURAL HISTORY OF BREAST CANCER

Lars Holmberg

INTRODUCTION

Randomized clinical trials and observational studies in breast cancer screening have provided us with much information relevant to a critical discussion of the natural history of breast cancer. Some of the scientific contributions from the screening studies have been of considerable interest, but so far researchers have taken little advantage of the opportunity to form testable new hypotheses or produce research ideas on the basis of these observations. In the following, data that shed light on the natural history of breast cancer will be discussed in relation to a few key problems.

1. Some cancers metastasize late in their preclinical phase or during the first part of their clinical course

Breast cancer screening lowers the mortality from breast cancer. When groups invited or not invited to screening are compared regarding breast cancer mortality, the observed differences cannot be explained by lead-time effects and diagnosis of nonlethal cancers (but of course these factors may still constitute essential clinical problems). Women with breast cancer detected at screening less often get recurrences and less often die of the disease, compared with unscreened women with breast cancer, and thus, by bringing forward the time of diagnosis, some women are prevented from developing clinically relevant distant metastases during their lifetime. This could imply at least three different possibilities:

1. Some women could have truly localized disease when they are diagnosed, with no micrometastases at the time of treatment.
2. Some women could have localized disease in a clinical sense; here micrometastases could be present at the time of diagnosis but would not survive treatment (with or without systemic adjuvant treatment).
3. Some women have localized disease in a clinical sense; here micrometastases may be present at the time of diagnosis, but these micrometastases remain dormant or progress so slowly that they never become manifest during the remainder of the patient's lifetime.

It cannot, of course, be ruled out that all three possibilities occur. Patients of the same kind are also present in the unscreened population, but the screening exerts its effect on

Breast Cancer Screening, edited by Ismail Jatoi. © 1997 Landes Biosience.

mortality by increasing the proportion of these women among the breast cancer patients. The reduced mortality in the screened population challenges the over-simplistic interpretation of the deterministic view of breast cancer biology—that breast cancer always is already a systemic disease from the time of its inception and hence that local treatment cannot alter its natural history. In fact, the screening studies have falsified this hypothesis and shown that early diagnosis and treatment do matter.

2. Does metastatic capacity parallel growth rate?

Breast cancers that are discovered between two screening examinations (interval cancers) constitute a group of more rapidly growing tumors.[1] Some interval cancers may be misdiagnosed, and such cases may have been present for a long time, but undoubtedly the interval cancer group as a whole must be a group which is "enriched" with fast-growing tumors. Studies of interval cancer cases have shown that the survival is similar to that in clinically detected cancers in the unscreened group.[1-3] This phenomenon may have at least two possible explanations:

1. The cell growth rate and metastatic capacity may be truly independent tumor characteristics.
2. The cell growth rate and metastatic capacity may be coupled to each other, but the growth rate of the tumor mass as a whole (i.e., its ability to become rapidly manifest as a mammographically detectable or a clinically evident cancer) may not reflect the tumor cell proliferation per se, but may be related to several different dimensions, such as the balance between cell production and cell death, production of new tumor stroma, attraction of inflammatory cells and so on. This latter hypothesis is supported by the finding that markers for proliferative activity in tumor cells seem to be coupled to the prognosis.

There is one interesting exception to the observations that interval cancers have a prognosis similar to that in clinically detected cancers in the unscreened group, namely the finding in the Malmö mammographic screening trial[4] (MMST) that women with interval cancer had a significantly poorer prognosis than those with tumors detected in an ordinary clinical setting, with the estimated relative hazard being 2.3. This observation challenges the notion that the tumor growth rate does not parallel the metastatic capacity. On the other hand, the results of the MMST trial may also be attributable to a differential sensitivity of the screening program. That is, the screening program in Malmö may have more readily identified slow-growing more highly differentiated lesions, while small, early, grade III cancers may have been missed, surfacing as interval cancer cases and explaining both the interval cancer finding and the rather small effects on mortality seen in the first rounds of the MMST trial.

3. Does tumor progression occur in the time window relevant for screening?

There has been a long-standing debate as to whether screening for breast cancer detects tumors not only at an earlier stage, when they are smaller, but also when they are less malignant. That is, tumor progression would occur in the time frame when screening exerts an effect by making the diagnosis earlier. The study of this phenomenon is hampered by several methodological difficulties: Firstly, in most studies addressing this problem there is as yet no means to eliminate the problem of length bias sampling. Thus, even after correction for tumor diameter, a finding of more benign tumors in the screened group could be due to the propensity of screening programs to find slow-growing tumors. Secondly, it is not clear how the increased proportion of in situ cancers detected by the screening program should be viewed. Are the in situ cancers really a measure of the ability of the screening program to detect potentially lethal cancers already at a preinvasive stage, or do they reflect a tendency to overdiagnosis (see below)? A parallel question to this is whether all small invasive cancers really have the ability to progress to lethal cancers. A third difficulty is that there is no unifying and well tested concept in breast cancer biology to tell us what tumor biological properties to use as markers for different stages of progression.

The authors of a Finnish report[5] have interpreted their findings as contradicting the hypothesis that screening also exerts its effect by detecting tumors when they are less aggressive. They concluded that "biological aggressiveness, as assessed by DNA flow cytometry, does not increase during the detectable preclinical phase." However, their results show that even in the repeated screens there is a tendency for a lower S-phase and a larger proportion of DNA-diploid cells among the screening detected cancers. Their conclusion is based on the *summary picture* for screen detected cancers and the cancers detected in nonattenders or in the interval, but tumor aggressiveness could not be expected to be influenced among those cancers detected clinically. The conclusions drawn from this study have also been criticized[6,7] on the grounds that they are based on relatively small numbers of cases and that there are indications that the Finnish pilot screening program had a low sensitivity. Thus, this study alone does not refute the hypothesis concerning tumor progression.

The study in which the most serious attempt has been made to circumvent the problem of length bias sampling rather indicates that tumor progression may occur.[8] In this study there was a strong correlation between malignancy grade and tumor size and, furthermore, the prognosis in screening-detected cancers (not including those detected by prevalence screening) was to a large extent dependent on tumor size, nodal status and malignancy grade. It thus seems that at least some of the cancers progress within the preclinical detectable phase. There were also indications that the ability of mammography to detect tumors when they were less malignant was greatest in the age group 50-69, which is compatible with the mortality reduction associated with that particular screening program. These indi-

cations that tumor progression occurs in the preclinically detectable phase are also supported by observational studies in France[9] and in the Netherlands[10] as well as by data from the Edinburgh trial.[11]

A remaining difficulty, however, is that in the Swedish trial,[8] the relative hazard for death was still considerably reduced in screening-detected cancers (RH = 0.66, CI = 0.43-1.00), even when adjustments were made for tumor size, node status and grade. The risk of having positive nodes as evaluated with the multivariate model was 0.50 (CI = 0.33-0.74) in incidence screens even with adjustments for tumor size and grade. It may therefore be concluded that histopathological tumor size, node status (positive vs. negative) and tumor grade do not give us the full picture either of the tumor burden or of the malignant potential of the tumor. Nor can the possibility be completely ruled out that detection of "innocent tumors" may play a role, despite the attempts made in the Swedish trial to create a set of tumors unbiased regarding length bias sampling.

No extensive attempts have been made to explain what the increased absolute and relative numbers of intraductal cancers in screening programs imply. Survival analyses based on a Swedish nation-wide population-based cancer registry have indicated that the prognosis in breast cancer in situ is extremely good in age groups and population segments that have been offered screening.[12]

A really convincing, strong test to challenge the theory concerning tumor progression even when the tumor is in its preclinically detectable phase or early in its clinical phase has yet to be undertaken. The most carefully constructed test carried out so far within the Swedish two-county study[8,13] has led to the conclusion that this question is worthy of thorough future investigation. One way to avoid a repetition of inconclusive ad hoc studies would be for a research team to construct as detailed a theory as possible, making very specific predictions of what will be found in a study based on data from randomized clinical trials. Presumably such a study would also have to incorporate modern genetic markers of tumor progression.

4. Overdiagnosis of invasive cancer occurs in less than 10%

In two, much-cited publications concerning autopsy findings, the prevalence of clinically undetected in situ or invasive breast cancer lesions was reported to be as high as 20-25%.[4,15] However, most of these lesions were cancers in situ. Furthermore, it is not known whether these lesions are of a kind that would ever become mammographically detectable. It is not unlikely that there are very slowly progressing histopathologically premalignant or malignant changes that are mammographically largely undetectable, and hence, constitute problems as side findings in surgery for benign lesions rather than as lesions detected in a screening program. Lobular cancer in situ is an example of this.[16]

As stated in section 3 above, our knowledge about tumor progression and about markers in relation to tumor progression is sparse and thus we do not yet have laboratory investigative instruments to quantify the degree of overdiagnosis. Another study from the Finnish screening program investigating tumor stage and tumor markers, much as the studies cited in section 3, has been taken to indicate detection of "harmless" cancers. However, that study does not include an empirical approach (other than adjustment for tumor size) to analyze the problems of length bias sampling, tumor progression and overdiagnosis and therefore remains difficult to interpret. We still have to rely on quantifiable epidemiological estimates of the incidence of breast cancer in a screened population compared with a control group. Up to now such estimates have indicated that the overdiagnosis rate may lie somewhere between 0% and 10%.[18,19]

There have also been attempts to elucidate the question whether increased utilization of screening mammography might be responsible for the increase in the incidence of breast cancer seen in the U.S.[20-23] The con-

clusions drawn from these studies vary, but three of them lend support to the possibility that increased diagnostic activity may be responsible for a rising trend in incidence which departs from the underlying increase in the incidence rate of about 1% per year that has been going on since the 1940s. Any interpretation of these data in terms of overdiagnosis, however, remains speculative.

In a screening program, the proportion of cancers detected as in situ is typically 10-15%, as compared with 3-5% in the average clinical setting. As indicated above, it is striking that few attempts have been made to analyze the long-term implications of this difference, both in terms of protecting some women from getting an invasive cancer and regarding overdiagnosis.

5. Does the natural history of breast cancer differ with age?

The fact that the screening effect differs by age group, and more specifically is lower in women below the age of 50, has attracted immense interest. The whole medico-political-ethical debate surrounding this issue is in itself a notable chapter in the history of medicine. The arguments for and against screening of women below 50 will be fully reviewed elsewhere in this book and the discussion in this chapter will be restricted to the question of whether the differential effects by age might possibly be explained by differences in the natural history of breast cancer between the respective age groups.

The screening studies have not refuted the theory that the natural history differs by age group. If the difficulty in interpreting the results in the youngest age group had depended only on study design (power, different test performance in different settings, imbalances in randomization, etc.), the uncertainty would have been decreased by the extensive overviews and meta-analyses that have been carried out.[24-26] The overviews and meta-analyses have so far helped us to better outline the most important issues regarding difference by age group, but they have not clarified them—this despite the fact that the same overviews have substantially diminished any uncertainty regarding the effects in the age group 50-69.

It is possible that the architecture of the breast in the young woman may make it more difficult to detect a small cancer. Screening studies have also shown that the tumor growth rate is more rapid in younger women, which thus is a feature of the natural history that has implications for the design of screening programs.[27] There is also some evidence—as partly discussed above—that screening alters the distribution of stage and grade to a lesser extent in younger women than in those aged 50-69. In an observational study[28] comedo cancers (low grade ductal invasive cancers) were less affected by screening, and such cancers were more common among the younger women. In another observational study,[29] the risk of having node metastases at the time of detection was much lower in younger than in older women, which could indicate both a differential sensitivity by age group and that there is a considerably smaller margin for therapeutic benefit in the younger group. This latter assumption is also supported by the finding in several studies that women around the menopause have the best breast cancer prognosis.[30-33]

It is quite clear that arbitrary division by chronological age has little to do with the biological understanding of how the tumors behave. Some variables may show a more continuous—though not necessarily linear—change with age. Studies of the prognosis and metastatic pattern rather indicate a complex biphasic relationship to age.[30,34] For other variables, there may be reasons for making the division not by age but by pre- and postmenopausal (or even pre-, peri-, or postmenopausal) status. Analyses of some outcomes in relation to age may be complicated by an intricate pattern of interaction between test performance, treatment response and host defense. In the perspective of the widespread debate concerning the optimal age for the start of screening, comparatively little has been done to formulate and test *biological* hypotheses relevant to screening effect by age.

Little is known as to whether the natural history of breast cancer differs qualitatively between the oldest women, say those aged 70 and above, and women aged 50-69. It is clear, however, that a long lead time in elderly women may give room for overtreatment, since competing risks of death may imply that normally the women would never have experienced the clinical cancer. Questions on screening and tumor biology in the elderly have been unfairly forgotten in the heated debate over the lower age limit.

SUMMARY

Screening studies have provided much interesting information regarding the natural history of breast cancer. The research opportunities created by mammography screening are interesting from several points of view; diagnosis reaches several years[35] into the preclinical phase which probably is an important period in tumor development; tumors are diagnosed on several different developmental stages; most programs are well structured creating an excellent situation for data collection; there are good possibilities to standardize treatment, etc. Many of the new insights provided are departing points for further speculations and investigations, rather than being facts. The possibilities for studies in tumor biology have, however, been relatively unexplored so far, mainly because of a lack of testable theoretical systems and also because of a lack of insight into what biological markers can be used to define factors such as progression and metastatic capacity. A lack of contact and mutual understanding between researchers from different fields may also have been an obstacle, e.g., between the complex epidemiology of screening and the new frontiers in breast cancer biology. More work on constructive scientific speculations based on the screening results obtained so far and on new developments in genetic and molecular biology should lead to rapid expansion of this field. The material is certainly out there!

REFERENCES

1. Holmberg L, Tabár L, Adami HO et al. Survival in breast cancer diagnosed between mammographic screening examinations. Lancet 1986; ii:27-30.
2. Frisell J, von Rosen A, Wiege M et al. Interval cancer and survival in a randomized breast cancer screening trial in Stockholm. Breast Cancer Res 1992; 24:11-16.
3. Peeters PHM, Verbeek ALM, Hendriks JHCL et al. The occurrence of interval cancers in the Nijmegen screening programme. Br J Cancer 1989; 59:929-32.
4. Andersson I, Aspegren K, Janzon L et al. Mammographic screening and mortality from breast cancer: the Malmö mammographic screening trial. Br Med J 1988; 297:943-8.
5. Hakama M, Holli K, Isola J et al. Aggressiveness of screen-detected breast cancers. Lancet 1995; 345:221-4.
6. Day NE, Tabar L, Duffy SW et al. Population breast-cancer screening. (Letters to the Editor). Lancet 1995; 345:853.
7. Alexander FE, Andersen TJ. Population breast-cancer screening. (Letters to the Editor). Lancet 1995; 345:854.
8. Duffy SW, Tabar L, Fagerberg G et al. Breast screening, prognostic factors and survival—results from the Swedish two county study. Br J Cancer 1991; 64: 1133-8.
9. Tubiana M, Koscielny S. Natural history of human breast cancer: recent data and clinical implications: Breast Cancer Res 1991; 64:108-13.
10. Uyterlinde AM, Baak JPA, Schipper NW et al. Prognostic value of morphometry and DNA flow-cytometry features of invasive breast cancers detected by population screening: comparison with control group of hospital patients. Int J Cancer 1991; 48:183-81.
11. Anderson TJ, Lamb J, Donnan P et al. Comparative pathology of breast cancer in a randomized trial of screening. Br J Cancer 1991; 64:108-13.
12. Wärnberg F, Holmberg L. Prognosis in patients with carcinoma in situ of the breast. A population-based study in Sweden. Abstract. Eur J Cancer 1996; 32A, suppl 2.
13. Tabár L, Fagerberg G, Day NE et al. Breast cancer treatment and natural history: new insights from results of screening. Lancet 1992; 339:412-4.
14. Nielsen M, Jensen J, Andersen J. Precancerous and cancerous breast lesions during lifetime and at autopsy. Cancer 1984; 54:612-55.
15. Nielsen M, Thomsen JL, Primdahl S et al. Breast cancer and atypia among young and middle-aged women: a study of 110 medicolegal autopsies. Br J Cancer 1987; 56:814-9.
16. Andersson JA, Fechner RE, Lattes R et al. Lobular carcinoma in situ (lobular neoplasia) of the breast (a syposium). Pathol Annu 1980; 15:193-223.
17. Klemi PJ, Joensuu H, Tuominen J et al. Aggressiveness of breast cancers found with and without screening. Br Med J 1992; 304:467-9.
18. Day NE. Screening for breast cancer. Br Med Bull 1991; 47:1-15.
19. Peeters PH, Verbeek AL, Straatman H et al. Evaluation of overdiagnosis of breast cancer in screening with mammography: results of the Nijmegen programme. Int J Epidemiol 1989; 18:295-9.
20. White E, Lee CY, Kristal AR. Evaluation of the increase in breast cancer incidence in relation to mammographic use. J Natl Cancer Inst 1990; 82:1546-52.
21. Lantz PM, Remington PH, Newcomb PA. Mammography screening and increased incidence of breast cancer in Wisconsin. J Natl Cancer Inst 1991; 83:1540-6.
22. Glass AG, Hoover RN. Rising incidence of breast cancer: relationship to stage and receptor status. J Natl Cancer Inst 1990; 82:693-6.
23. Feuer EJ, Wun LM. How much of the recent rise in breast cancer incidence can be explained by increased mammography utilization? Am J Epidemiol 1992; 12: 1423-36.
24. Hurley SF, Kaldor JM. The benefits and risks of mammographic screening for breast cancer. Epidemiol Rev 1992; 14: 101-30.
25. Elwood JM, Cox B, Richardson AK. The effectiveness of breast cancer screening by mammography in younger women.

The Online Journal of Current Clinical Trials 1993; 1993(Doc No 32).

26. Nyström L, Rutqvist LE, Wall S et al. Breast cancer screening with mammography: overview of Swedish randomized trials. Lancet 1993; 341:973-978.

27. Tabár L, Fagerberg G, Day NE, Holmberg L. What is the optimum interval between mammographic screening examinations? An analysis based on the latest results of the Swedish two-county breast cancer screening trial. Br J Cancer 1987; 55:547-51.

28. Lindgren A, Thurfjell E, Holmberg L. The influence of mammography screening on the pathological and clinical panorama of breast cancer, APMIS (in press).

29. Nordén T, Thurfjell E, Hasselgren M et al. Mammographic screening for breast cancer. What cancers do we find? Eur J Cancer (in press).

30. Adami HO, Malker B, Holmberg L et al. The relation between survival and age at diagnosis in breast cancer. N Engl J Med 1986; 315:559-63.

31. Rutqvist LE, Wallgren A. The influence of age on outcome in breast carcinoma. Acta Radiol (Oncol) 1983; 22:289-94.

32. The Cancer Registry of Norway. Survival of cancer patients: cases diagnosed in Norway 1953-1967. Oslo: The Norwegian Cancer Society, 1985.

33. Mueller CB, Ames F, Anderson GC. Breast cancer in 3,558 women: age as a significant determinant in the rate of dying and causes of death. Surgery 1978; 83:123-32.

34. Holmberg L, Lindgren A, Nordén T et al. Age as a determinant of axillary node involvement in invasive breast cancer. Acta Oncol 1992; 31:533-538.

35. Duffy S, Chen HH. Estimation of mean sojourn time in breast cancer screening using a Markov chain model of both entry to and exit from the preclinical detectable phase. Stat Med 1995; 14: 1531-1543.

CHAPTER 2

THE CASE IN FAVOR OF MAMMOGRAPHIC SCREENING FOR WOMEN IN THEIR FORTIES

Daniel B. Kopans

INTRODUCTION

There is no question that screening mammography can reduce the size and stage at detection of breast cancer.[1,2] The natural history of breast cancer can be interrupted for many women,[3] and this can result in reduced breast cancer deaths.[4] Controversy has arisen when analysts have tried to determine if this benefit is possible for women at all ages, or if it only applies to those in specific age groups.

Just as there is nothing magical that happens to the breast at the age of 50, there is nothing that happens at the age of 40. It is likely that women at any age can benefit from screening, but the absolute number of women who benefit will be in proportion to the numbers of women who develop cancer at that age. There is no question that the younger the population, the lower the incidence of breast cancer. Liberman et al have shown that the breast cancer detection rate for women ages 35-39 in their screening program does not differ from the rate for women ages 40-45.[5] Nevertheless, since most will not accept results from trials other than those that are randomized, with controls, and since none of the randomized, controlled trials (RCT) of breast cancer screening have included women under the age of 40, this chapter will confine itself to women ages 40-49. The reader should be aware, however, that mammography can detect breast cancers earlier, regardless of age, and that this would likely translate into reduced mortality.

THE SCREENING CONTROVERSY

A detailed description of the screening controversy can be found in ref. 6. In 1993, less than 4 years after agreeing to the Consensus Guidelines of 1989, the National Cancer Institute (NCI) withdrew its support for screening women ages 40-49 and initiated a period of major confusion for women and their physicians. The decision, by the NCI, began as a result of the belief among a few individuals that there was no evidence of benefit for these women, and, ultimately, culminated in a judgment determined by the pressures of politics.

Breast Cancer Screening, edited by Ismail Jatoi. © 1997 Landes Biosience.

The decision was, in the opinion of this author, based on inappropriate data analysis and flawed scientific reasoning. The NCI had required that the randomized, controlled trials of screening demonstrate a statistically significant mortality reduction for the subgroup of women ages 40-49, in the early years of follow up. What they neglected to tell women and their physicians was that it was mathematically impossible for the RCT either individually, or collectively, to provide statistically significant benefit in the early years of follow up. In addition to the fact that the trials were not performed to optimize early detection among these women (the screening intervals were too long, single-view mammography was the norm and the thresholds for intervention were too high), the trials were not designed to permit legitimate subgroup analysis of this age group. There were only one-third the number of women that would have been needed to permit an expected mortality reduction of 25% to be significant. Consequently, although five out of the eight trials were demonstrating a benefit that ranged from a 22% mortality reduction to as high as a 49% reduction for these women, the benefit was dismissed because the numbers did not reach statistical significance.

The new NCI guidelines were scientifically inconsistent

Not only was the NCI analysis of mammography erroneous, but their recommendations were scientifically inconsistent and unsupportable using their own criteria. Just as can be found in the 1989 Preventive Services Task Force (USPSTF) recommendations, the NCI had only singled out mammography in its official guideline change. Clinical breast examination continued to be encouraged[7] despite the fact that both the NCI and the USPSTF stated that only measures that had been shown to provide *statistically significant* breast cancer mortality reduction in randomized, controlled trials should be supported. If the available data supporting the mammographic screening of women ages 40-49 were not sufficient, it was inconsistent to continue to recommend

clinical breast examination. The data supporting the use of screening with mammography were more solid than the data supporting the use of clinical breast examination.

The NCI suggested that clinical breast examination had not been studied. They overlooked the fact that the Health Insurance Plan (HIP), Edinburgh trial, and the National Breast Screening Study of Canada (NBSS) screened women ages 40-49 with both mammography *and* clinical breast examination. If the data from these trials were used to deny women mammography screening, they also showed no benefit from clinical breast examination.

Although mammography does not detect all cancers, and does not detect all cancers earlier, studies have shown that mammography detects the majority of breast cancers at a smaller size and earlier stage than clinical breast examination. The only reason that the NCI would have included this recommendation was to avoid the perception that it was completely abandoning women ages 40-49.

The fact the NCI process and conclusions had been highly questionable was reaffirmed on October 20, 1994 when the Committee on Government Operations of the United States Congress published their report entitled *Misused Science: The National Cancer Institutes Elimination of Mammography Guidelines for Women in Their Forties*.[8] Their investigation confirmed the above summary and severely criticized the NCI for its lack of scientific balance and objectivity in its withdrawal of screening support for women in their forties.

The Committee concluded that:
1. The NCI had not adequately reviewed the data.
2. The report that formed the basis of the NCI decision was written by established opponents of screening.
3. Data, from nonrandomized trials, that supported screening were excluded from review.
4. The NCI overruled its advisory group.
5. The NCI did not follow proper procedures.

The Committee recommended that:

1. The NCI should revise its statement to provide balance.
2. The NCI should convene a consensus conference on the subject.

The fact is, if the trials had been analyzed as they were designed, there was statistically significant proof of the benefit for screening women beginning by the age of 40 that had been available for years. It was only the inappropriate use of subgroup analysis of trials lacking statistical power to permit such analysis, that confused the facts.

There is a statistically significant benefit for screening women ages 40-49

What is remarkable is that, with longer follow up, and the commensurate increased numbers of cancer deaths in the trials, the NCI requirement has now been met despite the fact that the trials were never meant to permit this type of subgroup analysis. In 1995, a meta-analysis by Smart et al demonstrated a 24% mortality reduction for women in their forties.[9] This was not accepted because the benefit just missed significance unless the data from the National Breast Screening Study of Canada (NBSS) were not included. Although there was good reason to not include the Canadian results, even if the NBSS was included, the benefit was significant using a single-tailed test of significance, but opponents required a two-tailed test.

The Canadian trial was actually much different from the other seven trials. The other trials first targeted a population of women, and then the women were, in a blinded fashion, randomly divided into "screens" and "controls" (either individually or by community residence or physician practices). Then those women allocated to be screened were invited to come in for screening (many actually refused, but are still counted as having been screened).

The Canadian trial differed significantly in that it solicited volunteers making it a population that was not representative of the general population. When the women agreed to participate they were *all given a clinical breast examination* prior to being assigned to be in the screened group or in the control group. Not only was the make up of the group different from the other trials, but there have been significant questions raised over the fact that the allocation process was not done in a blinded fashion and that there was a bias in the allocation of women.

With longer follow-up of the RCT, the benefit that had been evident in 1993 achieved statistical significance. In January of 1997 the updated results from the RCT were presented to a Consensus Development Conference (CDC) Panel of the National Institutes of Health. Not only was the new overview analysis statistically significant when the results from all of the trials (including Canada) were compared, but the Gothenberg trial has a 44%, statistically significant benefit, and the Malm trial has a 35%, statistically significant mortality reduction for these younger women (Fig 2.1). What many fail to realize is that there are only two trials for women ages 50 and over that are significant alone. Despite the hasty decision of the CDC Panel, which received widespread attention claiming it could find no reason to support screening women in their forties, in March of 1997, the American Cancer Society, on the basis of a review of the data by 30 experts, reaffirmed the recommendation that women should be screened in their forties but changed the recommendation to annual screening. The NCI and its national Cancer Advisory Board came to the same conclusion and reversed its position of 3 years by supporting screening for women, beginning at age 40 every 1-2 years.

BASIC STATISTICAL AND ANALYTICAL ISSUES IN BREAST CANCER SCREENING

SURVIVAL VS. MORTALITY

The problem of determining whether there is a benefit from screening would seem trivial. Superficially it would seem that if women whose breast cancers are detected by screening live longer than those whose are not, one might conclude that screening was beneficial. There are several reasons why the question is not so simple and why this approach may be misleading and cannot be used to confidently determine the efficacy of screening.

LENGTH-BIASED SAMPLING

Periodic screening has a greater likelihood of finding slower growing cancers than those growing rapidly (See Screening Interval below). Women whose cancers are detected by screening may have more indolent cancers. If screening selects for women with nonlethal cancers, then the observation that their survival is better than women who are not screened may merely be a reflection of this phenomenon. This is termed "length bias sampling" and it is one reason why

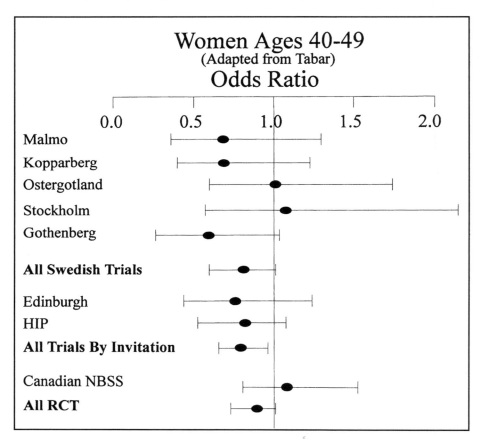

Fig. 2.1. These round dots are point estimates (the ratio of deaths in the screened group to deaths among the controls at a given time of follow up) for screening women ages 40-49 in the RCT. The horizontal bars bracket the 95% confidence intervals. If the entire bar is to the left of 1 this means that the results are statistically significant. In other words, no matter where along the bar the "truth" lies, the screened women had significantly fewer deaths than the controls. The smaller the number of women in a trial, the wider the confidence interval.

When all of the trials by invitation (similar design) are combined there is statistically significant benefit for screening women beginning by age 40. Even when the NBSS is included the results remain significant. Adapted from Tabar-Falun Meeting on Breast Cancer Screening with Mammography in Women Aged 40-49 Years: Report of the Organizing Committee and Collaborators. International Journal of Cancer (in press).

evaluating the survival of women whose cancers are detected by screening, and comparing them to others or to historical controls, can be misleading.

LEAD TIME BIAS

The use of survival statistics (how long an individual survives with the cancer) is also complicated by "lead time bias." By detecting a cancer earlier, the length of time between detection and death from breast cancer may be longer, but it may not be due to the fact that the date of death was deferred, but merely that the date of detection was earlier. A benefit is only real if the date of death is deferred.

This concept can be seen in the following, hypothetical situation. Assume that two identical women develop identical breast cancers at exactly the same time and that the cancers will grow at the same rate. If untreated, the cancers will affect both women equally, leading to death 15 years later (Fig. 2.2). If one of the woman was to take advantage of screening, her cancer might be detected 5 years after it began to grow. If she lived another 10 years, her *survival from the time of diagnosis* would be 10 years.

If the second woman waited until her lesion grew to palpable dimensions she may have her cancer diagnosed 7 years after it began to grow. If she lived another 8 years before succumbing to the cancer her *survival*, from the time of diagnosis to the time of death, of 8 years, would appear to be 2 years less than that of the first woman. Since the date that the cancer began can never be known, the only measurable data points would be the date of diagnosis and the time until death (survival time). Superficially, the screened woman would appear to have benefited from early detection, since her *survival* was longer. However, both women still died 15 years after the cancer began, and, consequently, their absolute *mortality* was unaffected, with no true benefit from the test. In this model, the apparent benefit was due to "lead time bias." The cancer was discovered earlier in the first woman in its inexorable course, and it was consequently "known about" for a longer period of time, but the

time of death, in this scenario, was not altered.

If, on the other hand, the screened woman outlived the unscreened woman then, since they had both been destined to die at the same time, her deferred mortality would represent an absolute benefit from screening, independent of lead time, and would prove that earlier diagnosis actually delayed her death. It is this demonstration of *mortality* reduction (actually delaying death) and not survival that is the best measure of a test's efficacy.

THE RANDOMIZED, CONTROLLED TRIAL

The model of identical women does not exist in real life, and the date at which a cancer begins to grow cannot be determined. Investigators, however, have recognized the importance of observing a mortality reduction and not using survival to measure benefit. The randomized, controlled clinical trial (RCT) simulates "the twins" by using the laws of probability. If the numbers of participants is large enough, randomly assigning women to be offered screening or to act as unscreened controls will produce two groups that will contain women whose cancer will behave identically. There will be the same number of women who develop breast cancer each year and will be the same number of women dying each year from breast cancer. Since the RCT only compares deaths each year from breast cancer, and, at least theoretically, if the numbers are large enough, each woman in the screened group will have a counterpart in the control group that will be her "twin." An RCT is not interested in "survival" and it eliminates the biases inherent in other types of analysis.

If, after screening, the women in the screened group have fewer deaths per year compared to the unscreened control group, and if that difference meets the test of significance, the efficacy of screening can be validated. The randomized, controlled trial is the only way that a test, such as screening for breast cancer, can be validated. The RCT eliminates the effects of lead time bias and length-biased sampling.

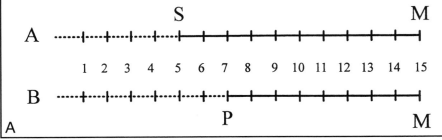

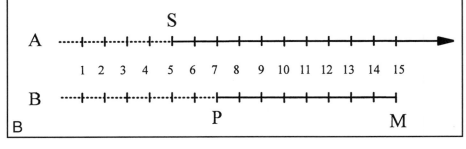

Fig. 2.2. Leadtime bias. (A) Assume there are two identical women whose cancers develop at the same time and grow at the same rate. Woman "A" is screened, and her cancer is detected at point "S", and woman "B" is not screened, and her cancer is not detected until it is palpable (point P). Woman "A"s *survival* (from the time of detection to death) is 10 years and appears to be 2 years longer than woman "B" whose *survival* is 8 years. Although she knew about her cancer 2 years earlier than woman "B", woman "A", in this scenario, actually did not benefit since both women still died 15 years after the cancers began. This is "leadtime bias."

If, however, woman "A" outlived woman "B" (Fig. 2.2B), then there would be a benefit from screening. Randomized, controlled trials simulate twins by having "identical" populations created by the process of randomization. Randomization and a large population should result in women "A" and women "B". Each woman and her cancer has a twin in the other group. The same number of women should die each year from breast cancer. If the screened group has fewer deaths then screening is effective, and leadtime bias is avoided.

THE "GOLD STANDARD" OF PROOF

Much of the controversy has revolved around the concepts of "evidence" of benefit vs. "proof" of benefit. There can be many sources of evidence of benefit. Since mortality is directly linked to the size and stage of a beast cancer, a reduction in the size and stage of cancers at the time of diagnosis is "evidence" that there is a benefit from screening. Improved survival from screening represents "evidence" of a benefit as long as one accounts for "lead time." "Proof," on the other hand, must eliminate lead time bias and length bias sampling and can come, therefore, only from randomized, controlled trials (RCT).

Even the demonstration of a reduction in breast cancer deaths among the screened women in an RCT may not be sufficient since the difference may be due to chance. Most analysts will not accept "proof" of benefit unless the difference in the number of deaths in the screened group vs. the number of control group deaths is "statistically significant" and, therefore, unlikely to be due to chance.

Even this is arbitrary because chance is always a factor, and "statistical significance" is chosen based on probabilities. It is generally accepted that a result is "statistically significant" if there is a 5% or smaller probability that the result was due to chance. Simply expressed, "proof" means that the results have a <5% probability of having been due merely to chance and a 95% likelihood that they represent a "true" relationship.

It is the issue of "statistical significance" that caused much of the disagreement in the screening debate since "evidence" was available early in the debate. Data from the Breast Cancer Detection Demonstration Project (BCDDP) showed that there is no significant difference between survival rates for screened women under age 50 and those ages 50-59, and no differences by age based on tumor size, grade and stage.[10] The Swedish, Kopparberg trial confirmed that there is no difference in survival for younger women compared to older women when their cancers are collated by size, stage and histologic grade.[11]

When the RCT were analyzed as they were designed, they demonstrated a statistically significant benefit for screening women beginning at age 40.[12] Older women have shown a statistically significant mortality reduction as a result of down-staging from screening. Mammography has been shown to down-stage tumors among younger women as well, and a mortality reduction can be expected when they are screened appropriately.

The evidence had always been available, what had been lacking was "proof" of benefit for the subgroup of women in their forties. With the passage of time and an increase in the number of cancer deaths, the mortality reduction, for the subgroup of women ages 40-49, is now "statistically significant," proving the benefit.

SIMPLY PERFORMING A RANDOMIZED, CONTROLLED TRIAL IS NOT SUFFICIENT

Unfortunately, the fact that a trial is randomized, with controls, does not guarantee the validity of its results. RCT can, themselves, be biased by poor design, flawed randomization or deficient execution. An RCT of screening derives its validity from the statistical power of the trial, the random allocation of participants to provide populations with identical characteristics, the quality of the screening and the actual benefit from screening. A deficiency in one or more of these factors will compromise the validity of the trial.

STATISTICAL POWER

Since a reduction in death from breast cancer is the desired benefit, statistical "proof" of benefit requires that there be enough women in the study to provide sufficient numbers of cancers and, more importantly, sufficient numbers of cancer deaths such that, if the screened women have fewer deaths, the difference between the deaths in the screened group versus the unscreened controls will be "statistically significant."

Insufficient numbers of women or more precisely, an insufficient number of cancer deaths among the control group can weaken the statistical validity of the results. There may be a true benefit from screening, but, if there are too few deaths, the differences will not be statistically significant, and a real benefit will be disregarded. This is exactly what happened in the analysis of the screening data with regard to women ages 40-49.

Design and Execution Are Critical

The design of and performance of RCT is critical. The necessary size of a trial will be influenced by the expected number of cancers that will develop in the population over the course of the trial (prior probability) and the rate of death from breast cancer that is to be expected among these women, in the absence of screening (death rate). In order to achieve the same statistical power, a trial in which there are fewer cancer deaths must be larger than a trial in which more women (in the control group) die of breast cancer. Stated simply, if there are no cancer deaths among the control group, then there can be no benefit from screening.

Standard algorithms (the power calculation) are used to estimate the size of the trial needed to prove a benefit. Planning for a trial must include an estimate of the expected reduction in breast cancer deaths among the screened women (benefit). If there is a large benefit from screening, then fewer women will be needed than if there is a smaller benefit. It is generally accepted that the trial should be sufficiently large so that the number of participants will provide a sufficient number of deaths from breast cancer to have an 80% power (higher would be better, but this is the usually accepted level) of showing a specified level of benefit with a 95% likelihood that the benefit is not due to chance (at the .05 level). The smaller the expected benefit, the larger the number of women needed in the trial.

It is the need for statistical power that requires clinical trials to be very large. This is especially true in the breast cancer screening trials since, although breast cancer is a common cancer, only a few women per thousand are diagnosed each year, and fewer than 50% of these die as a result of the breast cancer.

FOLLOW UP

The length of time that the women must be followed is determined by the time period in which the benefit is expected. If, as is true for women in their forties, the 5-year survival from breast cancers diagnosed without screening is high,[13] then the women must be followed long enough for the controls to die of breast cancer so that the benefit for the screens will become evident. This also influences the size of the trial. If investigators are seeking a demonstration of an early benefit, then they must screen appropriately (a short time interval between screens and a low threshold for intervention) and have a large number of women with rapidly growing cancers that will be lethal soon after the start of the trial. Since, for younger women, only a small number of women in the control group die rapidly from their cancers, a trial must be very large to demonstrate an early benefit.

It is more likely that screening will benefit women with moderately fast-growing cancers (see below). This is especially true if the time between screens is long. Since the survival for these is also better than for older women, longer follow up will be necessary to permit the accumulation of sufficient numbers of deaths so that the benefit can be demonstrated with statistical significance.

Finally the size of the trial is influenced by the degree of certainty that is needed to accept a benefit (statistical significance). A decision that 95% certainty is needed will require a larger trial than one where a 90% certainty is acceptable.

Any alteration in these factors that involves fewer participants or breast cancer deaths can reduce the ability of the trial to have the "statistical power" to "prove" a benefit.

RCT must be carefully designed to try to insure that all of these factors are taken into consideration. Variations alter the statistical ability (power) to prove a benefit. Since these trials are very expensive to run, investigators try to reduce the population size as much as possible to keep down costs. Insufficient numbers of participants is one of the major weaknesses in the RCT that have been performed. Most of the trials have had marginal power to "prove" a benefit from screening, and that power has been further compromised by breaking the data into even smaller numbers by retrospective subgroup analysis by age.

RETROSPECTIVE SUBGROUP ANALYSIS

The RCT of breast cancer screening that have been performed were designed to evaluate a wide range of ages and their power was predicated on the inclusion of all women studied. With the exception of the National Breast Screening Study of Canada (NBSS), none of the trials was prospectively designed or performed to evaluate women ages 40-49 as a separate subgroup. None of the trials, *including the NBSS*, has involved sufficient numbers of women under the age of 50 to expect a statistically significant benefit from screening in the early years of follow up of the participants. The retrospective analysis of trials by age subgroups, when they were not designed for this type of analysis, is the same as designing a trial that, to begin with, is too small. Experts such as Lachin warn against data that involve numbers that are too small:

> "...if the statistical test fails to reach significance, the power of the test becomes a critical factor in reaching an inference. It is not widely appreciated that the failure to achieve statistical significance may often be related more to the low power of the trial than to an actual lack of difference between the competing therapies. Clinical trials with inadequate sample size are thus doomed to failure before they begin and serve only to confuse the issue of determining the most effective therapy for a given condition."[14]

This was reinforced by Moher et al when they warned:

> "If a trial with negative results has insufficient power, a clinically important but statistically nonsignificant effect is usually ignored, or worse, is taken to mean that the treatment under study made no difference."[15]

The fact is that the screening trials, collectively as well as individually, lacked the statistical power to demonstrate a mortality reduction in the early follow up of the women under age 50. In order for a trial to have an 80% power to "prove" a 25% mortality reduction (with statistical significance, at 5 years following the first screen for women ages 40-49 assuming an 80% 5-year survival among the controls) the trial would have to involve a total population of close to 500,000 women.[16] In all the world's trials put together the total number of women who were under the age of 50 amounts to less than 175,000. In other words, if all of the women in the trials, who were under the age of 50, are included, there are only one third the number that would be needed to demonstrate a "statistically significant" benefit of 25% in the early follow up. By using retrospective age subgroup analysis, analysts made it *mathematically impossible* for the data to be statistically significant for women ages 40-49. To then argue that the benefits that have appeared do not support screening because they are not statistically significant is specious and scientifically erroneous.

Most analysts agree that screening can reduce the death rate by approximately 30% for women ages 50-69. They would likely find, that if the population were divided into an even smaller subgroup any mortality reduction for 57 year old women, for example, would not be statistically significant. If subgroup analysis of data lacking statistical power is acceptable, then, reduced to the absurd, trials would require only one participant. Breaking the trials into subgroups that lack statistical power and then making medical recommendations based on that subgroup analysis is scientifically misleading and medically unsupportable.

THE TRIAL DATA ARE DILUTED BY NONCOMPLIANCE AND CONTAMINATION

Not only have the trials not involved sufficient numbers of women, but their power has been further compromised by "noncompliance" and "contamination." In screening trials there are some women who are invited to be screened but refuse. These women are termed "noncompliers" (a woman cannot be forced to be screened). There are other women who are supposed to be "unscreened" controls who obtain mammograms on their own outside the screen (women cannot be prevented from obtaining mammograms on their own outside of the study) causing "contamination" of the control group. Since these women are still counted with the group to which they were allocated, "noncompliance" and "contamination" dilute the effects of screening. Noncompliers who die of breast cancer are still counted as having been screened, and women whose lives are saved by having their cancers detected by screening outside the trial are still counted as unscreened controls. Screening cannot affect those who are not screened, and if "control" women are screened, the trial merely compares screened women to screened women.

If the statistical power of the trial is to be maintained, these dilutional factors must be taken into account in designing a trial. The only way to compensate for dilution from noncompliance and contamination is to increase the number of women in the trial. The formula for increasing the number of women in the trial is:

> The Planned Sample Size *multiplied by the factor* (1 / (1 - The Rate of Contamination - The Rate of Noncompliance)2).

For example, if 25% of the women in the control group are expected to have mammograms on their own as contamination of the "unscreened" controls, the number of women needed in the trial, as originally estimated in the power calculation, must be increased by the factor $1/(1-.25)2 = 1.78$. Thus, if 25% of the control women "crossover" and have mammograms, in a trial in which 50,000 women are needed to prove a

specific, anticipated benefit, the number of women in the trial must be increased by 78% to 89,000 women to retain the same power to prove a benefit. The number would have to increase to 200,000 women if, in addition, 25% of the women offered screening refused to be screened.

OTHER FACTORS THAT INFLUENCE RCT

There are many other factors that influence an RCT including the characteristics of the population under study. If the study is designed based on an expectation that there will be a certain number of cancers developing over time, and a commensurate number of deaths, and the population proves to be more healthy, with fewer cancers and/or deaths, then the trial may provide misleading results. The frequency of the screen will also impact the results. If, for example, mammography can detect cancers, on average, 2 years before they would ordinarily be found, then screening every 2 years will not result in "earlier" detection and there will be little or no benefit.

The technical quality of the screen and the threshold for intervention will also influence the benefit. If the mammograms are of suboptimal quality for the detection of small cancers or if the radiologists decide that they must have a high percentage of biopsies where the diagnosis of cancer is made, then they, a priori, must permit small cancers to pass through the screen.[17] If the detection threshold is set too high, and results in little or no reduction in the size and stage of the cancers at diagnosis, then there will be no benefit from the screen.[18]

In many of the trials only single-view mammography was used. This has been shown to overlook as many as 20% of breast cancers.[19]

THE PARTICIPANTS IN A SCREENING TRIAL INFLUENCE ITS RESULTS

Screening trials must be designed with great care since errors in design can lead to misleading results. Ideally, a screening trial should involve women from the same population that is expected to participate if screening is shown to be beneficial. If the population studied is not representative of the general population, then the results of the trial may not apply to the general population (generalizability). If the population studied is selected in a nonrandom fashion, the results of the trial may not be applicable to the general population. For example, women who volunteer for trials usually have a different likelihood of disease (prior probability), and, because they may have a different level of health than the average woman, they may have a different course with the same disease. The results of a trial in which women select themselves for participation by volunteering may not apply, for example, to a population of women who are referred for screening by their doctor.

The National Breast Screening Study of Canada (NBSS), for example, solicited volunteers to participate in the study. These women were then randomized into two groups, a screened group, and controls (who were not offered mammography). Asking women to volunteer insured that there would be a high level of compliance, but it meant that the results of the trial could only be applied to women who volunteer. This seems, superficially, to be a trivial point, but there are clear biases that are the result of studying volunteers and not the general population. As noted earlier, the other seven randomized, controlled trials targeted general population groups, randomly divided them and then invited those allocated to the screened group in for screening. This approach more likely reflects what would occur in a general screening of the population. This screening by invitation suffers from the fact that many women who are invited to be screened, refuse (noncompliance), and as discussed above, the trial must compensate for noncompliance by involving more women to make up for the loss in statistical power that results.

INCLUDING WOMEN WITH CLINICAL SIGNS OF BREAST CANCER CAN DILUTE THE RESULTS OF THE TRIAL OR COMPROMISE ITS VALIDITY ALTOGETHER

Theoretically, in RCT, two identical groups are being compared with the only

difference between the groups being that one group is screened and the other is not. The results of an RCT may, however, be influenced by the inclusion of women with advanced breast cancer (node positive, incurable cancer) at the outset of the trial. Women who are allowed to participate, who already have undiagnosed, advanced breast cancer, are unlikely to benefit from screening since their fate was determined prior to their entry into the trial. The cancers that are advanced at the outset will dominate the early mortality statistics and can obscure any early benefit. Elwood has stated categorically that screening trials should not include women with "clinical symptoms" of breast cancer.[20] If these women are included and there is not an equal distribution of advanced cancers for which screening is a priori ineffective, then the trial may be compromised and its results in doubt by the overweighting of inevitable deaths in the group with the excess of these cancers.

The inclusion of women with advanced breast cancer is likely a major source of error in the NBSS. Instead of being divided equally between the screened group and the controls, there were almost four times more women with advanced breast cancer (four or more positive lymph nodes) who were allocated to the screened group than to the controls in the NBSS (this is statistically significant). This differed from the experience in all of the other trials, and the NCI's own biostatistics branch pointed out that this suggested an allocation imbalance.[21]

Not only had the NBSS investigators permitted women with "clinical symptoms" to participate in their screening trial, but they argued that they needed to include these women or they would not have had sufficient numbers of women with cancer in the trial to meet their "power" requirement. Including women with clinically evident cancers increases the overall "power" of the trial by including more cancers and "events" (deaths), but it dilutes the ability to measure the screening benefit. Although there has been surprisingly little criticism of this rationale, reduced to the absurd, it could be argued the "power" of a trial could be increased by including women who had already died of breast cancer. This would increase the number of women with breast cancer and the number of deaths and statistical power, but it would, obviously, dilute any benefit from screening. If women with advanced cancers are allocated evenly, then only dilution will result. If the allocation is imbalanced, then it can compromise the entire trial results as has occurred in the NBSS.

TRIAL DESIGNS

None of the eight RCTs have been properly designed to evaluate screening benefit for women ages 40-49 as a separate group. Seven of the trials were designed to assess a broader range of ages. For example, the Health Insurance Plan of New York study (HIP) was designed to evaluate the benefit of screening women aged 40-64.[22] The size of the population had a specified power (50%—not the usual 80%) to prove a screening benefit for this range of ages. Analysts have tried to separately evaluate the benefit for women 40-49 through retrospective segregation by age. Since the study was not designed for this, and its power for the total population was marginal at best, there was an insufficient number of women in the younger population to have the statistical power to prove a benefit. Although fewer women have died among the screened population relative to the controls for these ages, statisticians argue that, without sufficient numbers, it is not certain whether or not this apparent benefit is due to chance alone.[23] This is circular reasoning. Since there are insufficient numbers of women to be able to have the statistical power to "prove" a benefit, the data should not be analyzed as if they could be used, legitimately, to prove a benefit. Certainly they should not be used to suggest that there is no benefit. Similarly, all other the other studies have had insufficient statistical power individually and, even when grouped together, to be able to prove an expected benefit of approximately 25-30%.

Even the Canadian trial, which was purported to be designed to evaluate women

ages 40-49 separately was actually too small to evaluate women in this age group. It lacks the statistical power to demonstrate a statistically significant mortality reduction for these women. It turns out that the design of the NBSS was based on "feasibility." Because of limited resources, it was the largest trial that could be mounted. A review of the design reveals that if the NBSS design parameters had been met, it was only large enough to permit the demonstration of a 40% or larger benefit at 5 years.[24] It never had the power to show an expected benefit of 25%. The power of the NBSS was further reduced by a survival rate among the control group that was almost twice what was expected. Fewer deaths among the control women further weakens the power of the trial. In addition, 26% of the control women had mammograms. This contamination was unplanned for in the design of the NBSS. As noted earlier, in order to compensate for the effects of mammography in the control group (screening the controls), the NBSS would have had to involve almost 40,000 additional women ages 40-49.

The absence of statistical power in the trials is indisputable. Even Dr. Cornelia Baines, one of the investigators in the Canadian trial wrote:

> "Those who advocate screening of women ages 40-49 years are right when they say no study thus far (including the NBSS) has had adequate power for this age group."[25]

At a meeting of experts, in Atlanta, in April 1994, cosponsored by the American Cancer Society and the National Cancer Institute, there was unanimous agreement that the trials lacked the statistical power to permit the subgroup analysis that NCI has used to withdraw support for screening these women.[26]

The facts are that, by the time of the NCI review in 1993, five out of the eight trials had demonstrated a mortality reduction for women ages 40-49. This, however, was rejected by the NCI because the numbers of deaths involved were too small to be statistically significant. The lack of significance was clearly due to the lack of statistical power in the trials which was reflected in the wide confidence intervals around the "point estimates" of the benefits.

Given the lack of statistical power to permit the retrospective, accurate evaluation of women ages 40-49, as a separate subgroup, the question must be raised as to why the data were analyzed as if they had the statistical power, and why subgroup analysis, with insufficient statistical power, was used to make medical recommendations. The only conclusion that can be reached for this major compromise of proper scientific analysis is that the issues were influenced by politics and economics. In light of the available data, the trends in the data and the expectation of additional information with longer follow up of the RCT, there was no reason to alter the guidelines.

IF ONLY "HIGH RISK" WOMEN ARE SCREENED, MOST BREAST CANCERS WOULD BE MISSED

The NCI suggested that there was no benefit from screening women ages 40-49, but they recommended that high risk women (those with a first degree relative with breast cancer), continue to be screened. Using their own analytic requirements for efficacy, this approach has no scientific support. If the data supporting the screening of all women, ages 40-49, are not acceptable, *there are no data that show that screening high risk women will decrease mortality*. A frequently cited analysis showed, as would be expected, that there will be a higher yield of cancers if women ages 40-49, who have a first degree relative with breast cancer, are screened.[27] This does not, however, mean that screening these women will reduce their mortality. Furthermore, the Kerlikowske et al analysis biased the conclusion by comparing women ages 30-49 with women ages 50-70+ skewing the results to the extremes. When women ages 40-49 are compared to women ages 50-59 in the same study, the differences in detection rate are not statistically significant[28] (although there is almost certainly a small difference due to the increasing incidence with increasing age).

The Kerlikowske study also reconfirmed, that, as with all risk factors, only a small percentage of women who develop breast cancer are at high risk.[29] If the authors had only screened high risk women, they would have overlooked 77% of the breast cancers that they detected among women under the age of 50. Screening only high risk women will not benefit the vast majority of women who develop breast cancer since, depending on the definition of high risk, as few as 5% of women who develop breast cancer may be included. The overwhelming majority of women who develop breast cancer (60-95%) are not among the group at high risk.

THE BENEFIT FOR WOMEN AGES 40-49 IS NOT A RESULT OF THEIR HAVING REACHED THE AGE OF 50 DURING THE TRIALS

Some analysts have suggested that the benefit, which seems to appear later for women ages 40-49, than for older women, is due to the fact that the women who entered the trials in their late forties turned 50 during the trials and were saved by screening because they were older. There is no scientific basis for this assumption, and its invocation is medically irresponsible. It implies that age 50 is "magical" and that the body, and cancers, somehow know that the "magic age" has been attained.

In order to avoid biases in analyzing trial data, strict criteria must be observed. Just as noncompliers must still be counted as having been screened, and contaminators are still counted as unscreened controls, RCT must be analyzed by the age at allocation and not the age at diagnosis. This is required to avoid biasing the trial since the age at diagnosis is a pseudo-variable that is influenced by the intervention under study. If the age at diagnosis is used, then women whose cancers are detected while in their forties whose counterparts in the control group are not diagnosed until they are in their fifties, will appear in the data analysis as insignificant cancers. Cancers that could have been prevented by screening women in their forties will be attributed as deaths among women in their fifties. It is unclear why analysts would insist on following some requirements of RCT analysis, but then ignore the requirement that analysis be based on the age at allocation to avoid introducing biases. Despite this fact, in the three trials that have analyzed the data by age at diagnosis, the majority of the benefit is for women whose cancers were detected while in their forties.

AN EARLY BENEFIT REQUIRES EXPLANATION

Unless the time between screens is very short, it is unclear how an early benefit can occur. A delayed benefit is, biologically, more likely.

Opponents of screening have argued that, since the benefit from screening younger women did not begin to appear until 5-7 years after the first screen, screening was, therefore, less effective among younger women. It must be remembered that the randomized, controlled trials were not optimized for screening women ages 40-49. The interval between screens was too long, and many of the trials used single-view mammography which has been shown to miss as many as 20% of breast cancers. It is, in fact, difficult to explain how an immediate benefit can occur from screening. Breast cancer has a long natural history. Most cancers are not diagnosed until the later years of a trial. Furthermore, lead times for mammographic detection range from 2-4 or more years before a lesion becomes clinically evident. The time at which a benefit appears is a reflection of how quickly the control group's cancers successfully metastasize (the screened group's cancers must be found before this occurs) and how quickly those metastases grow sufficiently to kill the control women. In order for an immediate benefit to occur, the screened woman, with rapidly growing cancer, must be fortuitously detected early in the trial (this is unlikely because of length bias sampling) just prior to the successful establishment of metastatic disease (so that she will not die). Her control group counterpart's cancer must successfully metastasize very soon after that time

so that when her cancer is detected a year or more later she will die rapidly. This is a highly unlikely scenario. It is not scientific to reject a "delayed" benefit. A "delayed" benefit makes more sense biologically than does an immediate benefit.

WHY DON'T ALL OF THE TRIALS SHOW A BENEFIT?

The majority of the trials have demonstrated a benefit for screening women under the age of 50. Instead of looking only at the numbers, analysts should also review the potential explanations for the three trials that have not, as yet, shown a benefit. The Canadian trial (NBSS) has been severely criticized for its design and execution as more investigators review the parameters of its performance.[30,31] In addition to its insufficient statistical power, the NBSS involved volunteers that produced a control group whose survival was far superior to that anticipated in the study protocol, there was a major problem with the allocation process resulting in an imbalance of women with advanced cancers placed in the screened group, and the quality of the mammography was shown, in an objective review organized by the investigators, to be poor. A recent review by Bailar and MacMahon[32] failed to interview the nurses and clerks performing the randomization and, thus, we may never know how the process was compromised. The continued excess cancer deaths in the NBSS remain enigmatic. It differs from all the other trials and is likely the result of faulty randomization.

In the Ostergotland trial in Sweden, almost 50% of the women who died in the screened group had refused screening. As noted above, the rules of randomized, controlled trial analysis require that these deaths still be counted as being in the screened group. Nevertheless, women in that trial, who availed themselves of screening, enjoyed a benefit.

The third trial that has not yet shown a benefit is the Stockholm trial. Women, in that trial, ages 40-49, were screened with single-view mammography. Single-view mammography has been shown to miss more than 10% of cancers.[33] The women in Stockholm were also screened at an interval of more than 2 years. This has been shown to be too long a time between screens.[34,35] The trial also appears to have had a high threshold for intervention with a high interval cancer rate (cancers not detected at screening that come to clinical detection during the time between screens). Furthermore, the Stockholm trial only went through two screening cycles before all women (including controls) were offered screening.

There are good explanations as to why these few trials have not shown a benefit. These factors should have been taken into account before the NCI concluded that there is no benefit from screening women ages 40-49.

SCREENING INTERVAL

The frequency of screening (time between screens) is not a trivial question. The fact that the mortality from breast cancer can be reduced proves that the natural history of breast cancer can be interrupted. This suggests that there is a period of time in the growth of many, if not all, cancers before they reach a "level of lethality." As can be seen (Fig. 2.3) the screening interval may determine the types of cancer detected and can impact on how soon a benefit can be expected. Only cancers that are slow to reach the "level of lethality" will be detected, and the patient may derive little benefit, if the time between screens is long. If the interval is shortened, then the tumors with moderate growth rates can be influenced, and it is likely many of these have been "cured" in the screening trials and account for the mortality reduction. The only way to interrupt cancers that reach the "level of lethality" faster is to shorten the time between screens. If women ages 40-49 are to be screened, the available data suggest that it should be every year. The lead time for mammography for women ages 40-49 is approximately 2 years. If women this age are screened every 2 years the advantage of early detection will be diminished. Screening should be on an annual basis.

Despite the fact that the requirements for benefit have been achieved, opponents of screening continually change their arguments and requirements

With the achievement of a statistically significant benefit in the randomized, controlled trials, the point should be moot, but the arguments opposing screening continue to mutate. The arguments in support of screening have remained constant, but the arguments opposing screening have changed as each has been shown to be scientifically invalid. In 1992, based on the early results of the NBSS, women and their physicians were told that screening was actually causing an increase in cancer deaths among the screened women.[36] When it became clear that this was likely either statistical fluctuation, or, more likely, due to the randomization imbalance in the NBSS where incurable cancers were more heavily allocated to the screened group than the control group,[37] the argument shifted, in 1993, to the NCI position that there was no statistically significant benefit.[38] In 1994, when the benefit began to become apparent, opponents began to suggest the possible "harms" associated with screening,[39] and when the benefit became irrefutable, the argument shifted to the "costs" of screening.[40]

Now that the benefit is "significant," opponents of screening argue that the benefit among women ages 40-49 is due to the fact that they became age 50 during the period of screening and suddenly screening began to save their lives. In addition to being a biologically untenable hypothesis (the body has no idea when it turns age 50), as noted earlier the analysis suggested by opponents would require the violation of a basic principle of RCT. In order to avoid bias RCT data must be analyzed by the age the patient was at the time of allocation. The age at diagnosis is considered a pseudo-variable that is dependent on intervention being investigated. Its use would, a priori, bias the results against detection among the younger women. de Konig et al attempted to analyze the question using a computer model,[41] but since the model was based on results for a

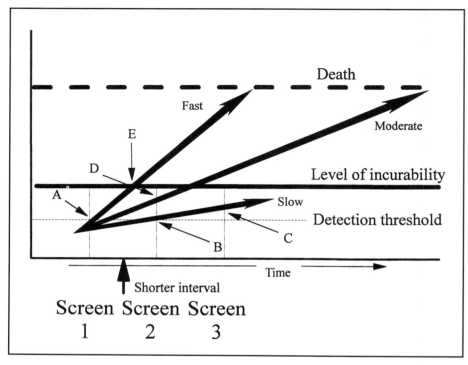

Fig. 2.3. The growth rate of cancers likely follows a bell-shaped, Poisson distribution. Assume that the thick horizontal line is the "Level of Incurability." When a cancer reaches this level, it is incurable. This may be the second cell that has developed the necessary changes to become invasive and metastatic, and even earlier detection will not save the individual. However, it is clear that the natural history of breast cancer can be interrupted, and this level is directly related to cancer size.

The detection threshold is the level at which mammography can detect a cancer. Anything below this line cannot be detected. Any cancer above the line is detectable. The vertical lines represent a screen.

If slow-growing cancers are evaluated it can be seen that, perhaps, at the first screen (A) they are missed since they are just at the detection threshold. They are detectable at the second screen (B), but even if missed again, they are detectable at the next screen (C) before they reach a level of lethality. In fact, some of these may never be lethal in the patient's lifetime. The fact that periodic screening is more likely to find slower growing cancers is called "length bias sampling."

Cancers with moderate growth patterns may not be detected at the first screen, but they can be detected at the next screen (D) before they reach the level of lethality and it is likely the detection of these cancers that have resulted in the RCT demonstrating decreased mortality. It should be noted that it may take many years for the control counterpart to die and the benefit of early detection become apparent.

Cancers with rapid growth patterns may not be detected at the first screen, and if the time between screens is too long (screening interval) they may reach the level of incurability (E) before the next screen. The only way to interrupt faster growing cancers is to screen more frequently (small arrow).

nonRCT case-controlled study in Nijmegen, which was poorly executed and had particularly bad results for women ages 40-49,[42] the model has little bearing on reality. Furthermore, this argument could be reduced to the absurd by suggesting that women in their fifties benefited because they reached the age of 60 and that women in their sixties benefited because they reached the age of 70, etc.

Despite the fact that it is inappropriate to analyze the data by age at diagnosis, this has been done for three of the trials. In the HIP, Kopparberg and Gothenberg trials, the majority of the benefit for women ages 40-49 was for cancers detected while the women were still in their forties.

Despite the fact that it has been clearly demonstrated that women in their forties can benefit from mammographic screening, opponents continue to try to find reasons to deny the benefit. The basic concern of opponents is the potential cost of screening, but they recognize that it would be politically untenable to tell women that screening can save lives but that it is not worth the cost. Hence, numerous, scientifically unsupported arguments have been made to justify the opposition to mammographic screening. Many of these fallacies and their associated facts are discussed below.

FALLACIES AND FACTS IN BREAST CANCER DETECTION AND DIAGNOSIS

Fallacy: Screening is a public health issue.

Fact: Screening, first and foremost, benefits the woman who avoids premature death from breast cancer. It is secondarily a public health issue.

Because of the desire to provide screening for all women, the debate has been viewed, primarily, from the public health perspective. This has resulted in a compromise of scientific analysis by the economic issues. King has written:

> "Screening is a public health activity concerned not with individuals, but with populations...."[43]

This is a fundamental misconception. Immunization for communicable diseases is a public health issue because immunity in the population directly influences the likelihood that members will contract the disease. Screening for a communicable disease, such as tuberculosis, is a public health issue because it may reduce the potential for us all to contract the illness. On the other hand, screening for breast cancer is of primary benefit to the individual, her family and friends. Preventing her death does have some benefit to society, but it is difficult to measure that benefit. The major public health issue involved revolves around who will pay for screening. As a consequence the medical and scientific benefit from screening should be determined and kept separate from the cost. Women and their physicians should be provided the most accurate analysis from a scientific and medical perspective so that an individual can decide for herself whether or not to participate. "Society" can then decide whether to provide screening as a benefit. Unfortunately, the economic issues have been allowed to compromise the scientific and medical analysis.

Opponents of screening women in their forties have raised one factually incorrect issue after another to support their position. They have inappropriately grouped data to make women in their forties appear to be different from those over the age of 50. One of the biggest mistakes has been the comparison of women in their forties with *all other women* and the use of a single age (50) as a point of analysis. This has resulted in a serious misrepresentation of the facts concerning women ages 40-49.

Fallacy: Breast cancer is not a significant problem for women in their forties.

Fact: Breast cancer is not a trivial problem for women in their forties.

The incidence of breast cancer increases with increasing age. Approximately 1.3-1.6 women in 1000 will develop breast cancer each year between the ages of 40-49. This rises to 2.2-2.6 for women ages 50-59, and

3.3-3.9 for women ages 60-69. Opponents of screening these women have used these incidence ratios to suggest that women in their forties comprise only a small percentage of the women who develop breast cancer each year. For example, according to SEER estimates (The Surveillance, Epidemiology, and End Results program of the National Cancer Institute) there were 28,900 women who were diagnosed with invasive breast cancer in the United States in 1993. Opponents of screening argued that this comprised only 16% of the total breast cancers diagnosed that year.[44] They argued that we should concentrate on the 86% that occurred among the other women age 50 and over. Superficially this appears to be quite compelling, but it is an analysis that is misleading since it is provided without any context. Women in their forties are compared to *all other women* combined. The weakness of the argument becomes apparent when women in other decades of life are evaluated the same way. Most agree that women in their fifties should be screened, yet, in 1993, women in their fifties only accounted for 17% of all of the breast cancers diagnosed (31,500). It could be easily argued that we should not screen women in their fifties, but rather concentrate on the 87% of cancers that occurred among all the other women. In fact, in 1993, no decade accounted for >24% of the breast cancer cases (Fig. 2.4). Because the "baby boomers" are moving through their forties, there were actually *more cancers diagnosed among women in their forties* than among women in their fifties in both 1995 and 1996.

Breast cancer is not a trivial issue for women in their forties. More than 40% of

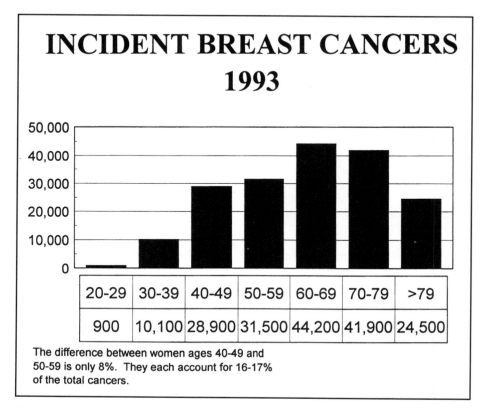

INCIDENT BREAST CANCERS
1993

20-29	30-39	40-49	50-59	60-69	70-79	>79
900	10,100	28,900	31,500	44,200	41,900	24,500

The difference between women ages 40-49 and 50-59 is only 8%. They each account for 16-17% of the total cancers.

Fig. 2.4. This graph provides the absolute number of invasive cancers, by decade, diagnosed in 1993 according to the American Cancer Society.

the years of life lost to breast cancer are from women diagnosed before the age of 50.[45] Breast cancers diagnosed while women are in their forties account for 30% of the years of life lost to these malignancies. In addition, the number of women with breast cancer who are in their forties is higher than the available data suggest since, in the absence of screening, cancers that may be detectable while a woman is in her forties are presently not diagnosed until she is in her fifties. The number of cancers diagnosed among women in their forties will likely be even higher with appropriate mammographic screening.

DILUTIONAL NIHILISM

The benefit of an intervention that saves an individual's life can be trivialized by diluting over the entire population. Although Lindfors and Rosenquist have shown that screening women beginning by the age of 40 is similar in cost per year of life saved as numerous medical interventions that are well accepted, opponents continue to make arguments involving scale. There is no question that, out of the approximately 50 millions women in the United States, only a very small number will benefit from breast cancer screening since, fortunately, the vast majority of women do not develop breast cancer in a given year. Opponents of screening women in their forties have used this to trivialize the problem. For example, if we assume that approximately 1 woman in 1000 will develop breast cancer each year while in her forties (a slight under estimate), 10,000 women must be screened to find 10 cancers. Assuming 4 of them will die of their cancer and that this can be reduced by 25% using screening, then 10,000 women must be screened to save a single life.

This certainly seems like an unreasonable ratio. What is interesting, however, is that the analysis is only performed for women in their forties. Using the same analysis for women in their fifties 10,000 women would have to be screened to save two lives and 10,000 women in their sixties must be screened to save three lives. It may be that "society" decides that screening is not worthwhile, but women in their forties should not be singled out as, somehow, being different. When the above analysis s reviewed it should be remembered that there are 12 times as many women who develop breast cancer each year in comparison to cervical cancer and 10 times as many deaths from breast cancer as from cervical cancer yet cervical cancer screening is an accepted part of health care.

Fallacy: Women in their forties differ from women ages 50 and over and should be compared as a group.

Fact: There are very few objective differences between cancers among "younger" women and those among "older" women. None of the parameters of screening change abruptly at the age of 50, or at any age, and comparing women ages 40-49 with all other women creates an artificial threshold.

Unfortunately, a number of misunderstandings have occurred by grouping data without recognizing how that might influence the analysis of those data. By using the age of 50 as the point of analysis, and comparing women under the age of 50 to those age 50 and over, many factors are, spuriously, made to appear to change abruptly at age 50.

Fallacy: The breast turns to fat at the age of 50.

Fact: The breast does not turn to fat at age 50 or at any other specific age.

Most of the arguments against screening women under the age of 50 describe the fact that the breast tissues in younger women are radiographically dense and can hide small cancers. Some analysts, who have decided that there is no benefit from screening women ages 40-49, have tried to rationalize this position by suggesting that the breast is dense in women under the age of 50 and then turns to fat and becomes more radiolucent at age 50 permitting the detection of cancers earlier among women ages 50 and over. It is true that younger women tend to have a higher percentage of fibrous connective tissue and glandular tissue than older women, but the percentages do not change at the age of 50 or any other age.

Although a higher percentage of "young" women have dense breast tissue, this is not a phenomenon that has an abrupt change at any age. There is a gradual progression in the percentage of women with dense breasts by mammography. The percentage of women with dense breasts decreases gradually with increasing age. We have analyzed our data by each individual age and have found that at age 30 approximately 90% of women have radiographically dense breast tissue. The percentage changes by about 1-2% each year of age so that by the age of 50 approximately 50% of women have dense tissues and 50% fatty. The change continues steadily until around the age of 60 where the patterns appear to stabilize and level out (Fig. 2.5A). The misinterpretation of the data have come as a result of age grouping. If our same data are grouped to compare women ages 40-49 to those ages 50 and over then there appears to be a major change at the age of 50 when this is merely an artifact of inappropriate data grouping (Fig. 2.5B).

The fact that the breasts do not turn to fat at menopause or at age 50[46] was actually demonstrated many years ago. Prechtel demonstrated that the percentage of women with dense breasts decreases steadily with increasing age with no abrupt alteration at age 50, or at menopause.[47]

Another misconception is that the radiographic density of the breast is related to its firmness. Two studies have shown that the density of the breast on mammograms has no relationship to the size of the breast, its compressed thickness or its firmness.[48,49]

THE "HARMS" OF BREAST CANCER SCREENING

Opponents of screening have suggested that women in their forties should not be screened using mammography because of the associated "harms" that screening produces. These include the anxiety from being recalled for additional evaluation, and the biopsies that result from abnormal mammograms where the pathology proves to be benign. The latter have been termed "unnecessary" biopsies. There is no question that screening for any cancer results in false positive calls, and that these cause anxiety and biopsies cause physical trauma. What has been misleading is that opponents have implied that somehow this is confined to women in their forties and that, suddenly, at the age of 50 these become less significant. In fact, women of all ages should be apprised of the negative aspects of screening in an accurate fashion so that they can decide whether or not to participate.

Fallacy: There is a high percentage of women in their forties who are recalled for additional study based on a screening mammogram.

Fact: The recall rate for an abnormal mammogram is approximately the same regardless of age.

Opponents of screening have suggested that if women in their forties are screened, too many will be recalled for additional evaluation and will be unnecessarily alarmed. The fact is that approximately the same percentage of women (5-7%) are recalled for additional evaluation following a screening mammogram, regardless of age.[50] There is no abrupt change at the age of 50 or any other age. This is similar to other screening tests such as the evaluation of

Fig. 2.5. (A) Breast patterns were analyzed by individual age and divided into dense and predominantly fat. The percentage of women at each age who have dense tissues decreases steadily with increasing age with no abrupt change at any age. (B) The same data, grouped into women under the age of 50 and age 50 and over make the tissue densities appear to change suddenly at the age of 50.

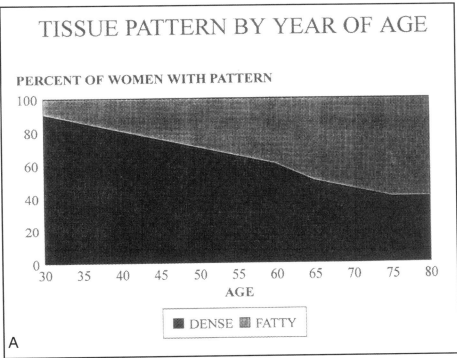

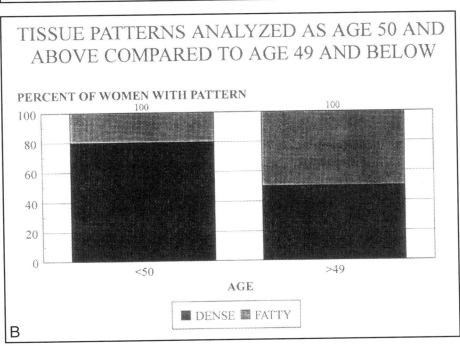

women who have an abnormal cervical cancer screen.

Fallacy: The rate of biopsies recommended based on mammography changes abruptly at the age of 50.

Fact: The recommendation for a biopsy based on mammography is the same regardless of age.

Opponents of screening have suggested that mammography leads to too many biopsies with benign results among women in their forties, but that somehow this changes for women after the age of 49. In our screening program the percentage of women recommended for a breast biopsy is virtually the same 1-2% regardless of age.[50] There is no sudden change in the rate at which biopsies are recommended.

Fallacy: Mammography leads to too high a percentage of biopsies recommended that prove to be benign (unnecessary).

Fact: There is a higher percentage of biopsies with benign results recommended on the basis of clinical breast examination than as a result of mammography and when these palpable masses prove to be cancer they are at a latter stage than those detected by mammography.

If the goal is to reduce "unnecessary" biopsies, then clinical examination should be eliminated. A higher percentage of biopsies performed on the basis of a clinical examination are benign, than for those performed based on an abnormal mammogram. Cancers detected by clinical examination are generally at a larger size and more advanced stage than those detected by mammography.[51]

Fallacy: Breast biopsy leads to scarring of the breast that will confuse future mammography.

Fact: The breast usually heals with little or no scarring evident on subsequent screening mammograms.[52]

It is very rare that postsurgical change will be evident on the mammogram a year after a biopsy with benign results (at the time of the next screen). It is exceptional that post surgical change following a benign breast biopsy is confusing. It is a myth that mammographic analysis is compromised by post surgical change when the biopsy has been for a benign process.

Some have suggested that mammography be reserved for the analysis of a palpable abnormality. This too is false. By the time a cancer is palpable the benefit of mammography has been lost. It is primarily a screening test and has little value as a diagnostic test.

Fallacy: The yield of breast cancers detected by mammography changes suddenly at age 50 and screening should be concentrated on women at these ages.

Fact: The yield of breast cancers detected by mammography does not change abruptly at age 50, but increases steadily with increasing age reflecting the prior probability of cancer in the population.

Additional arguments have been made to try to buttress the NCI decision. In 1993, Kerlikowske et al published a review of the results from the screening program at the University of California at San Francisco.[27] That review urged that screening be concentrated on women ages 50 and over. They concluded this based on what they suggested was a major change in the detection of breast cancer at this age. The authors reported a cancer detection rate of 2 per 1000 for women under the age of 50 as compared to 10 per 1000 for those over the age of 50. This was quite misleading as evidenced by a subsequent analysis by Sox who clearly failed to realize the deception in stating:

"The yield (of cancers) of the first mammogram was five times higher in women 50 years of age and older (10 cancers per 1000 studies compared with 2 cancers per 1000 studies)... Clearly mammography is much more efficient in detecting breast cancers in older women."[53]

In fact, a careful review of the Kerlikowske data reveal that the authors grouped women ages <u>30</u>-49 and compared them to women ages 50-70[+]. Including women in their thirties lowered the detection rate for women under the age of 50 while including women in their sixties and seventies inflated the rate for women in their fifties. When the data are evaluated for women ages 40-49 as compared to 50-59 (a more appropriate comparison) the detection rates are 3 per 1000 compared to 6 per 1000 with overlapping confidence intervals that suggest that these are not significantly different. Clearly the detection rate of cancer increases with age, but there is no abrupt change at the age of 50 or at any age. This misperception is merely an artifact of inappropriate age grouping.

Our own review of the cancer detection rate, in a similar screening program, in which we analyzed the rates at each, individual age, rather than by grouping, demonstrates a steady increase in the yield of cancers with increasing age with no abrupt change at the age of 50, or any other age.[50] The detection of breast cancer by mammography is a reflection of the prior probability of breast cancer in the population.

SUMMARY

Virtually every argument that has been used to support the position of those who oppose screening women in their forties has been shown to be fallacious. Although it has been argued that the age of 50 is merely a surrogate for menopause, opponents have used the age of 50 as if it has some biological significance which it clearly does not. There are no parameters of screening that change abruptly at the age of 50. In fact, there is no evidence that these parameters change abruptly at any age. Health planners

may not wish to provide screening as a benefit, but women should be informed of the facts so that they can decide for themselves whether or not to participate.

There is clear proof of benefit from mammographic screening. It is likely that the benefit will be greatest if mammography is performed on an annual basis. The only reason to go to a longer time between screens is economic, and women should be so informed.

CONCLUSION

Compelling evidence has been available for years that screening, using mammography, on a periodic basis, is just as effective in reducing mortality for women ages 40-49 as for women ages 50-59. With the latest data from the RCT, there is now statistically significant "proof" of benefit.

The argument should be moot. Nevertheless, the controversy has raised significant issues that will likely bear on future analysis. Medical and scientific organizations have an obligation to analyze all the scientific evidence concerning breast cancer screening and to provide the best medical guidance. The ability of the health care system and the available resources to provide the recommended care should be a separate discussion and the public should participate in the decision.

Although cost/benefit analysis is beyond the scope of this review, if the analysis by Rosenquist and Lindfors is correct,[54] then the cost per year of life saved from screening women beginning by the age of 40 is well within the costs from other accepted interventions such as coronary artery bypass surgery.[55]

The data strongly suggest that women ages 40-49 should be advised to be screened every year rather than every 2 years. Screening by mammography and clinical breast examination, if performed properly, can be expected to reduce the death rate from breast cancer for women in this decade by at least 25-30%.

REFERENCES

1. Carter CL, Allen C, Henson DE. Relation of tumor size, lymph node status, and survival in 24,740 breast cancer cases. Cancer 1989; 63:181-187.
2. Clay MG, Hiskop G, Kan L, Olivotto IA, Burhenne LJW. screening mammography in British Columbia 1988-1993. Am J Surg 1994; 167:490-492.
3. Tabar L, Duffy SW, Krusemo UB. Detection method, tumor size and node metastases in breast cancers diagnosed during a trial of breast cancer screening. Eur J Cancer Clin Oncol 1987; 23(7): 959-962.
4. Fletcher SW, Black W, Harris R, Rimer BK, Shapiro S. Report of the International Workshop on Screening for Breast Cancer. J Natl Cancer Inst 1993; 85: 1644-1656.
5. Liberman L, Dershaw DD, Deutch BM, Thaler HT, Lippin BS. Screening mammography: Value in women 35-39 years old. AJR 1993; 161:53-56.
6. Kopans DB. Mammography screening and the controversy concerning women aged 40-49. Rad Clin N Am 1995; 33: 1273-1290.
7. Goldberg KB, Goldnerg P. NCI drops breast screening guidelines, issues "summary of scientific fact." The Cancer Letter Vol. 19 No. 48 Dec. 10, 1993.
8. House Committee on Government Operations. Misused Science: The National Cancer Institutes Elimination of Mammography Guidelines for Women in Their Forties. Union Calendar No. 480. House Report 103-863. October 20, 1994.
9. Smart CR, Hendrick RE, Rutledge JH, Smith RA. Benefit of mammography screening in women ages 40-49: Current evidence from randomized, controlled trials. Cancer 1995; 75:1619-1626.
10. Smart CR. Highlights of the evidence of benefit for women aged 40-49 years from the 14 year follow up of the Breast Cancer Detection Demonstration Project. Cancer 1994; 74:296-300.
11. Tabar L. New Swedish breast cancer detection results for women aged 40-49. Cancer 1993; 72:1437-1448
12. Shapiro S. Screening: Assessment of current studies. Cancer 1994; 74:231-238.
13. Adami H, Malker B, Holmberg L, Persson I, Stone B. The relation between survival and age at diagnosis in breast cancer. New Engl J Med 1986; 315: 559-563.
14. Lachin JM. Introduction to sample size determination and power analysis for clinical trials. Controlled Clin Trials 1981; 2:93-113.
15. Moher D, Dulberg C, Wells GA. Statistical power, sample size, and their reporting in randomized controlled trials. JAMA 1994; 272:122-124.
16. Kopans DB, Halperin E, Hulka CA. Statistical power in breast cancer screening trials and mortality reduction among women 40-49 with particular emphasis on The National Breast Screening Study of Canada. Cancer 1994; 74:1196-1203.
17. D'Orsi CJ. To follow or not to follow, that is the question. Radiology 1992; 184:306.
18. Peer PG, Holland R, Jan HCL, Hendriks, Mravunac M, Verbeek ALM. Age-specific effectiveness of Nijmegen Population-Based Breast Cancer-Screening Program: Assessment of early indicators of screening effectiveness. J Natl Cancer Inst 1994; 86:436-441.
19. Wald NJ, Murphy P, Major P, Parkes C, Townsend J, Frost C. UKCCCR multicentre randomized controlled trial of one and two view mammography in breast cancer screening. BMJ 1995; 311: 1189-1193.
20. Elwood JM, Cox B, Richardson AK. The effectiveness of breast cancer screening by mammography in younger women. Online J Curr Clin Trials 1993; 32.
21. Tarone RE. The excess of patients with advanced breast cancers in young women screened with mammography in the canadian national breast screening study. Cancer 1995; 75:997-1003.
22. Shapiro S, Venet W, Strax P, Venet L. Periodic Screening for Breast Cancer: The Health Insurance Plan Project and Its Sequelae, 1963-1986. Baltimore, Maryland: The Johns Hopkins University Press, 1988.
23. Chu KC, Smart CR, Tarone RE. Analysis of breast cancer mortality and stage distribution by age for the Health Insur-

ance Plan Clinical Trial. JNCI 1988; 80:1125-1132

24. Miller AB, Howe GR, Wall C. The national study of breast cancer screening. Clinical and Investigative Medicine 1981; 4:227-258.

25. Baines CJ. The Canadian National Breast Screening Study: A perspective on criticisms. Ann Intern Med 1994; 120: 326-334.

26. Joint Meeting on the Feasibility of a Study of Screening Young Women for Breast Cancer. Atlanta, Georgia: April 20-21, 1994.

27. Kerlikowske K, Grady D, Barclay J, Sickles EA, Eaton A, Ernster V. Positive predictive value of screening mammogrpahy by age and family history of breast cancer. JAMA 1993; 270:2444-2450.

28. Kopans DB. The use of mammography for screening. JAMA 1994; 271:982.

29. Seidman H, Stellman SD, Mushinski MH. A different perspective on breast cancer risk factors: Some implications of nonattributable risk. Cancer 1982; 32(5): 301-313.

30. Kopans DB, Feig SA. The Canadian National Breast Screening Study: A critical review. AJR 1993; 161:755-760.

31. Burhenne LJW, Burhenne HJ. The Canadian National Breast Screening Study: A Canadian critique. AJR 1993; 161:761-763.

32. Bailar JC and MacMahon B. Randomization in the Canadian National Breast Screening Study: a review for evidence of subversion. Can Med Assoc J 1997; 156(2):193-9.

33. Muir BB, Kirkpatrick A, Roberts MM, Duffy SW. Oblique-view mammography: Adequacy for screening. Radiology 1984; 151:39-41.

34. Moskowitz M. Breast cancer: Age-specific growth rates and screening strategies. Radiology 1986; 161:37-41.

35. Tabar L, Faberberg G, Day NE, Holmberg L. What is the optimum interval between screening examinations?— An analysis based on the latest results of the Swedish Two-county Breast Cancer Screening Trial. Br. J. Cancer 1987; 55:547-551.

36. Wald NJ, Murphy P, Major P, Parkes C, Townsend J, Frost C. UKCCCR multicentre randomized controlled trial of one and two view mammography in breast cancer screening. BMJ 1995; 311: 1189-1193.

37. Kopans DB, Feig SA. The Canadian National Breast Screening Study: A critical review. AJR 1993; 161:755-760.

38. Fletcher SW, Black W, Harris R, Rimer BK, Shapiro S. Report of the International Workshop on Screening for Breast Cancer. J Natl Cancer Inst 1993; 85: 1644-1656.

39. Harris R. Breast cancer among women in their forties: Toward a reasonable research agenda. J Natl Cancer Inst 1994; 86:410-412.

40. Kattlove H, Liberati A, Keeler E, Brook RH. Benefits and costs of screening and treatment for early breast cancer: Development of a basic benefit package. JAMA 1995; 273:142-148.

41. de Konig HJ, Boer R, Warmerdam PG, Beemsterboer PMM, van der Maas PJ. Quantitative interpretation of age-specific mortality reductions from the Swedish Breast Cancer-Screening Trials. J Natl Cancer Inst 1995; 87:1217-1223.

42. Kopans DB. Mammography screening for breast cancer. Cancer 1993; 72: 1809-1812.

43. King J. Mammography screening for breast cancer. Letter to the Editor. Cancer 1994; 73:2003-2004.

44. Smith RA. Epidemiology of breast cancer in a categorical course in physics: technical aspects of breast imaging. Second Edition. Oak Brook, Illinois: RSNA Publications, Radiological Society of North America, 1993:21-33.

45. Shapiro S, Venet W, Strax P, Venet L. Periodic Screening for Breast Cancer: The Health Insurance Plan Project and its Sequelae, 1963-1986. Baltimore, Maryland: The Johns Hopkins University Press, 1988.

46. Kopans DB. "Conventional Wisdom": Observation, experience, anecdote and science in breast imaging. AJR 1994; 162:299-303.

47. Prechtel K. Mastopathic und altersabhangige brystdrusen verandernagen. Fortschr Med 1971; 89:1312-1315.

48. Swann CA, Kopans DB, McCarthy KA, White G, Hall DA. Mammographic density and physical assessment of the breast. AJR 1987; 148:525-526.

49. Boren WL, Hunter TB, Bjelland JC, Hunt KR. Comparison of breast consistency at palpation with breast density at mammography. Invest Radiol 1990; 25: 1010-1011.

50. Kopans DB, Moore RH, McCarthy KA, Hall DA, Hulka CA, Whitman GJ, Slanetz PJ, Halpern EF. Biasing the interpretation of mammography screening data by age grouping: Nothing changes abruptly at age 50. Presented at the Radiological Society of North America Meeting (Chicago, Illinois, 1995).

51. Bassett LW, Liu TH, Giuliano AE, Gold RH. The prevalence of carcinoma in palpable vs impalpable mammographically detected lesions. AJR 1991; 157:21-24.

52. Sickles EA, Herzog KA. Mammography of the postsurgical breast. AJR 1981; 136:585-588.

53. Sox H. Screening mammography in women younger than 50 years of age. Ann Inter Med 1995; 122:550-552.

54. Rosenquist CJ, Lindfors KK. Screening mammography in women aged 40-49 years: Analysis of cost-effectiveness. Radiology 1994; 191:647-650.

55. Tengs TO, Adams M, Pliskin JS, Safran DG, Siegel JE, Weinstein MC, Graham JD. Five-hundred life-saving interventions and their cost-effectiveness. Risk Analysis June 1995; 15 No. 3.

CHAPTER 3

THE CASE AGAINST MAMMOGRAPHIC SCREENING FOR WOMEN IN THEIR FORTIES

Ismail Jatoi*

Mammographic screening for women between the ages of 40-49 is extremely controversial and one of the most frequently debated topics in medicine.[1] In the United States, mammographic screening for younger women is common practice. However, this is not true in Europe. The rift between the American and European views was highlighted within a few months after the publication of the National Breast Cancer Screening Study of Canada. In February, 1993, the American Cancer Society (ACS) and the European Society of Mastology (EUSOMA) met in New York and Paris, respectively, to review the results of the Canadian study and other clinical trials on mammographic screening for younger women.[2,3] After reviewing the same data, the two organizations arrived at opposite conclusions: the ACS reaffirmed its longstanding recommendation for screening women starting at age 40 while EUSOMA recommended that screening begin at age 50. Why, in general, do Americans and Europeans have such strongly differing views on this subject? Are American investigators reluctant to accept the results of clinical trials that fail to support a common sense view, while others accept such trials at face value? Does the medico-legal climate or fee-for-service system in the United States influence physicians' views on this subject? Or, alternatively, does pressure to contain costs influence some organizations and governments to recommend against mammographic screening for younger women? There are no simple answers to these questions. However, it is important to note that, for over a decade, the United States has stood alone among the major industrialized countries in having encouraged mammographic screening for women under the age of 50.[4] Yet, the U.S. mortality rates for breast cancer continue to mirror those of the other industrialized nations.[5-6]

Even though the ACS guidelines are generally followed in the United States and the EUSOMA recommendations generally accepted in Europe, opponents and proponents of

---

*The opinions or assertions contained herein are the private views of the authors and are not to be construed as reflecting the views of the Departments of the Army, Air Force or Defense.

Breast Cancer Screening, edited by Ismail Jatoi. © 1997 Landes Biosience.

mammographic screening are found on both sides of the Atlantic. For instance, several major American organizations have, in recent years, issued guidelines on mammographic screening that are often at odds with one another.[7] These conflicting guidelines have set off a heated debate within the United States. In 1993, the National Cancer Institute of the United States (NCI) elected to make no recommendation on mammographic screening for younger women, but instead issued the statement that "randomized, controlled trials had not shown a statistically significant reduction in mortality in women under the age of 50."[8] In addition, a consensus development panel called by the National Institutes of Health (NIH) recently issued a report which states that "At the present time, the available data do not warrant a single recommendation for mammography for all women in their forties."[9] Other influential organizations such as the American College of Physicians and the United States Preventive Task Force have gone on record as opposing the use of mammographic screening for women below the age of 50. In contrast, the American College of Radiology and the American Medical Association favor mammographic screening for women below the age of 50. The recommendations of several major organizations (as of January, 1997) in regard to screening younger women is summarized in Table 3.1.

The persistent controversy over mammographic screening for younger women is not entirely unexpected. Although several studies over the past 30 years have evaluated the efficacy of mammographic screening, only one randomized prospective study was specifically designed to test the effectiveness of screening women under the age of 50. Furthermore, the various types of studies on mammographic screening have potential shortcomings. These include three biases that I shall discuss below. Ultimately, the success of mammographic screening should not be measured by its ability to extend survival from time of diagnosis, but rather by its ability to reduce mortality. In addition, the potential for benefit must we weighed against the potential for harm.

OVERVIEW OF THE SCREENING TRIALS

Historically, there have been two schools of thought concerning the natural history of breast cancer.[10] One school has maintained that breast cancer is systemic at inception and that events in the breast are merely a local manifestation of a systemic problem. A proponent of this school has recently argued that we are missing the forest (the systemic disease) because our efforts are primarily directed at the tree (the breast).[11] Thus, it has been suggested that early detection and timely extirpation of the primary breast tumor should have little impact in reducing breast cancer mortality. However, another school of thought maintains that breast cancer is a progressive disease and that the cancer begins as a cell or clone of cells in the breast which multiplies and grows in size. At some point during the

---

Table 3.1. Recommendations of various organizations in regard to mammographic screening for women below age 50

Recommend Routinely	Do Not Routinely Recommend
1. American Cancer Society	1. American College of Physicians
2. American College of Radiology	2. U.S. Preventive Services Task Force
3. American Medical Association	3. American Academy of Family Physicians
4. American College of Obstetricians and Gynecologists	4. American College of Surgeons
5. College of American Pathologists	5. Canadian Task Force on the Periodic Health Examination

development of the tumor mass, metastasis occurs and the resulting metastatic deposits lead to the death of the patient. Within this cascade of events, a "window of opportunity" exists: if the cancer is detected and treated before the onset of metastasis, the natural course of the disease can be arrested and death averted.

Those who believe that breast cancer is a progressive rather than systemic disease have long maintained that mammographic screening can result in the detection of breast cancers within the "window of opportunity." Thus, the proponents of mammographic screening believe that screening will ultimately result in a significant reduction in breast cancer mortality. Over the past 30 years, numerous studies were designed to test this hypothesis: case-control, retrospective and prospective. As a result, we now know more about screening for breast cancer than about screening for any other type of cancer. However, before evaluating the merits of these studies, we must consider three biases pertinent to any screening studies: lead time, length and selection.

Lead time bias is the interval between the diagnosis of cancer on mammography and the time when the cancer becomes clinically apparent. Lead time bias may make it appear that screening prolongs life when it simply extends the period of time over which the cancer is observed. This was shown in the lung cancer screening trials.[12] These trials demonstrated an improved survival for patients with screen-detected lung cancers, but no reduction in lung cancer mortality. Screening, therefore, simply moved the time of diagnosis backward, but had no real impact on the length of life. This should not be confused with better prognosis and lower mortality. Indeed, retrospective studies comparing survival between screened and unscreened populations fail to account for lead time bias and are therefore flawed. This can be illustrated by comparing the retrospective study of Stacey-Clear et al with the Canadian prospective breast cancer screening trial.[13,14] Both showed good 5-year survival for younger women who underwent mammographic screening.

However, at 7 years, the Canadian study showed a nonsignificant excess in mortality in the screened group. This could only be explained by assuming a lead time bias of up to 4 years.

Screening tends to detect those cancers that are slower growing and biologically more favorable. Such tumors will have a better prognosis than the clinically detected cancers and this is termed length bias.[15] Slower growing tumors will exist for a longer period of time in the preclinical phase and are therefore more likely to be diagnosed by mammographic screening. In contrast, the faster growing tumors exist for a shorter period of time in the preclinical phase and are more likely to be detected clinically in the intervals between the screening sessions. Comparisons of tumors detected by screening mammography with those detected by physical examination fail to account for length bias. Indeed, some comparisons of screen-detected cancers with interval cancers (those detected by physical examination between screening sessions) have shown that the interval cancers have a poorer prognosis.[16]

Clinical trials often recruit volunteers. Volunteers for clinical trials tend to be health conscious and, therefore, have a lower all-cause mortality. Thus, any comparison between such volunteers and nonvolunteer controls will contain a selection bias. The impact of selection bias was illustrated in a case-control evaluation of the effect of breast cancer screening in the United Kingdom, comparing attenders and nonattenders for screening.[17] Populations from two separate districts were compared: a screening district and a comparison (nonscreening) district. It was found that breast cancer mortality was higher among the nonattenders of the screening district when compared to women in the comparison district. The investigators attributed this to selection bias.

Prospective, randomized, controlled clinical trials take into account the biases discussed above. There have been eight randomized trials that have examined the efficacy of mammographic screening and seven of these have included women below the age of 50.[18] A total of 500,000 women of all age groups were recruited into these trials and nearly 170,000 of these were between the ages of 40-49 at the start of the trials. The seven trials that have included women between the ages of 40-49 are the Health Insurance Plan (HIP), Swedish Two County, Malmo, Gothenberg, Stockholm, Edinburgh and Canadian National Breast Screening Study I (NBSS I). Of these seven trials, only the NBSS I was specifically designed to study the efficacy of screening women between the ages of 40-49, while in the remainder, the value of mammographic screening for women of this age group was derived from subset analysis.

The first randomized clinical trial was the HIP study.[19] This study involved 62,000 women between the ages of 40-64 at entry, enrolled in the HIP medical insurance plan of New York. These women were randomly assigned to either a study or control group. The study was initiated in 1963 and showed a possible benefit to screening women below the age of 50 after long term follow up. However, it has been suggested that the main reason for an apparent mortality reduction in the screened group is a poorer survival of Stage I breast cancers in the control arm of the trial, when compared to both the screen-detected and nonscreen-detected cancers in the study group. Furthermore, the 25% reduction in mortality was not seen until 10-18 years after the start of the study. The possible reason for this delayed benefit remains wide open to speculation. As most trials show a benefit to screening women above the age of 50 within 7-9 years after initiation of the trial, why is a much longer time interval required to see a benefit for screening women under the age of 50? One might speculate that, as the HIP trial progressed, many women who were below the age of 50 at the start of the trial, passed their 50th birthday. Thus, the possible long term benefit of screening younger women in the HIP may be attributed to screening those women beyond the age of 50. I further discuss this hypothesis below.

Attention should also be drawn to the design of the HIP trial. While many of the screening trials have randomized women to screening with mammography alone or no screening, the HIP trial randomized to screening with mammography and physical examination (PE) or no screening. Ultimately, only 19% of the breast cancers in women aged 40-49 were detected by mammography alone and 57% were detected by PE alone. Thus, the HIP trial can not be used to support the argument that mammographic screening is effective for this age group. If anything, the trial suggests that PE plays an important role in reducing breast cancer mortality and merits additional investigation as a screening tool.

The Edinburgh trial was initiated in 1978 and involved 44,288 women between the ages of 45-64 at the start of the trial.[20] Like the HIP trial, these women were randomized to screening with mammography and PE or no screening. For women between the ages of 45-49 at the start of the trial, there were 11370 in the study group and 10269 in the control group. At 7 years of follow up, the relative risk of death in the screened group in comparison to the control group was 0.98 (95% CI: 0.45-2.11) for women below the age of 50 at the start of the trial. At 10 years of follow up, that relative risk was 0.78 (95% CI: 0.46-1.31). Thus, a statistically significant benefit to screening women under the age of 50 was never demonstrated.

An overview of the four Swedish randomized clinical trials has been reported.[21] The four trials included in the overview were the Two-County, Malmo, Stockholm and Gothenberg. These trials involved a total of about 90,000 women under the age of 50. A nonsignificant 13% (95% CI: 37% to -20%) decrease in mortality was demonstrated for younger women in the screened group after 12 years of follow up. Even if this figure were to represent the actual benefit of screening women under the age of 50, what would it mean in absolute terms? If we assume that the risk of a 40 year old woman developing breast cancer over a 10 year period is 1.0% and her risk of dying from it is 0.5% (worst case scenario), then the Swedish overview suggests that mammographic screening for women between the ages of 40-49 results in an absolute reduction in breast cancer mortality of 0.5% x 13%, or 0.065%.

The only study that was specifically designed to test the effectiveness of mammographic screening for women between the ages of 40-49 was the Canadian National Breast Screening Study (NBSS I).[14] The NBSS I was designed with enough statistical power to detect at least a 40% reduction in mortality with screening. The total number of women included in the NBSS I study was 50,430. After 7 years of follow up, there was a nonsignificant excess mortality in the screened group, the relative risk in the screened group being 1.36 (95% CI: 0.84-2.21).

Kerlikowske et al have undertaken a meta-analysis of the eight randomized, controlled trials and four case-control studies on breast cancer screening.[22] Although a significant reduction in breast cancer mortality was seen after 7-9 years of follow up for women who were above the age of 50 at the start of the studies, this was not the case for younger women. Indeed, for women aged 40-49 years of age who were followed for 7-9 years, there was a nonsignificant increase (2%) in breast cancer mortality (95% CI: -18% to +27%), but after 10-12 years of follow up, there was a nonsignificant reduction (17%) in breast cancer mortality (95% CI: -24% to 13%). Breast cancer is much less common in women below the age of 50 than in women above that age and mortality associated with breast cancer is also much greater in older women. Thus, it has been suggested by some who advocate screening for younger women that longer follow up allows the screening trials to accumulate sufficient numbers of breast cancer deaths, thereby providing the statistical power necessary to show a reduction in breast cancer mortality. However, Kerlikowske et al suggest that this is not so. Indeed, if the explanation is simply a lack of statistical power, then the percentage reduction of breast cancer mortality reported at 7-9 years should be similar to that at 10-12 years, only with wider confidence intervals. As this is not the case, then the difference in

mortality reduction between the two interval groups may either simply be due to chance, or, alternatively, the delayed benefit of screening younger women may be attributed to the effect of screening these younger women beyond the age of 50. In contrast, Kerlikowske et al reported a significant reduction in breast cancer mortality associated with screening women over the age of 50, the relative risk being 0.74 (95% CI: 0.66-0.83). The magnitude of this benefit was similar, whether measured with short term or long term follow up.

The mortality reduction seen after long follow up of women between the ages of 40-49 was further assessed by de Koning et al.[23] These authors used a computer simulation model known as MISCAN (Microsimulation Screening Analysis) and included the results from the Swedish randomized trials in their analysis. The computed simulation model suggested that about 70% of the 10% observed reduction in breast cancer mortality for women between the ages of 40-49 at the start of the screening trials was indeed due to screening these women after they passed the age of 50.

In view of the persistent controversy surrounding the efficacy of mammographic screening in younger women, another large, randomized prospective trial has been initiated in the United Kingdom.[24] In this study, women will be aged 40-41 at entry. A study group of 65,000 women will be offered mammographic screening at the first visit and annually thereafter for seven or eight rounds, while a comparison group of 135,000 women will be offered the usual care with no screening. Upon reaching the age of 50, both groups will be offered regular screening. These women will be followed for 14-15 years. The trial has been designed with 80% power to detect a mortality reduction of 20%, assuming that 70% of the women accept the offer to undergo screening.

CRITICISM OF THE SCREENING TRIALS

Historically, those clinical studies that support common sense views are generally well received. In contrast, studies that fail to support such views are often severely criticized. For example, until recently, most surgeons believed that breast cancer was a locally progressive disease and that the dissection of the axilla and the extent of the mastectomy influenced survival. This paradigm was promulgated by Halsted in the late 19th century and was intuitively very appealing to most surgeons.[25] When the results of the National Surgical Adjuvant Breast and Bowel Project (NSABP-04 and 06) clinical trials failed to support this paradigm, the trials were severely criticized and their conclusions were not initially accepted.[26] Thus, it should come as no surprise that the screening trials have been criticized for failing to demonstrate the effectiveness of screening in younger women. After all, the notion that the early detection of breast cancer benefits all women, regardless of age, has been inculcated in the minds of clinicians since the late 19th century. I shall now address some of the criticisms that have been directed against the screening trials and against the National Breast Cancer Screening Study (NBSS) of Canada in particular.

As breast cancer is less common in younger than older women, some critics have charged that all the screening trials to date lack the statistical power to show a significant mortality reduction in younger women. Indeed, Kopans has calculated that a trial that could prove a 25% mortality reduction at 5 years for women ages 40-49 years would require 500,000 women.[27] To date, the Canadian study is the largest trial to recruit women in their forties and it only contained about 50,000 women of this age group. A trial involving 10 times that number will probably never be feasible. Furthermore, if such large numbers of women are required to show a benefit, then the benefit in absolute terms must be very small indeed. The potential for harm in screening such large numbers of asymptomatic women must then be weighed against the potential for a very small benefit. I shall discuss the potential for harm later in this chapter.

The proponents of mammographic screening for younger women also argue

that technology has improved in recent years and that the mammographic equipment used in the clinical trials to date do not represent the state of the art equipment that is available today. Dupont maintains that "it is quite possible that today's mammography may produce meaningful savings in lives of women in their forties, even though yesterday's mammography was unable to demonstrate this benefit. This provides an argument for conducting a new clinical trial using modern methods."[28] Yes, technology is constantly improving, but are we to conduct a new trial every time there is an advancement in mammographic technology? Between 1963-1980, eight randomized, controlled trials on mammographic screening were initiated. If improvements in mammographic technology were to translate directly into greater reductions in breast cancer mortality, then the later trials should have shown a greater reduction in breast cancer mortality for women over the age of 50 than did the earlier trials. But this is not the case. Indeed, Wright and Mueller point out that just the opposite is true: the later trials showed less of a benefit than did the earlier trials![29]

Much criticism has been directed against the Canadian National Breast Screening Study I (NBSS).[14] This was the only trial that was specifically designed to test the effectiveness of mammographic screening for women between the ages of 40-49 and it showed a nonsignificant excess in mortality in the screened group after 7 years. Critics have charged that the quality of mammography was poor, particularly during the early years of the trial and that the screening arm of the trial therefore does not represent what can be achieved with state of the art technology.[30] However, when compared to earlier screening trials and even with current screening programs in Canada that are judged state of the art by most American radiologists, the NBSS breast cancer detection rates compared very favorably.[31] It is also ironic that no criticisms concerning quality of mammography have been leveled against the HIP study, which used techniques and standards of mammography that are now considered obsolete. Many proponents of mammographic screening for younger women believe that the results of the HIP study justify their position. Thus, it appears that the proponents of screening have applied a double standard when identifying trials for criticism!

In the NBSS, women were randomized to either the screened or control group after an initial clinical breast examination.[14] Thus, some critics charge that the randomization process in the NBSS was flawed and that a greater number of women with breast lumps (and hence, advanced cancers) were assigned to the screened group, thereby contributing to the excess of breast cancer mortality attributable to the screened group.[32] Support for this criticism comes from the observation that a greater number of advanced (node positive) cancers were detected in the first screening round of the study group.[14] However, the charge concerning randomization has never been substantiated.[33] Furthermore, other trials, most notably the Swedish Two County Study, have also reported an excess of node-positive cancers in the screened group.[34] Indeed, these findings may have relevance to our understanding of the biological significance of nodal metastasis. Perhaps nodal metastases are not simply indicative of tumor chronology as many clinicians have long assumed, but more indicative of the tumor phenotype.[35] There is some evidence to support this hypothesis.

The NBSS has also been criticized on the grounds that there was contamination of the control group.[27] Indeed, it has been reported that 26% of the women in the control group had mammograms. Thus, it has been suggested that the NBSS compared screened women with other screened women, thereby diluting out any benefit attributable to mammographic screening. However, it must be remembered that the control group in the NBSS was considered the "usual care" group.[36] The objective of the study was to compare an established screening program with good clinical care, as is generally practiced in most communities in Canada. Therefore, it would be expected that any woman in the control group who was found clinically to have a breast mass would receive a mammogram as part of her diagnostic work up. This represents the standard of care and if the implementation of mammographic screening does indeed reduce breast cancer mortality, it must do so above and beyond that which can be achieved under the generally established methods of usual care. Miller has pointed out that all other trials have compared screening with nothing, a highly artificial situation.[36]

WHY AGE 50?

If we accept the results of the randomized clinical trials at face value, then an important question arises: why does mammographic screening benefit older but not younger women? And, in particular, why does the age of 50 separate those who do and do not benefit from screening? The age of 50, of course, approximately corresponds to the time of the menopause and differences in the biology and epidemiology of breast cancer have been reported between pre- and postmenopausal women.[18] For example, there are changes in the incidence of breast cancer associated with the menopause: a steep rise occurs until about the age of 45-55 and this is followed by a less rapid increase in incidence thereafter.[37] The characteristics of the primary tumor are also influenced by the menopause. Thus, younger women have a lower proportion of estrogen receptor positive tumors and a higher labeling index.[38] Additionally, the risk factors for breast cancer change with the menopause. Indeed, some studies have shown that obesity is associated with a higher risk of postmenopausal breast cancer but a lower risk of premenopausal cancer.[39] Therefore, the changes noted in the effectiveness of screening is consistent with other studies showing differences in the biology and epidemiology between pre- and postmenopausal breast cancer. Indeed, one might speculate that, if participants of the screening trials had been categorized by menopausal status rather than age, a more significant difference in the effectiveness of screening between younger and older women might have become apparent. The screening trials may, therefore, be providing us with important insights into the natural history of breast cancer. The relevance of the screening trials to the natural history of breast cancer is further discussed in a separate chapter in this book.

Several other hypotheses have been proposed to account for the difference between screening older and younger women and we can only mention a few. For example, Van Netten et al have proposed an intriguing hypothesis based on the observation that in situ breast cancers are fairly common in younger women.[40] Many investigators have long assumed that invasive breast cancers are derived from in situ cancers, but the mechanism is not known. Thus, Van Netten et al suggest that tissue injuries in areas of the breast containing the in situ cancers may have some significance. Blows to the breast or severe compression could result in spillage or dislocation of in situ carcinoma cells into the surrounding stroma, where these cells could then interact with macrophages, resulting in invasion or distant spread. As much as 25 kg of pressure is applied to the breast during mammography and younger women are more vulnerable to this sort of trauma than are older women. After all, the breasts of younger women are more dense than that of older women and therefore require more compression force during mammography. Furthermore, as women grow older, the chances of external trauma to organs such as the breast increase and therefore trauma from mammography may become less of an issue. Although this hypothesis may seem far fetched, it is of interest that Egan found that breast cancer mortality was twice as high among women with mammographically dense breasts (Dy and P2 groups of Wolfe's parenchymal patterns) when compared to those with less dense breasts and Levallius postulates that this could be due to the greater compression force required during mammography.[41,42]

Tabar et al have reported that, in the Swedish Two County study, the rate of interval cancers (cancers arising between mammographic screens) was much higher in the 40-49 age group than for the other age groups.[43] Thus, it has been suggested that interval cancers may account for the failure of the screening trials to show a benefit for screening women under the age of 50. Tabar therefore advocates reducing the intervals between screening sessions for younger women. However, the high rate of interval cancers in younger women is contrary to what one might expect. For instance, Adami et al have shown that breast cancers arising in women between the ages of 40-49 have the best overall prognosis[44] which would suggest a slower rate of growth for these cancers relative to older women and lead one to expect a lower incidence of interval cancers in women between the ages of 40-49. Nonetheless, interval cancers are important to consider in any screening program. In the Nijmen project, for instance, after seven rounds of screening, the interval cancer rate peaked at 24.9/10,000 whereas the rate of cancer detected by screening was between 29.5-38.9/10,000.[45] Furthermore, the high rate of interval cancers recently documented in an NHS screening program will probably mean that the stated target of reducing breast cancer mortality in the U.K. by 25% by the year 2000 will not be met.[46]

HAZARDS OF SCREENING

There is as yet no evidence to support the efficacy of mammographic screening for younger women. Indeed, in contrast to older women, no benefit from screening women in their forties is seen in the immediate years after the initiation of screening. The presence of a marginal benefit after screening for 10 years is, at best, uncertain. These facts are quite clear from data derived from the screening trials. Yet, some argue that screening for women in their forties should continue until the evidence to support this practice becomes available. Those who apply this logic often fail to appreciate the potential hazards of screening. Should we subject large numbers of asymptomatic younger women to the hazards of screening, with no proof of benefit and only the reassurance that such proof is forthcoming? In light of the potential for harm, the onus of proof of benefit must rest with the proponents of screening and, ethically, such proof must be obtained before screening is applied to younger women. At least five potentially harmful effects of screening merit particular attention: lead time, false positives, cost, radiation exposure and overdiagnosis.[1] These potential hazards of screening are summarized in Table 3.2 and I shall discuss them in detail below.

LEAD TIME

Screening clearly advances the time of diagnosis. However, if this does not translate into a reduction in breast cancer mortality, then some women are given advanced notice of impending death with no tangible gain. For women over the age of 50, screening reduces breast cancer mortality by 30%.[22] Thus, even among women of this age group, the majority will gain lead time but no benefit. Nonetheless, as screening does save some lives for women over age 50, it seems appropriate for women of this age group. But for women below the age of 50, there is as yet no clear evidence of benefit. Therefore, younger women with screen-detected breast cancers may gain lead time with no benefit. What impact does this have on quality of life? It has been estimated that the diagnosis of breast cancer is advanced by 2-4 years with screening.[1] If this is indeed the case, then younger women will suffer an additional 2-4 years of anxiety, stress

and perhaps, even financial hardship (resulting from loss of insurance coverage or an increase in their insurance premiums) as a result of their early diagnosis. And for all of this, they will gain nothing. The adverse effects of lead time therefore merit careful consideration when recommending screening mammography for younger women.

FALSE POSITIVES

False positives are those cases reported as suspicious or malignant on the screening mammogram that, on subsequent evaluation, prove to be benign. False positives are more common in the United States than in Europe, probably owing to the medico-legal climate in the United States and hence the greater unwillingness of American radiologists to commit themselves to a benign diagnosis.[47] Analysis of the American Breast Cancer Detection Demonstration Project (BCDDP) revealed that the positive predictive value of mammographic screening was only 10%, meaning that nine women had a false positive result on screening for every cancer found.[48] On the other hand, European studies have indicated positive predictive values ranging from 30-60%.[49] Furthermore, it has been reported that the false positive rate is higher in younger compared to older women. Indeed, Kerlikowske et al reported a false positive rate of 96% for women in their forties and 81% for those in their seventies.[50] False positives result in

Table 3.2. Hazards of screening younger women

Harmful Effect	Consequences
Cost	Increased expenditures on intervention of no proven value
Lead Time	Advanced notice of impending death
Radiation Exposure	Increased risk of breast cancer in women who carry the gene for ataxia-telangiectasia
False Positives	Unnecessary breast biopsies
Overdiagnosis	Financial/emotional consequences of being falsely labeled as a cancer patient

Reproduced with permission from Jatoi I, Baum M. Mammographic screening in women under age 50: a critical appraisal. In: Querci della Rovere G, Morgan MW, Warren R, eds. Breast Screening and the Management of Early Breast Cancer. Graffam Press: Edinburgh (in press).

unnecessary biopsies and contribute to anxiety and cancerphobia. Lidbrink et al recently reviewed the impact of false positives on the overall cost of the Stockholm mammography screening trial.[51] Even though only 10% of all breast cancers occur in women between the ages of 40-50, 41% of the costs of false positives (in terms of additional work up and biopsies) in the Stockholm screening trial was attributed to women of this age group. It has also recently been estimated that, among those women in the United States who obtain annual mammography between the ages of 40-50, approximately 30% will have a false positive mammogram over a 10 year period that will result in an unnecessary biopsy.[52]

RADIATION EXPOSURE

Exposure to relatively low doses of radiation might be detrimental. An estimated 1.4% of the general population are carriers of a single gene for ataxia-telangiectasia (AT).[53] These carriers are predisposed to developing breast cancer after exposure to relatively low doses of radiation. Indeed, Swift et al estimate that relatively modest doses of radiation, such as a woman might receive from x-ray fluoroscopic procedures involving the chest or abdomen leads to an almost six-fold excess risk of breast cancers for AT blood relatives.[54] Thus, it appears that even low doses of radiation may increase the risk of developing breast cancer in AT heterozygotes. Swift estimates that the proportion of AT heterozygotes among women with early breast cancer onset is greater than 7%.

OVERDIAGNOSIS

Peters et al define overdiagnosis as "a histologically established diagnosis of invasive or intraductal breast cancer that would never have developed into a clinically manifest tumor during the patient's normal life expectancy if no screening examination had been carried out."[55] Since the advent of mammographic screening, the incidence of ductal carcinoma in situ (DCIS) has increased dramatically.[56] DCIS is rarely palpable and these lesions are almost exclusively discovered by mammographic screening. Prior to the introduction of mammographic screening, DCIS accounted for only 1-2% of all breast cancers. Today, over 8% of all breast cancers and 22% of those discovered by mammographic screening are identified as DCIS. Many clinicians have long assumed that DCIS is a preinvasive cancer that, if untreated, invariably leads to invasive breast cancer. This assumption is based on two observations: DCIS is often found adjacent to invasive cancers and, with simple excision of DCIS, recurrences frequently occur and these recurrences are often invasive cancer.[57] A woman with a mammographically detected DCIS is therefore regarded by most insurance companies and employers as a breast cancer patient. This can have a very adverse effect on her quality of life.

There is now considerable evidence to suggest that not all DCIS progresses to invasive breast cancer. Nielsen et al reported the results of 110 medico-legal autopsies of women between the ages of 20-54 who died of accidents.[58] DCIS was found incidentally in 15% of these women, a prevalence four to five times greater than the number of overt cancers expected to develop clinically over 20 years. Thus, contrary to conventional wisdom, occult DCIS is fairly common in younger women. Additionally, in autopsies of women with a previous diagnosis of breast cancer, Alpers and Wellings found DCIS in 48% of contralateral breasts even though only 12.5% of breast cancer patients develop contralateral breast cancer after 20 years of follow up.[59] Finally, in two separate studies, Rosen et al and Page et al retrospectively reviewed benign breast biopsy findings and discovered a number of instances where DCIS had been overlooked by the initial pathologist.[60,61] In the series reported by Rosen et al, 30 patients with DCIS were identified and after an average follow up of 18 years, clinically manifest breast cancer developed in only 8 patients. Similarly, Page et al identified 28 women with DCIS and found that clinically apparent breast cancer developed in only 7 women after 15 years of follow up. All these studies suggest that most women diagnosed with

DCIS by means of mammographic screening probably would not develop clinically manifest breast cancers during their lifetime. Thus, the diagnosis of DCIS through the use of mammographic screening contributes significantly to the overdiagnosis of breast cancer.

Nonetheless, for purposes of obtaining insurance, loans and employment, women with mammographically detected DCIS often face the same challenges that confront those women with invasive cancer.[56] These include the outright refusal of insurance coverage or coverage with inflated premiums, the offer of only high-risk types of policies and denial of life insurance. Women who are diagnosed with DCIS may encounter difficulties when seeking employment. Although the Americans with Disabilities Act of 1992 prohibits employers from discriminating against persons with serious illnesses, many companies continue to do so (many are unaware of the Act).[62] Small companies, in particular, have misgivings about employing a woman diagnosed with DCIS. Indeed, a single patient with a mammographically detected DCIS can pose a financial burden for a small company by significantly raising that company's health insurance premium. Thus, the overdiagnosis of breast cancer by means of mammographic screening may have a very adverse impact on the quality of life.

The overdiagnosis of breast cancer results in overtreatment. It is ironic that many surgeons in the United States advocate total mastectomy for the treatment of situ cancer (with the rationale that total mastectomy for DCIS is 100% curable) and yet consider lumpectomy and axillary lymph node dissection as a viable alternative to modified radical mastectomy for the treatment of invasive breast cancer. Now, hopefully, with the publication of the results of the National Surgical Adjuvant Breast Project-17 (NSABP-17), surgeons will resort to less radical surgery for the treatment of DCIS.[63] The NSABP-17 study demonstrated that radiation therapy combined with lumpectomy effectively controlled the risk of recurrence for DCIS.

COST

The overall cost of health care has risen dramatically in recent years and governments around the world are attempting to limit those costs. Rosenquist and Lindfors have determined that, if the estimated mortality reduction from mammographic screening is 15% or greater, then the marginal cost per year of life saved would be comparable to that of other generally accepted medical procedures.[64] However, such a benefit for screening women below the age of 50 has not been shown. Kattlove et al have recently conducted a cost-effective analyses using data from the Swedish screening trials.[65] These authors determined the cost to save one potential life at 10 years with mammographic screening. If the nonsignificant 13% reduction in screening women between the ages of 40-49 (from the Swedish Overview analysis) represented the true benefit of screening women of this age group, then to save one potential life at 10 years for women of this age group would cost $1,480,000. In contrast, the cost of mammographic screening to save one potential life for women aged 60-69 would be $146,000 and for women aged 50-59 the cost would be $183,000. Of course, no one can place a price on a human life. Nonetheless, these figures should be considered along with the potential hazards of screening when deciding how best to appropriate scarce resources.

INFORMED CONSENT

Annas writes that "the structure of medical practice—including factors such as cost containment, the profit motive, government regulations, fear of malpractice suits, media hype and risk management schemes—probably influences actual practice more than professional standards. This seems especially true in medical screening, including breast cancer screening."[66] Katz argues that, in situations where physicians do not know what course of treatment is best for their patients, they are obligated to share the uncertainty with their patients.[67] Why should the same criterion not apply to the uncertainty surrounding the efficacy of mammographic screening for younger women? Yet, promotional campaigns launched by major local and national cancer organizations urge younger women to obtain screening mammograms, but do little to inform them about the screening controversy or the potential hazards of screening.

Few investigators have addressed the possible impact of obtaining informed consent prior to mammographic screening. Black et al surveyed 200 women between the ages of 40-50 and found that most grossly overestimated their breast cancer risk and the benefit of screening.[68] For example, younger women overestimated their risk of dying of breast cancer within 10 years by more than 20-fold. Furthermore, if a 10% relative risk reduction in mortality was assumed from screening younger women, then the respondents overestimated the relative risk reduction of mortality by six-fold and the absolute risk reduction by 100-fold. Additionally, most women are completely unaware of the hazards of screening that I have outlined above. Advertising campaigns have been launched by local and national cancer organizations to encourage mammographic screening, but often mislead women into thinking that every cancer detected by screening equals a life saved and that there are no hazards associated with screening. Indeed, Baum maintains that true informed consent for an invitation to screening might reduce rather than increase the acceptance of mammographic screening among women.[69] Lee has also outlined the need to discuss the basic risks of disease and the risks associated with screening procedures with patients.[70] He argues that "this byproduct of informed consent will reduce the paradox of health that emanates from our advanced technology: we are healthier, but because we worry more about the possibility of disease, we are unhappier." Thus, in the continuing controversy over mammographic screening for younger women, informed consent should perhaps be viewed as the middle ground.

As many women grossly overestimate their risks of developing breast cancer, it might be appropriate to tell a 40-year-old woman with no significant family history of breast cancer that her chances of developing breast cancer over a 10-year period is 13 per 1000.[70] The potential risks/benefits of mammographic screening should also be discussed. This was computed by Harris for a group of 1000 women between the ages of 40-49 in the United States.[52] Annual mammography for this group of women would result in a total of 10,000 mammograms (the frequently ordered "6 month follow up" mammograms are ignored in this calculation). Harris calculates that about 300 women (30%) during this period would have false positive mammograms that would result in unnecessary biopsies. Additionally, 30 women would be reassured that they do not have breast cancer when in fact they do. For purposes of this calculation, Harris assumes a mortality reduction of 20% from screening and estimates that this will result in one woman's life being prolonged from screening 1000 women, but only after the women approach the age of 60. He calculates that 125 breast cancers will be diagnosed during this period. It seems appropriate to point out that many of these "cancers" would be in situ cancers that in most instances would not develop into a clinically manifest invasive cancer during the lifetime of these women.

CONCLUSION

The controversy over mammographic screening for women in their forties is likely to continue unabated for the foreseeable future. Much has been said and written about this subject, but we are no closer to a consensus now than we were 10 years ago. Blanket recommendations by major physicians' organizations either favoring or opposing mammographic screening for younger women do little to resolve the controversy. If anything, these recommendations are often conflicting and add to the confusion in the minds of patients and physicians alike. Most clinicians and epidemiologists have focused on what impact, if any, mammographic screening has on the reduction of breast cancer mortality. Yet, during these discussions, the impact of screening on quality of life has received little attention. There are clearly hazards associated with screening and many have a profound effect on quality of life. Women have a right to know the facts concerning mammographic screening and should be urged to make an informed decision concerning its merits. Ultimately both the proponents and critics of mammographic screening for younger women share the same goal: to reduce breast cancer mortality and improve the quality of life for all women. The controversy centers over the best means by which to achieve these goals.

REFERENCES

1. Jatoi I, Baum M. American and European recommendations for screening mammography in younger women: a cultural divide? Br Med J 1993; 307: 1481-3.
2. Jenks S. ACS keeps mammogrpahy guidelines for women under 50. J Natl Cancer Inst 1993; 85(5):348-49.
3. Vanchieri C. Europeans say screen only women age 50 and older. J Natl Cancer Inst 1993; 85(5):350.
4. Davis DL, Love SM. Mammographic screening. JAMA 1994; 271(2):152-3.
5. Chu KC, Tarone RE, Kessler LE et al. Recent trends in U.S. breast cancer incidence, survival and mortality rates. J Natl Cancer Inst 1996; 88:1571-9.
6. Beral V, Hermon C, Reeves SG, Peto R. Sudden fall in breast cancer death rates in England and Wales. (Letter) Lancet 1995; 345:1642-3.
7. Fletcher SW. Why question screening mammography for women in their forties? Radiol Clin North Am 1995; 33(6): 1259-71.
8. Kaluzny AD, Rimer B, Harris R. The National Cancer Institute and guideline development: lessons from the breast cancer screening controversy. J Natl Cancer Inst 199; 86:901-2.
9. Marwick C. NIH consensus panel spurs discontent. JAMA 1997; 277(7):519-20.
10. Van Netten JP, Ross AS, Cann SA, Derry DM, Ashwood Smith MJ. Is breast cancer a progressive or systemic disease? (Letter) Lancet 1995; 345:319-20.
11. Devitt JE. Breast cancer: have we missed the forest because of the tree? Lancet 1994; 344:734-5.
12. Eddy DM, ed. Common Screening Tests. Philadelphia: American College of Physicians, 1991.
13. Stacey-Clear A, McCarthy KA, Hall DA et al. Breast cancer survival among women under age 50: is mammography detrimental? Lancet 1992; 340:991-4.
14. Miller AB, Baines CJ, To T, Wall C. Canadian national breast screening study I. Breast cancer detection and death rates among women aged 40 to 49. Can Med Assoc J 1992; 147:1459-76.
15. Miller AB. Is routine mammography screening appropriate for women 40-49 years of age? Am J Prev Med 1991; 7:55-62.
16. Miller AB. Mammography in women under 50. Hem Onc Clin N Amer 1994; 8:165-77.
17. Moss SM, Summerley ME, Thomas BJ, Ellman R, Chamberlain JOP. A case-control evaluation of the effect of breast cancer screening in the United Kingdom trial of early detection of breast cancer. J Epidemiol Comm Health 1992; 46: 362-4.
18. Elwood JM, Cox B, Richardson AK. The effectiveness of breast cancer screening by mammography in younger women. Online J Curr Clin Trials, 25 Feb 1993 (Doc No 32).
19. Shapiro S, Venet W, Strax P, Venet L. Periodic screening for breast cancer: the Health Insurance Plan project and its sequelae, 1963-86. Baltimore: Johns Hopkins University Press, 1988.
20. Roberts MM, Alexander FE anderson TJ, Chetty U, Donnan PT, Forrest P et al. Edinburgh trial of screening for breast cancer: mortality at seven years. Lancet 1990; 335:241-6.
21. Nystrom L, Rutquist LE, Wall S, Lindgren A, Linquist M, Ryden S et al. Breast cancer screening with mammography: overview of Swedish randomized trials. Lancet 1993; 341:973-8.
22. Kerlikowske K, Grady D, Rubin SM, Sandrock C, Ernster VL. Efficacy of screening mammography. A meta-analy-

sis. JAMA 1995; 273-149-54.

23. de Konig HJ, Boer R, Warmerdam PG, Beemsterboes PMM, van der Maas PJ. Quantitative interpretations of age-specific mortality reductions from the Swedish breast cancer screening trials. J Natl Cancer Inst 1995; 87:1217-1223.

24. Breast screening in women under 50. Lancet 1991; 337:1575-6.

25. Halsted WS. A clinical and histological study of certain adenocarcinoma of the breast and a brief consideration of the supraclavicular operation and of the results of operation for cancer of the breast from 1889 to 1898 at the Johns Hopkins Hospital. Ann Surg 1898; 28:557-576.

26. Fisher B. Personal contributions to progress in breast cancer research and treatment. Sem Onc 1996; 123(4): 414-427.

27. Kopans DB. Screening for breast cancer and mortality reduction among women 40-49 years of age. Cancer 1994; 74: 311-22.

28. Dupont WD. Evidence of efficacy of mammographic screening for women in their forties. Cancer 1994; 74:1204-6.

29. Wright CJ, Mueller CB. Screening mammography and public health policy: the need for perspective. Lancet 1995; 346: 29-32.

30. Kopans DB. The Canadian screening program: a different perspective. Am J Roentgenol 1990; 155:748-9.

31. Baines CJ. A different view on what is known about breast screening and the Canadian national breast screening study. Cancer 1994; 74:1207-11.

32. Kopans DB, Feig SA. The Canadian national breast screening study: a critical review. Am J Roentgenol 1993; 161:755-60.

33. Baines CJ. The Canadian national breast screening study: a perspective on criticisms. Ann Intern Med 1994; 120: 326-334.

34. Tabar L, Fagerberg G, Duffy SW, Day NE, Gad A, Grontoft O. Update of the Swedish two-county program of mammographic screening for breast cancer. Radiol Clin North Am 1992; 30:187-209.

35. Jatoi I, Clark GM, de Moor C, Hilsenbeck SG, Osborne CK. Axillary lymph node metastasis in primary breast cancer: an indicator of tumor chronology or biology? Proc Am Soc Clin Onc 1995; 14:100 (Abstr)

36. Miller AB. Should screening mammography be performed for women 40-49 years of age? Presented at the 31st Annual Meeting of the American Society of Clinical Oncology, May, 1995.

37. Clemmensen J. Carcinoma of the breast. Results from statistical research. Br J Radiol 1948; 21:583.

38. Henderson IC. Biologic variations of tumors. Cancer 1992; 69:1888-95.

39. Willett W. Nutritional epidemiology. New York: Oxford University Press; 1990.

40. van Netten JP, Morgentale T, Ashwood Smith MJ, Fletcher C, Coy P. Physical trauma and breast cancer. Lancet 1994; 343:978-79.

41. Egan RL. Mammographic patterns and breast cancer risk. JAMA 1980; 244:287.

42. Levallius B. Screening mammography. Lancet 1994; 343:793.

43. Tabar L, Fagerberg G, Day NE, Holmberg L. What is the optimum interval between mammographic screening examinations?—An analysis based on the latest results of the Swedish two-county breast cancer screening trial. Br J Cancer 1987; 55(5):547-51.

44. Adami HO, Malker B, Holmberg L, Persson I, Stone B. The relationship between survival and age at diagnosis in breast cancer. N Engl J Med 1986; 315: 559-563.

45. Field S, Michell MJ, Wallis MGW, Wilson ARM. What should be done about interval breast cancers? Br Med J 1995; 310:203-4.

46. Woodman CBJ, Threlfall AG, Boggis CRM, Prior P. Is the three year breast screening interval too long? Occurrence of interval cancers in NHS breast screening programmes north western region. Br Med J 1995; 310:224-6.

47. Kopans DB, Swann CA. Observation on mammographic screening and false positive mammograms. Am J Roentgenol 1988; 150:785-6.

48. Baker LH. Breast cancer detection demonstration project: 5-year summary re-

port. CA 1982; 42:1-35.

49. Reidy J, Hoskins O. Controversy over mammography screening. Br Med J 1988; 297:932-3.

50. Kerlikowske K, Grady D, Barclay J et al. Positive predictive value of screening mammography by age and family history of breast cancer. JAMA 1993; 270: 2444-2450.

51. Lindbrink E, Elfving J, Frisell J, Jonsson E. Neglected aspects of false positive findings of mammography in breast cancer screening: analysis of false positive cases from the Stockholm trial. Br Med J 1996; 312(7026):273-6.

52. Harris R. Efficacy of screening mammography for women in their forties. J Natl Cancer Inst 1994; 86:1722-24.

53. Swift M. Ionizing radiation, breast cancer and ataxia-telangiectasia. J Natl Cancer Inst 1994; 86:1571-72.

54. Swift M, Morrell D, Massey RB et al. Incidence of cancer in 161 families affected by ataxia-telangiectasia. N Engl J Med 1991; 325:1831-1836.

55. Peeters PHM, Verbeek ALM, Straatman H et al. Evaluation of overdiagnosis of breast cancer in screening with mammography: results of the Nijmegen programme. Int J Epidemiol 1989; 18:295-9.

56. Jatoi I, Baum M. Mammographically detected ductal carcinoma in situ: are we overdiagnosing breast cancer? Surgery 1995; 118:118-20.

57. Van Dongen JA, Fentiman IS, Harris JR et al. In-situ breast cancer: the EORTC consensus meeting. Lancet 1989; 2:25-7.

58. Nielsen M, Thomsen JL, Primdahl S, Dyreborg U andersen JA. Breast cancer and atypia among young and middle aged women: a study of 110 medicolegal autopsies. Br J Cancer 1987; 56:814-9.

59. Alpers CE, Wellings SR. The prevalence of carcinoma in situ in normal and cancer-associated breasts. Human Pathol 1985; 16:796-807.

60. Rosen PR, Braun DW Jr, Kinne DE. The clinical significance of pre-invasive breast carcinoma. Cancer 1980; 40:919-25.

61. Page DL, Dupont WD, Rogers LW, Landenberger M. Intraductal carcinoma of the breast: follow up after biopsy only. Cancer 1982; 49:751-8.

62. Berkman BJ, Sampson SE. Psychosocial effects of cancer economics on patients and their families. Cancer 1993; 72: 2846-9.

63. Fisher B, Constantino J, Redmond C et al. Lumpectomy compared with lumpectomy and radiation therapy for the treatment of intraductal breast cancer. N Engl J Med 1993; 328:1581-6.

64. Rosenquist CJ, Lindfors KK. Screening mammography in women aged 40-49 years: analysis of cost-effectiveness. Radiology 1994; 191:647-50.

65. Kattlove H, Liberati A, Keeler E, Brook RH. Benefits and costs of screening and treatment for early breast cancer. JAMA 1995; 273(2):142-8.

66. Annas GJ. Breast cancer screening in older women: law and patient rights. J Gerontol 1992; 47:121-125.

67. Katz J. The silent world of doctor and patient. New Haven, CT: Yale University Press, 1984.

68. Black WC, Nease RF, Tosteson ANA. Perceptions of breast cancer risk and screening effectiveness in women younger than 50 years of age. J Natl Cancer Inst 1995; 87:720-31.

69. Baum M. Informed consent may increase non-attendance rate. (Letter) Br Med J 1995; 310:1003.

70. Lee JM. Screening and informed consent. N Engl J Med 1993; 328:438-40.

CHAPTER 4

MAMMOGRAPHIC SCREENING IN WOMEN 50 AND OLDER

D. David Dershaw

Mammographic screening for women 50 and older has been accepted as a basic component of the health care of these women. It has been extensively tested in multiple populations and its impact on reducing the mortality of breast cancer is essentially universally accepted. Although evaluated in multiple studies, the full impact of mammographic screening in this population is difficult to estimate because of the variables in study designs, inherent biases in some studies and differences in technology in many studies.

To understand the outcome of studies of screening mammography in women 50 and older it is important to be cognizant of the criteria for a good screening test, the possible limitations in study design and the end goal of the screening intervention.[1] A screening test is designed to identify women with preclinical disease. Those who are free of disease should test negative; those who are positive may have the disease. Optimally, those who test positive should have a high likelihood of having the disease, that is the test should have a high positive predictive value. The test should be acceptable to those who undergo it and who order it. The test should be cost-effective. The test will only be of value if it detects a disease for which a treatment intervention will change the outcome of the disease process.

A variety of biases may prejudice results of studies and these need to be understood when interpreting results of published studies.[2] *Lead time bias* is the amount of time a diagnosis has been advanced by early diagnosis. This can result in longer survival after diagnosis of a disease, but if early diagnosis does not result in cure, there will be no difference in overall mortality rate. For example, if mammography can diagnose breast cancer 4 years earlier than other methods but this early diagnosis does not result in more frequent cure, women diagnosed by mammography will live 4 years longer but the mortality rate for these women will be the same as those diagnosed by other methods. This bias can be overcome by selecting mortality not survival as an endpoint. *Selection bias* is the self-selection of women who have volunteered to participate in a screening program. They may be more conscientious about their health care and therefore may have a better outcome than others in the population. This bias can be overcome by randomized, controlled studies. *Length bias* results from the fact that fast-growing tumors may not be impacted by preclinical detection because they grow too quickly to be detected by the screening modality, whereas slower growing tumors with less biological impact will be more readily detected. Therefore, slower growing tumors with a better prognosis are more often detected. Long-term follow up to detect the impact of these tumors may be necessary. *Overdiagnosis bias* is the detection of tumors of questionable biological importance, tumors which may never have been diagnosed without screening and which have no medical significance. Detection of these tumors, obviously, has a very good prognosis. Again, long-term follow up may be necessary to detect any biological impact from the detection of these tumors.

Finally, the reader must be aware of certain shortcomings of any study design. Although studies are designed to test results of an intervention with full participation of the study population in the intervention, this is never the case. Less than 100% participation by the study population always occurs. Additionally, in controlled studies, the control group is designed to never undergo the intervention being tested. This has never been the case in controlled studies of mammography in which part of the control group has always undergone mammographic testing. Also, studies of mammography have been conducted with varying numbers of mammographic views, varying intervals at which mammography was performed and differing qualities of mammographic examinations. Data from available studies, therefore, represent a compilation of results from differing study designs, differing degrees of participation by the study groups, varying amounts of contamination of the control groups and different qualities and quantities of mammography. The results of these studies do not, therefore, indicate the maximal impact possible by high quality screening mammography done at optimal intervals for women who have been studied. Despite this limitation, overwhelming evidence demonstrates the desirability of mammographic screening for women 50 and older. The data supporting this conclusion are based on a variety of studies, the most important of which will be reviewed.

HEALTH INSURANCE PLAN OF NEW YORK STUDY

The first and perhaps the most important of all the mammography screening trials was that conducted by the Health Insurance Plan (HIP) of New York. This study was designed to determine if routine physical examination and screening mammography could decrease the mortality rate of breast cancer. The HIP study began in 1963 and consisted of study and control groups, each of approximately 31,000 women aged 40-64 years. The study group was invited for an initial examination and followed by three more examinations done annually, unless earlier follow up or biopsy was warranted on clinical grounds. The control group received routine clinical care. Of women in the study group, 65% appeared for the initial examination. Of the four examinations offered, 88% of the study group participated in at least one.[3] Only about one half of the group participated in all four screenings. The study was not designed for subset analysis by age, although this analysis has been performed.

During the HIP study 295 breast cancers were diagnosed in the control group and 225 in the study group. At 18 years of follow up there were 163 breast cancer deaths among the controls and 126 among the study group, a 23% reduction in mortality in the study group.[4] Among women 50-59 in the study group, 60.0% of breast cancers were detected by mammography and 41.5% of breast cancers detected were found only by mammography. Among all women 50 and older, 37.6% of the screen-detected cancers were found only by mammography. With the primitive mammography that was available in the 1960s, 40.0% of breast cancers found in women in their fifties in the study group were only detectable by physical examination. In the HIP study screening detected cancers were node negative in 70.5%, consistent with the greater likelihood of cure for those cancers that were detected at an early stage. The cancer survival rate was greatest for those whose cancers were detected only by mammography. At 12 years after diagnosis, the cancer survival rate (per 100) was 67.8 for those women whose cancers were detected only by mammography, 59.7 for those with screen-detected cancers, 62.5 for those in the control group with node negative tumors and 27.4 for node positive cancers diagnosed in the control group.

The results of the HIP study demonstrated that screening for breast cancer with mammography and physical examination could reduce the mortality of breast cancer by about one quarter and that those cancers detected by mammography alone had the best prognosis. The long follow up of this study has eliminated any lead time bias in the results. However, the contribution of other biases to the results is difficult to exclude. More importantly, a significant difference in the advantage of mammography in women under 50 versus older women was raised by the HIP results. Subset analysis by age demonstrated little advantage to screening women in their forties. At the completion of the HIP study significant technical advances in mammography had been made, raising the possibility of improved mammography for younger women with newer equipment. This prompted the National Cancer Institute and the American Cancer Society to sponsor the second, major American breast screening study to test newer technology and to disseminate techniques for the early detection of breast cancer to the medical profession and the public.

THE BREAST CANCER DETECTION DEMONSTRATION PROJECT

The Breast Cancer Detection Demonstration Project (BCDDP) was composed of 29 centers in 27 cities around the United States. More than 280,000 women volunteered to participate in the program which began in 1973.[5] In this noncontrolled study women were recruited over a 2 year period and were screened with mammography and physical examination, asked to return for five additional annual screenings and were then to be followed for another 5 years. Screening was completed in 1981. At the time of enrollment, women between the ages of 35-74 years were accepted and the median age of participants was 49.5 years. More than half of the women who entered the study participated in all five screenings. Study results are based on 1,074,019 screening events.

At the completion of the BCDDP in 1981, 4,443 breast cancers were recorded and another 886 were detected outside the screening program. For women 50-59 years old, only 6.7% of screen-detected cancers were found by physical examination only. In the HIP study this group made up 40% of screen-detected cancers. Cancers detected by mammography alone were not appreciably changed between the two studies (41.5% vs. 42.1%), but of all cancers detected in women in this age group 91.8% could be identifiable mammographically in BCDDP versus only 60.0% in HIP. This demonstrated improved mammographic detection of breast cancer among women in their fifties in BCDDP compared with those studied with the less advanced technology available a decade earlier. More dramatic advances were found in younger women.

Because BCDDP was not a controlled study, assessment of mortality reduction has been more difficult to evaluate than with results from HIP. For all women participating in BCDDP, the relative 5-, 8- and 10-year survival rates were 88%, 83% and 79%, respectively.[6] For similar tumor size and invasive class, survival rates were comparable with those for women in the National Cancer Institute's Surveillance, Epidemiology End Results (SEER) program. However, when all invasive cancers from BCDDP were compared with those from SEER data, 5- and 8-year survival improved from 74% and 65% in SEER to 87% and 81% for those detected by screening in BCDDP. Improved survival was largely due to the diagnosis of node negative invasive carcinomas smaller than 2 cm and intraductal carcinomas. Among women 50 years old or older at the time of diagnosis, the 5-year survival rate for those 417 diagnosed with intraductal carcinoma was 98% and for those 672 diagnosed with stage I (< 2 cm, node negative) cancer was 95%.

In analyzing data from BCDDP, lead time bias was addressed by making an allowance of one year's time in comparing survival for screen-detected cancers versus those not detected in the study. A similar calculation was used in HIP. Length time bias was addressed by comparing survival rates for those cancers detected at the initial screening (prevalence cases) with those detected in later screens (incident cases). Prevalence cases can be accumulating in the population for many years and could consist of slow-growing cancers as well as more aggressive histologies. The incidence yield for the 3 year follow up period was almost equal to the prevalence yield at initial diagnosis, indicating that slow-growing, biologically unimportant tumors did not account for an important percentage of breast cancers discovered.

BCDDP is flawed by its lack of a control group and by possible selection bias, due to the voluntary enrollment of women into this study. However, both of these issues had been previously addressed in the study design of HIP. BCDDP again demonstrated a reduction in breast cancer mortality for women over 50 with screening. This advantage was largely due to the early detection of breast cancers using mammography, a technique that was demonstrated to be more effective with the technology available in the 1970s that used a decade earlier in the HIP study.

THE SWEDISH STUDIES

Five studies have been conducted in Sweden, including randomized trials in Malmo, Kopparberg, Ostergotland, Stockholm and Gothenberg. Follow up has been reported for up to 13 years on 282,777 women.[7] For all women invited to be screened, there has been a 24% reduction in breast cancer mortality (95% confidence interval, 13-34%) with a 29% reduction in mortality for women 50-69 years old and was essentially identical for women 50-59 and 60-69 years old. The impact on women aged 70-74 years old has been marginal with the relative risk of death for those screened

slightly less than that for those unscreened but with a large confidence interval.

The study design for these five trials has varied. Two-view mammograms were used in the Malmo and Gothenberg trials, which also had the shortest intervals between screenings with 18-24 months in Malmo and 18 months in Gothenberg. Single-view mammograms and screening intervals of 24 months or longer were used in the other three trials. The maximum age of women accepted into the trials was 59 years in Gothenberg, 65 years in Stockholm, 70 years in Malmo and 74 in the two-county study conducted in Kopparberg and Ostergotland.

As in the previous studies, improved survival in the Swedish studies is related to detection of earlier stage cancers.[8] In the two-county trial, breast cancers detected by mammography as compared to those found in the nonscreened, control group were more frequently node negative (68.2% vs. 54.5%), more frequently under 1 cm (18.0% vs. 7.1%) and more frequently histologically grade I (21.3% vs. 16.8%). These data strongly suggest that mammography is capable of detecting smaller, curable breast cancers than those detected without mammographic screening. The Swedish experience is also important because it implies that mammographic screening done at 24 month intervals, rather than the annual screening schedule utilized in HIP and BCDDP, is effective in reducing breast cancer mortality in women 50-69 years old.

OTHER EUROPEAN TRIALS

Several other European trials of mammographic screening have been reported. The Edinburgh randomized trial recruited 44,288 women from 1978-1981.[9] The study group included 22,944 women, ranging in age from 45-64 years at entry into the study. Screening consisted of a baseline physical examination and two-view mammogram with follow up physical examination done annually for 7 years and done at 2 yearly intervals. Various definitions of breast cancer mortality were reported in this study. Depending on the definition, breast cancer mortality was reduced by 14-21%, but statistical significance was not reached. The study has been criticized because of randomization of women on the basis of the physician who cared for them, causing significant socioeconomic differences to occur between those in the screening and control groups. Differences in mortality from all causes in the Edinburgh study can be at least partially explained on the basis of these socioeconomic disparities. Overall, only 489 breast cancers with 105 breast cancer deaths occurred in the study group and 400 breast cancers with 120 breast cancer deaths in the control. These small numbers may account for the lack of statistical significance in this study. The numbers for women 50 and older are, of course, even smaller making significant analysis of these data impossible.

Beginning in 1975 in Nijmegen in the Netherlands a single-view mammography study with screening done every other year has analyzed data on over 40,000 women who have been invited to participate.[10] This was a case-control study comparing those who died from breast cancer in the screening program with comparable persons derived from the source population. This is not considered to have the statistical strength of a randomized, controlled study. Fifteen thousand women 50-69 and 7,000 women 70 and older were invited to participate. Results have been reported for the first eight rounds. About 60% of women in their fifties and sixties have participated; for women 70 and older the percentage has been considerably smaller, with only about 25% participating in the last four screens. Among the population 50-69 years old, 48% of breast cancers diagnosed were found at screening, 26% were interval cancers and 26% occurred in nonparticipants. In women 70 and older, due to the large numbers of nonparticipants, 52% of breast cancers occurred in this group; 35% of the remaining cancers were found at screenings. Screen-detected cancers were significantly smaller than those detected by other methods. For women 50-69 among screen-detected cancers 29% were less than or equal to 1 cm in

maximum diameter and 6% were intraductal. For cancers found in the same age group in nonparticipants these numbers were 10% and 3%, respectively. Also in this age group, breast cancers found in nonparticipants were lymph node positive in 53%, whereas they were node positive in only 33% of those found at the initial screen and 22% of those discovered at follow up examinations. Among women participating in the Nijmegen study the relative risk of death from breast cancer versus those not participating has been estimated at 0.48 (95% confidence interval 0.23-1.0) or a 52% reduction in the risk of death from breast cancer.[11]

Two-view mammographic screening with an average interval between screens of 2.5 years has been tested in Florence, Italy.[12] Beginning in 1970 women 40-70 years old were invited to participate and 60% attended the first round of screening. Results were also analyzed using a case-control approach. The odds ratio of death from breast cancer for women screened versus those not screened was 0.53 (95% confidence interval 0.29-0.95) with the entire benefit of screening essentially limited to women 50 and older. The study size was small with only 57 breast cancer deaths in the study population.

THE CANADIAN NATIONAL BREAST SCREENING STUDY

The Canadian National Breast Screening Study (NBSS) was a randomized, controlled trial designed to detect the impact of annual, two-view mammography beyond annual physical examination on the reduction of mortality from breast cancer on women aged 50-59 on entry into this study. At the time of the first report of results of this study in 1992, 39,405 women had been enrolled and were followed for a mean of 8.3 years.[13] The rate of participation of women with follow up was high with over 85% attending follow up screenings. Although slightly more node negative breast cancers were found in the study group (217) versus the control group (184), there were more node positive breast cancers (98 vs. 90) discovered in the study group, including 32 cancers with metastatic disease involving at least four nodes. Among women involved in the study, there were 38 breast cancer deaths in the study group and 39 in the control group. Although women whose cancers were detected by mammography alone had the highest survival rate in the study, the authors concluded that there was no benefit to the addition of mammography to physical examination to reduce breast cancer mortality.

The NBSS has been surrounded by controversy since shortly after its inception. Critics have questioned both the study design and its execution, concluding that the results of this study are not valid.[14-17] The study as designed has the power to detect a reduction in mortality of 40% in those women 50-59. If, for example, there were a 30% reduction in the death rate from breast cancer by the addition of mammography to physical examination, there are insufficient numbers of women enrolled to demonstrate this fact.[17] The length of follow up of women has been questioned.[14] Analysis of follow up procedures indicates that although a mean follow up time of 8.5 years is reported for the study, one third of women have been followed for less than 5 years. This may be too soon for the advantage of mammographic screening to become evident. Problems in randomization have also been noted. Randomization was not performed at the time of entry into the study but rather after a physical examination was done. This may have resulted in the placement of women with advanced, palpable cancers into the study arm requiring mammography rather than into the control arm. This explanation has been suggested to help understand the randomization of a large number of women with advanced, palpable cancers into the study arm evaluating women 40-49 years old. It may also explain how a large number of advanced cancers were found in women in their fifties.

In addition to these issues, the NBSS, which was designed to assess the impact of screening mammography, has been strongly criticized for the quality of mammography used in the study. From early in the program,

external reviewers had criticized the quality of mammography in NBSS.[15,18] At the end of 3 years, two external reviewers resigned because their concerns over inferior mammography did not result in any changes. The quality of mammography equipment was judged by radiation dose; film quality was not considered to be important. Although those who conducted physical examination of the breast were required to undergo special training, expertise in mammographic positioning or film interpretation was not required of centers participating in NBSS. The reference physicist for the study noted that for mammography "quality was far below state of the art."[16] The poor quality of film interpretation has been demonstrated by the occurrence of 2.4 interval cancers per 1,000 women screened in the older group of NBSS. In a screening program conducted in British Columbia during the same period but with extensive quality control for mammography, the interval cancer rate was 0.97 per 1,000 in the same age group.[19] Because of these issues, it is not inappropriate to at least question the validity of the results of NBSS as published in 1992. Unlike other screening studies that support its use, the conclusion from this Canadian study that mammography has no impact on breast cancer mortality for women 50-59 years old may not be appropriate. As will be seen below, when looked at in the context of all available data, the results from NBSS are not upheld.

LIMITATIONS IN THE DATA FROM SCREENING STUDIES

Determination of the true impact of mammographic screening from available studies is underestimated. This is due to the problems of compliance of the study population and contamination of the control group.[20]

Compliance, the actual participation of the study group as described in the study design, has varied considerably. Anything less than 100% compliance, of course, results in an underestimation of the effectiveness of the intervention being studied, in this case, screening mammography for women

50 and older. Of the population invited to screening, those who actually participated in the first screen varied from 89% in the Swedish two-county trial[21] to 61% in the Edinburgh study. Because they were volunteers, compliance in the first round of the Canadian NBSS was essentially 100%. First round compliance for other trials described above has been 67% for HIP, 74% for Malmo and 81% for Stockholm.[20]

Contamination occurs when the control population undergoes the intervention being tested. In this discussion it is when members of the control group have screening mammography. This diminishes the impact of screening as tested in the study group by decreasing the differences between these two populations. In the Malmo trial 24% of women in the control group underwent either screening or diagnostic mammography.[23] In the Canadian NBSS 26% of women in the control group were screened outside the study and 1.5% of this group underwent diagnostic mammography at entry into the study.[20] In Stockholm and Edinburgh the extent of contamination is unknown.

ANALYSIS OF DATA FROM SCREENING STUDIES

Although studies on mammographic screening have varied considerably with differing qualities of mammography, numbers of views and intervals of screening, combined analysis of data from available studies is of value. The larger numbers of women available when a combined analysis is performed add statistical significance to the results. However, such an analysis does not specify the decrease in likelihood of death from breast cancer under specific screening conditions, such as annual screening beginning at age 50 with two-view mammography.

Kerlikowske and colleagues[24] subjected 13 studies to meta-analysis. These included all the studies listed above except for BCDDP. In addition to the nine randomized, controlled studies and the case-control studies from Florence and Nijmegen,

the entire United Kingdom study, a case-control study of which the Edinburgh study was a component and the DOM project,[25] another case-control study, were included in the analysis. For women aged 50-74 years, the relative risk of death from breast cancer for those screened versus those not screened was 0.74 (95% confidence interval 0.66-0.83). This analysis concluded that this one quarter reduction in mortality for women in this age group was independent of screening interval, length of follow up and number of mammographic views.

In a study sponsored by the National Cancer Institute in 1993, eight randomized trials were analyzed.[20] These included the four Swedish trials, HIP, Edinburgh and the Canadian NBSS trials for women 50-59 and 40-49.[26] These authors concluded that all studies demonstrated some mortality reduction by screening for women 50-69 with most studies demonstrating a 30% reduction at 10-12 years. They concluded that in this age group this is an appropriate approximation of the impact of screening mammography on breast cancer mortality. However, data on women 70 and older were felt to be inadequate to decide whether or not screening mammography was effective in this age group.

Also in 1993 the European Society of Mastology held a consensus conference to evaluate breast cancer screening.[27] This group looked at data from the Edinburgh and HIP trials and the Swedish studies. Analysis of data was done including and excluding results of the Canadian NBSS study. For women 50-74 years old the group concluded that the reduction in cancer mortality from screening was 24% without inclusion of data from Canada (relative risk = 0.76, 95% confidence interval 0.67-0.87). If the Canadian results are included, mortality reduction is calculated at 22% (relative risk = 0.78, 95% confidence interval 0.69-0.88). The authors noted that if there were a comparable risk for the disease in both the study and control groups, the actual reduction in mortality through screening in this age group would be 31%. Because of the large numbers of women included in this analysis, the results are statistically significant at the 95% confidence interval.

On the basis of these data and analyses it is generally assumed by the medical community and lay population that mammographic screening for women 50 and older is a valuable intervention. However, screening mammography for these women is still not without controversy. Issues of cost-effectiveness and frequency of screening remain issues about which there continues to be argument. The upper age limit at which routine screening should be performed is also a subject of debate. Finally, it is important for both the physician recommending screening mammography and the women who undergoes it to understand that there may be some disadvantages to this procedure.

THE UPPER AGE LIMIT FOR BREAST CANCER SCREENING

The incidence of breast cancer increases with increasing age. It is rare before the age of 25, increases until 45 years, where its incidence levels off until 55. It then again increases in incidence until 75 years, after which it seems to decline.[28] This decreasing incidence after 75 has been argued to be due to patterns of data accumulation rather than the true incidence of the disease.[29] For women aged 65-74 the incidence of breast cancer has been reported at 200 per 100,000, compared with 160 per 100,000 in women 50-64. Mortality rates also increase with increasing age with 125 deaths from breast cancer per 100,000 for women 65-74 compared with 100 per 100,000 in the younger group. Despite the greater risk of breast cancer mortality in older women, the inclusion of these women in screening programs has been variable. In the United Kingdom women up to the age of 65 years are invited for screening.[30] In the Netherlands the upper age is 70 years.[31] No upper limit has been specified by most institutions in the United States.[32]

The ability of mammography to detect breast cancers in older women is clear cut. With the postmenopausal involution of glandular tissue, breast cancers are more readily detected in the increasingly fatty replaced breast. Also, based on data from the Florence program, the sensitivity of mammography in older women is greater. It has been estimated in women 65-69 at 94% versus 89% in women 60-64 and 84% in women 55-59.[33] Therefore, it seems that mammography should be an efficient method for the diagnosis of breast cancer in these women. However, does mammography reduce the mortality rate from breast cancer in older women?

Randomized screening trials have included women as old as 74 years at entry (HIP and two-county Swedish study), although most studies have been limited to women younger than 70 at entry into the program. Data from the two-county Swedish study showed an identical reduction in mortality for women 50-59 years old and those 60-69 years old, both of whom had a 29% reduction in mortality.[20] However, for women 70-74 only a 6% reduction in mortality from breast cancer was found and this was not statistically significant. However, participation of women in this age group was poor with few women older than 69 having mammograms. No other data specifically addressing this age group are available. The International Workshop on Screening for Breast Cancer concluded that the data were inadequate to make any conclusions about screening these women, but suggested that an individual woman's health should be considered in determining at what age breast cancer screening should cease.[20]

The Forum on Breast Cancer Screening has also considered this issue.[34] The group noted that for women over 65 the death rate from breast cancer was greater than in those 40-65 years old. Even with comorbidity factors, ambulatory women 85 years old have an overall mortality rate from all causes of only 53% in 4 years. In general, healthy women in this age group can be expected to live longer. These data were felt to indicate that older women live long enough and have a high enough mortality rate from breast cancer to benefit from mammographic screening, although the group acknowledged that no data are available to support the use of mammography in this age group.

In an analysis using optimistic and pessimistic assumptions about breast cancer screening in older women, Boer and colleagues[35] attempted to identify the best upper age limit for breast cancer screening. They noted that while arguments have been made about differences in the incidence and biology of breast cancer in women younger than 50 years old, there are not similar arguments that can be invoked to justify an upper age limit on screening. In fact, they argued, higher breast cancer mortality rates in older women are all the data necessary to suggest that screening these women may result in greater numbers of deaths being prevented in this population. Using two models that assumed different preclinical durations for breast cancer, the authors concluded that screening would have net benefit in mortality reduction for women at least until the age of 80 years, although cost-effectiveness may be questionable after age 69 and even more so after age 75.

The issue of the upper age limit for mammographic screening, however, is unsettled. There is no doubt that mammography can continue to detect preclinical, curable breast cancer in women 70 and older. For those with a life expectancy of four or more years it may improve mortality.

FREQUENCY OF SCREENING

The frequency at which screening should be done remains unsettled. The appropriate interval for screening depends upon the growth rate of breast cancer.[36] When breast cancers are detected as stage I tumors, patient survival is similar, regardless of the growth rate of the cancer. Improved survival from screening, therefore, depends upon detection of early cancers. The window of time available for detection at an early stage depends upon the growth rate of the tumor. For women 70 and older, no studies have focused on the appropriate interval for screening. In this age group, effective screening has been found in intervals ranging from 12-33 months.[34] In an analysis of data from

the Swedish two-county study for women 50 and older, the rate of development of interval cancers was relatively low in the first 2 years after screening, but it increased to almost 50% of the rate of cancers developing in the control group thereafter.[37] This is consistent with an analysis of screening data that suggested that the lead time gained from the mammographic diagnosis of breast cancer in women over the age of 50 years is 3.5-4.0 years.[38] A single screening event can therefore have an extended impact on breast cancer detection and survival.

Variable screening intervals in screening trials support the comparable impact on mortality made by 12- or 24-month screening intervals. For women 50-64 screened annually in HIP, the relative risk of breast cancer death compared to the control group was 0.68 (95% confidence interval 0.49-0.96). In Kopparberg the relative risk of death for all women screened at 24-month intervals was also 0.68 (95% confidence interval 0.52-0.89). The risk of breast cancer death does not appear to be greatly impacted by prolonging screening in women 50 and older to 2-year intervals. However, in the United States where screening for these women has been recommended annually, some cancers now detected at an early, curable stage would undoubtedly be more advanced at the time of detection with biannual screening. The most viable excuse for converting screening guidelines for women 50 and older to biannual examinations is economic.[36]

COST-EFFECTIVENESS

The demonstrated effectiveness of screening mammography in reducing breast cancer mortality can be considered significant enough for its cost-effectiveness to be a moot point. However, with increased concern by government and health care insurers over cost of care, evidence for cost-effectiveness of mammographic screening is considered increasingly important. Cost-effectiveness can be defined in a variety of ways. It is most compelling when an intervention improves survival and decreases the overall cost of care. An intervention may be defined as cost-effective if it has significant benefit at acceptable cost. An intervention can also be accepted as cost-effective if the additional investment it requires produces at least as many years of life saved as competing interventions.[39] Analysis of the cost-effectiveness of mammography depends upon a variety of data, including frequency of mammography, cost of mammography, costs incurred by excluding malignant disease when indeterminate findings are discovered at screening, cost of treating early and late breast cancer and the financial value of each year of life saved. Estimation of these figures can vary considerably. For example, in 1991 dollars the estimation of cost per year of life saved through screening varied from $3,400 to $28,700.[40] The former figure is based on data from Sweden with biannual screening; the latter is Scottish data based on annual screens. In a review by Mushlin[39] of four studies of the cost of screening including annual two-view mammography with physical examination using effectiveness as demonstrated in HIP and BCDDP, annual single-view mammography and physical examination and biannual single-view mammography, no cost savings could be demonstrated. The direct and induced costs of screening, including treating breast cancer at an earlier stage, outweighed the most expensive treatment of women with terminal breast cancer.

A recent analysis by Lindfors and Rosenquist[42] calculated the induced costs of screening by performing 50% of breast biopsies surgically and the other half as needle biopsies. The positive predictive value of mammography was estimated at 31% and 91% of cancers were considered mammographically detectable. It was assumed that annual mammography would reduce mortality in women 50 and older by 32%. Biannual mammography would reduce mortality by 30% in women 50-59, 27% in women 60-69 and 23% in women 70-79. For mammography done every other year in women 50-79, the mean cost per year of life saved was $16,000. A calculation of the cost of annual screening for women 50-79 was not included in the report. The authors concluded that this was the most cost-effective strategy for breast cancer screening, but they noted that the choice of a screening protocol depends upon the desired effectiveness of screening, as well as financial considerations.

Moskowitz has undertaken a cost-benefit analysis based on data derived from HIP and using 1987 dollars.[43] Screening costs included the actual cost of screening, time off from work to be screened and the "induced costs" for finding cancers in a screening setting. Induced costs included inpatient and outpatient biopsies and assumed a ratio of benign to malignant findings at biopsy of 4:1. These costs were compared to the costs of treating breast cancers at a more advanced stage in a nonscreened population, long-term and short-term disability costs and replacement costs for the excess women who would die of breast cancer in the nonscreened group. Using the HIP model of annual mammography and physical examination, Moskowitz estimated the cost per cancer found at $23,403 and cost per death averted at $123,400. The cost-effectiveness ratio was 0.73, indicating a decreased cost for treating breast cancer using screening than without screening. In the same analysis, using BCDDP data, Moskowitz calculated that screening by mammography alone was less expensive in all age groups than screening by physical examination alone. It is interesting to note that although the cost per cancer diagnosed was less in women 50 and over, due to the greater incidence of disease in the older population, the cost per year of life saved increased with each decade of age, due to the decreased life expectancy of older women.

A variety of maneuvers can be used to increase the cost-effectiveness of a screening program. The cost per mammogram can decreased by maximizing the number of women screened per day per facility, segregating screening from diagnostic populations and optimizing utilization of expensive personnel (for example, batch processing of screening mammograms by technologists and batch reading of these studies by radiologists).[44] Expertise in mammographic interpretation resulting in a lower call back rate for additional studies and a higher positive predictive value for biopsy recommendations can also significantly decrease the cost of screening. Mobile programs that can perform screening at the worksite can reduce the cost of screening to women who would otherwise need to leave work for a mammogram, although the cost to operate these programs may be greater than those of a fixed site facility.[45] Successful recruitment strategies are also necessary to encourage women to participate in screening. This can often be effectively done by individual mailings inviting women to undergo screening.[46]

DISADVANTAGES OF MAMMOGRAPHIC SCREENING

Because mammographic screening is offered to healthy women, it is important that negative consequences should not outweigh its benefits.[1] In considering the incorporation of screening mammography into the routine medical care of women it is, therefore, important to understand the negative impacts it may have.

Although screening is capable of detecting at least 90% of breast cancers, this is possible because of the detection of a large number of indeterminate lesions that need to undergo biopsy to determine if they are benign or malignant. The likelihood that a mammographic lesion sent for biopsy is a cancer, the positive predictive value of mammography is approximately 30%.[47] Therefore, for every three cancers sent to biopsy on the basis of a suspicious mammogram, seven benign lesions will be sampled. With increasing age, however, this ratio improves as cysts, fibroadenomas and other benign entities become less common and new lesions in the breast are more often caused by malignancy. However, surgery for benign entities results in emotional stress, time lost from normal activities including work and family and considerable expense. Even for those women for whom surgery is not needed, additional imaging work up may include special mammographic views and sonography. It is expected in a screening program that about 12% of women will need to undergo some additional test beyond the screening mammogram.[48]

The psychological impact of these events can be profound. In one study it was found that women who had abnormal mammograms that were found not to be due to cancer frequently had considerable anxiety even three months after the event.[49] Their symptoms were similar to those of posttraumatic stress disorder and included excessive worry and intrusive thoughts. Women with false-positive mammograms also may view themselves as different from the norm or not entirely healthy.[50] Additionally, this may be perceived negatively by insurers, who place these women in a higher risk pool.[1]

Women may also be found to have lesions that are histologically malignant but biologically unimportant. This can lead to overtreatment. Autopsy studies have suggested that 70% of lesions that found at cadaver examination may never become biologically significant.[51] Criticism has also been leveled at screening programs because some cancers that are discovered are overdiagnosed and overtreated. It has been suggested that all in situ and node negative cancers may not progress to clinically significant disease. However, at the present time it remains impossible to differentiate those with a capacity to grow and metastasize from those that are unimportant.

Finally, the issue of possible radiation carcinogenesis from mammography should be addressed. Negative publicity about this issue has resulted in fear of some women to undergo mammography. This fear is, of course, ungrounded. Radiation sensitivity of the breast for women old enough to participate in a screening program, especially those who are 50 years old or older, is minimal, at best. It has been estimated that for women 45 years of age the likelihood of death from a radiation-induced breast cancer caused by mammography is comparable to risk of death from lung cancer induced by smoking three cigarettes.[52]

SUMMARY

Screening mammography has been demonstrated in studies conducted on hundreds of thousands of women 50 years old and older to be an effective method of reducing mortality of breast cancer through early diagnosis. Mortality reduction of at least 30% is possible with this intervention. It is optimally performed as an annual examination, but significant mortality reduction can be achieved in the screened population with biannual screening. The cost-effectiveness of screening can be argued, but numbers are available that indicate it can save health-care dollars. Individual mammography programs can be customized to improve their cost-effectiveness. The upper age limit for women who should undergo screening has not been established. There is no doubt it should be offered to women up to age 69 years, but probably it is an effective intervention for mortality reduction for ambulatory women at least up to the age of 85. Women who undergo screening may be sent for additional imaging studies or biopsy to determine whether or not they have breast cancer and participation in a screening program may lead to considerable anxiety. However, routine screening mammography for women 50 and older should be an integral part of the routine health care of this segment of the population.

REFERENCES

1. Rimer BK. Breast cancer screening. In: Harris JR, Lippman ME, Morrow M, Hellman S, eds. Diseases of the Breast. Philadelphia: Lippincott-Raven, 1996: 307-322.

2. Miller AB. Screening and detection. In: Bland KI, Copeland EM, eds. The Breast: Comprehesive Management of Benign and Malignant Diseases. Philadelphia: WB Saunders, 1991:419-425.

3. Shapiro S. Evidence on screening for breast cancer from a randomized trial. Cancer 1977; 36(suppl 6):2772-2782.

4. Shapiro S, Vanet W, Strax P et al. Ten- to fourteen-year effect of screening on breast cancer mortality. J Natl Cancer Inst 1982; 69:349-355.

5. Baker LH. Breast cancer detection demonstration project: 5-year summary report. Ca-a Cancer Journal for Physicians 1982; 32:194-225.

6. Seidman H, Gelb SK, Silverberg E et al. Survival experience in the breast cancer demonstration project. Ca-a Cancer Journal for Clinicians 1987; 37:258-291.

7. Nystrom L, Rutqvist LE, Wall S et al. Breast cancer screening with mammography: overview of Swedish randomized trials. Lancet 1993; 341:973-978.

8. Tabar L, Fagerberg G, Duffy SW et al. Update of the Swedish two-county program of mammographic screening for breast cancer. Radiol Clin N Amer 1992; 30:187-210.

9. Alexander FE anderson TJ, Brown HK et al. The Edinburgh randomized trial of breast cancer screening: results after 10 years of follow up. Br J Cancer 1994; 70:542-548.

10. Peer PGM, Holland R, Hendriks JHCL et al. Age-specific effectiveness of the Nijmegen population-based breast cancer-screening program: assessment of early indicators of screening effectiveness. J Nat Cancer Inst 1994; 86:436-440.

11. Verbeek ALM, Hendriks JHCL, Holland R et al. Reduction of breast cancer mortality through mass screening with modern mammography: first results of the Nijmegen project 1975-1981. Lancet 1984; 1:1222-1224.

12. Palli D, del Turco MR, Buiatti E et al. A case control study of the efficacy of a non-randomized breast cancer screening program in Florence (Italy). Int J Cancer 1986; 38:501-504.

13. Miller AB, Baines CJ, To T et al. Canadian national breast screening study: 2. breast cancer detection and death rates among women aged 50 to 59 years. Can Med Ass J 1992; 147:1477-1488.

14. Burhenne LJW, Burhenne HJ. The Canadian national breast screening study: a Canadian critique. AJR 1993; 161: 761-763.

15. Kopans DB. The Canadian screening program: a different perspective (commentary). AJR 1990; 155:748-749.

16. Yaffe MJ. Correction: Canada study (let-

ter). J Natl Cancer Inst 1993; 85:94.

17. Mettlin CJ, Smart CR. The Canadian national breast screening study: an appraisal and inplications for early detection policy. Cancer (suppl) 1993; 72: 1461-1465.

18. Baines CJ, Miller AB, Kopans DB et al. Canadian national breast screening study: assessment of technical quality with external review. AJR 1990; 155:743-747.

19. Burhenne HJ, Burhenne LW, Goldberg F et al. Interval breast cancers in the screening mammography program of British Columbia: analysis and classification. AJR 1994; 162:1067-1071.

20. Fletcher SW, Black W, Harris R, Rimer BK, Shapiro S. Report of the international workshop on screening for breast cancer. J Natl Cancer Inst 1993; 85: 1644-1656.

21. Tabar L, Fagerberg CL, Gad A et al. Reduction in mortality from breast cancer after mass screening with mammography. Randomized trial from the breast cancer screening working group of the Swedish national board of health and welfare. Lancet 1985; 1:829-832.

22. Roberts MM, Alexander FE anderson TJ et al. Edinburgh trial of screening for breast cancer: mortality at seven years. Lancet 1990; 335:241-246.

23. Andersson I, Aspegren K, Janzon L et al. Mammographic screening and mortality from breast cancer: the Malmo mammographic screening trial. Br Med J 1988; 297:943-948.

24. Kerlikowske K, Grady D, Rubin SM et al. Efficacy of screening mammography: a meta-analysis. JAMA 1995; 273: 149-154.

25. Collette HJA, de Waard F, Collette C et al. Further evidence of benefits of a (non-randomized) breast cancer screening programme: the DOM project. J Epidemiol Community Health 1992; 46:382-386.

26. Miller AB, Baines CJ, To T et al. Canadian national breast screening study, 1: breast cancer detection death rates among women ages 40 to 49 years. Can Med Assoc J 1992; 147:1459-1476.

27. Wald NJ, Chamberlain J, Hackshaw A. European society of mastology consensus conference on breast cancer screening: report of the evaluation committee. Br J Radiol 1994; 67:925-933.

28. Kessler LG. The relationship between age and incidence of breast cancer. Population and screening program data. Cancer (suppl) 1992; 69:1896-1903.

29. Horton DA. Breast cancer screening of women aged 65 or older-a review of the evidence on specificity, effectiveness and compliance. Breast 1993; 2:64-66.

30. Chamberlain J, Moss SM, Kirkpatrick AE, Michell M, Johns L. National health service breast screening program results for 1991-2. Br Med J 1993; 307:353-356.

31. de Koning H, Fracheboud J, Boer R et al. Nation-wide breast cancer screening in the Netherlands: support for breast-cancer mortality reduction. Int J Cancer 1995; 60:777-780.

32. Costanza ME. Breast cancer screening in older women. Cancer 1992; 69: 1925-1931.

33. Paci E, Duffy SW. Modelling the analysis of breast cancer screening programmes: sensitivity, lead time and predictive value in the Florence district programme (1975-1986). Int J Epidemiol 1991; 20:852-858.

34. Costanza ME. Issues in breast cancer screening in older women. Cancer 1994; 74:2009-2015.

35. Boer R, de Koning HJ, van Oortmarssen GJ, van der Maas PJ. In search of the best upper age limit for breast cancer screening. Eur J Cancer 1995; 31A:2040-2043.

36. Moskowitz M. Guidelines for screening for breast cancer: is a revision in order? Radiol Clin N Am 1992; 30:221-233.

37. Tabar L, Faberberg G, Day NE et al. What is the optimum interval between mammographic screening examinations?-an analysis based on the latest results of the Swedish two-county breast cancer screening trial. Br J Cancer 1987; 55: 547-551.

38. Moskowitz M. Breast cancer: age-specific growth rates and screening strategies. Radiology 1986; 161:37-41.

39. Mushlin AI, Fintor L. Is screening for breast cancer cost-effective? Cancer 1992; (suppl) 69:1957-1962.

40. Day NE, Chamberlain J. Screening for

breast cancer workshop report. Cancer 1988; 61:55-59.

41. Clarke PR, Fraser NM. Economic analysis of screening for breast cancer report. For Scottish home and health department, February, 1991.

42. Lindfors KK, Rosenquist CJ. The cost-effectiveness of mammographic screening strategies. JAMA 1995; 274:881-884.

43. Moskowitz M. Costs of screening for breast cancer. Radiol Clin N Am 1987; 25:1031-1037.

44. Sickles EA, Weber WN, Galvin HB et al. Mammographic screening: how to operate successfully at low cost. Radiology 1986; 160:95-97.

45. Dershaw DD, Liberman L, Smolek B. Mobile mammographic screening of self-referred women: results of 22,540 screenings. Radiology 1992; 184:415-419.

46. Hurley SF, Jolley DJ, Livingston PM et al. Effectiveness, costs and cost-effectiveness of recruitment strategies for a mammographic screening program to detect breast cancer. J Natl Cancer Inst 1992; 84:855-863.

47. Bassett LW, Liu TH, Guiliano AE et al. The prevalence of carcinoma in palpable vs impalpable mammographically detected lesions. AJR 1991; 157:21-24.

48. Linver MN, Osuch JR, Brenner RJ et al. The mammography audit: a primer for the mammography quality standards act (MQSA). AJR 1995; 165:19-25.

49. Lerman C, Trock B, Rimer BK et al. Psychological and behavioral implications of abnormal mammograms. Ann Inter Med 1991; 114:657-661.

50. Peeters PH, Verbeek ALM, Straatman H et al. Evaluation of overdiagnosis of breast cancer in screening with mammography: results of the Nijmegen programme. Int J Epidemiol 1989; 18: 295-299.

51. Hurley SF, Kaldor JM. The benefits and risks of mammographic screening for breast cancer. Epidemiol Rev 1992; 14: 101-130.

52. Rothenberg LN, Feig SA, Haus AG et al. Benefits and risks of mammography. In: Mammography—A User's Guide. Bethesda: National Council on Radiation Protection and Measurements, 1986: 95-121.

SCREENING MAMMOGRAPHY: BALANCING THE HARM, THE COST AND THE BENEFIT

Charles J. Wright

INTRODUCTION

The present climate surrounding women's issues, especially in North America, is not conducive to a balanced public discussion and evaluation of mammography as a screening procedure for breast cancer. It has been widely and eagerly adopted as the only glimmer of light in a tunnel that is otherwise very dark. Breast cancer is a bad disease with serious physical and psychological consequences, high mortality and a persistently high long-term relapse rate. Breast cancer is a leading cause of premature death for women and the overall results of surgery and intensive management with hormonal and chemotherapeutic agents have not been encouraging in terms of changing the population mortality from the disease. In a very large study of women with breast cancer, unselected for stage of disease, method of therapy or any other consideration, 8% of the residual population died of breast cancer annually.[1] This rate of dying was continued out to 20 years from diagnosis, resulting in the fact that 80-85% of women who had breast cancer diagnosed eventually died of the disease. These are depressing figures and it is understandable that any potential course of action that might improve them would be enthusiastically pursued. Screening mammography is the only intervention that has been shown to reduce the mortality from breast cancer in certain groups of women, but there has been little publicity, and as a result very little public awareness, of how small the benefit actually is and how substantial the harm caused in the process.

Now that we have effective means of local control including surgery and radiotherapy, death from breast cancer occurs because of metastatic disease in the bones, liver, brain, lungs, and elsewhere throughout the body. If only the cancer could be detected at a stage before metastases have occurred, then local treatment would bring about complete cure. It is therefore logical to diagnose the disease as early as possible in order to remove the breast tumor during the interval before metastases develop that has been called the "cancer control window." Figure 5.1 is a graphic representation of this concept. Obviously, any successful screening test must be capable of finding a cancer both before the onset of metastases (after which it would be useless) and before clinical detection (after which it is unnecessary). As discussed below, there is no question concerning the ability of mammography to diagnose breast cancer, at least in most cases, earlier than would be possible clinically, but the requirement of the diagnosis to predate metastases underlies all the clinical trials that have been conducted and all the resulting controversy.

This chapter does not present a formal cost-effectiveness analysis of screening mammography, although such economic analyses are reviewed and discussed. Rather, this is an overview of the currently available evidence on all those aspects of screening mammography that must be weighed in the balance before making a public health policy decision, namely the benefits offered, the harm caused and the costs incurred. Formal cost-effectiveness analysis can bring useful information to the table, but in the real world that we currently inhabit such decisions tend to be made on a very subjective basis. It is essential therefore that all of the evidence on outcomes be reviewed, including desirable, undesirable, foreseen and unforeseen effects.

There are several disturbing aspects about the history and implementation of screening mammography that have received remarkably little attention and that require careful consideration:

- the increasingly conflicting evidence in historical sequence
- the size of the benefit in relation to the harm being caused
- the generation of false hope through public misinformation
- the huge opportunity cost, that is the diversion of valuable resources that may achieve better results in alternative uses.

WHAT DOES A SUCCESSFUL SCREENING PROGRAM LOOK LIKE?

Long lists of the generic requirements for any successful screening program can be found in clinical epidemiology textbooks, but they distill down to three essential elements.

1. The screening test must work, that is, it must be capable of detecting the target disease before clinical detection is possible.
2. The earlier diagnosis achieved by the screening test must be shown to benefit the population screened.
3. The benefit offered must be deemed to justify the harm (if any) caused and the financial cost.

There is no question that mammography "works" in terms of permitting

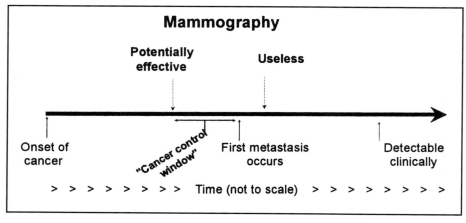

Fig. 5.1. Model of cancer development showing the "cancer control window" in relation to potential effectiveness of mammography

earlier diagnosis of breast cancer in many cases than would be possible on clinical examination. All of the screening trials and programs have demonstrated this. For example, the Breast Cancer Detection Demonstration Project (BCDDP)[2] demonstrated a 0.5% incidence of breast cancer among over a quarter of a million women screened. The data from the first year of the BCDDP are summarized in Table 5.1. Many of these lesions were clinically undetectable and therefore there is little doubt that the diagnosis would have been delayed in the absence of screening. Table 5.2, also derived from the BCDDP first year data, demonstrates in a population of women with breast cancer prevalence of 0.62% that the sensitivity of mammography was 87% and the specificity 95%. (For this calculation, it is assumed that women who had a negative mammogram but developed proven breast cancer within 12 months were false negative and should be included in the prevalence figure.) Results of similar magnitude have been found in all screening programs. These figures demonstrate that mammo-

graphy works, therefore, in terms of detecting breast cancer in many cases earlier than would otherwise be possible.

The second crucial question is whether the earlier diagnosis leads to any benefit for the patient. The most important potential benefit is a reduction in the mortality rate from the disease. Note that it is crucial to distinguish between mortality and "survival" in this context. Health care professionals and the public alike usually understand "survival" to represent the interval from diagnosis to death. Unfortunately, this commonly used outcome measure is of no value or interest in relation to a screening program. The major reason for this is lead-time bias which is the bias introduced by moving the diagnosis to an earlier point on the time scale, thus automatically increasing the case "survival" even when there is no benefit whatsoever. The concept of lead-time bias is illustrated in Figure 5.2. In this particular example, a woman who died 6 years after clinical diagnosis of breast cancer would have been considered a seven-year survival if the diagnosis had been made one

Table 5.1. Breast cancer detection demonstration project: cancer detection rate

	Number	%
Total number of women screened	268,141	100
Positive screening result	14,851	5.54
Cancer detected *	1,460	0.54

* Includes invasive cancer and carcinoma in situ

Table 5.2. Breast cancer detection demonstration project: 2 by 2 table

	Breast Cancer*		
Screening Result	**+**	**−**	**Total**
Positive	1,460	13,391	14,851
Negative	210**	253,080	253,290
Total	1,670	266,471	268,141

* Plus sign indicates proven breast cancer
** Proven breast cancer developed within 12 months of a negative mammogram

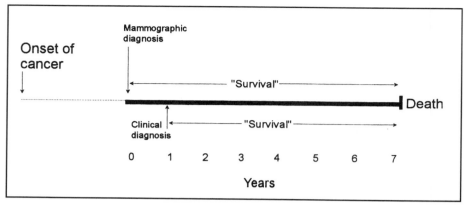

Fig. 5.2. Early diagnosis leads to longer "survival" even if the natural history of the disease is unchanged in any way.

year earlier on mammography, but she would have derived no benefit from this. In fact and this is discussed later, the extra year of knowing the diagnosis would only have added to her burden.

Another problem that is inevitably introduced in the analysis of screening programs is length bias. There is a large biological range of activity in breast cancer, some being very rapidly growing and some having very slow progression. A "snapshot" of cases at screening mammography is bound to include a higher proportion of the slow-growing type, as it is the faster growing examples that are more likely to turn up as "interval" cancers between screening episodes. This is another reason for the irrelevance of case survival statistics in the results and evaluation of screening programs. The outcome to be evaluated must be the mortality from the target disease. In the context of randomized, controlled trials, this means measuring the mortality from breast cancer over time in a screened population of women to compare with the breast cancer mortality in an unscreened but otherwise similar population.

Another potential advantage of screening is that earlier diagnosis could facilitate more conservative surgery for local control of the disease. Other measures, such as the proportion of node positive patients

diagnosed, or tumor size or grade, are only of interest as surrogate measures for the important outcomes of mortality and treatment choice. More and more women are now choosing more surgically conservative treatment plans in any case in view of the overwhelming evidence that the extent of local treatment has no effect on the eventual outcome and that conservative surgery with radiation therapy controls the local disease as effectively as more radical surgery. The prospect of less aggressive surgery with earlier diagnosis has often been stated as one of the reasons for screening with mammography, but this has not occurred in practice.[3] At the time screening programs were being introduced, conservative surgery for breast cancer was already becoming widely accepted as being equally effective and much more desirable from the patient's point of view.

THE CONFLICTING EVIDENCE FOR BENEFIT

It is not unusual to deal with conflicting evidence when assessing claims of benefit for health care interventions—witness the questions surrounding cholesterol and mortality, routine fetal monitoring in labor, dental amalgam, coronary artery stents and beta-carotene to name but a few. There have now been seven randomized prospective controlled clinical trials published on the effect of mammographic screening on breast cancer mortality. These are the Health Insurance Plan (HIP) Study,[4,5] the Swedish National Board of Health Study (SNBH)[6,7] (often recorded as two separate components in the Counties of Kopparberg and Ostergotland), the Malmo Study,[8,9] the Edinburgh Study,[10,11] the Canadian National Breast Screening Study (CNBSS),[12,13] the Stockholm Study[9,14] and the Gothenburg Study.[9,11] Curiously, there has not yet been any direct publication from the Gothenburg trial. The two references cited include limited data from Gothenburg in combining results from multiple studies.

As screening programs were reviewed, it soon became apparent that there was a difference in the results between older and younger women. If an arbitrary point of separation were taken at around the time of the menopause, it was noted that some benefit was demonstrable in some trials for the older but not the younger women. In most of the trials this issue has been handled by retrospective analysis in the different age groups, but the Canadian study was specifically designed to assess the results in the different age groups separately.

The trial results are summarized in Table 5.3. Figures 5.3 and 5.4 use the convention of displaying the results of each randomized trial separately in terms of the relative risk and 95% confidence interval (RR and 95% CI) of death from breast cancer in the screened population when compared with controls. A relative risk of 1.0 indicates no difference between the screened and control groups. This kind of display gives a better sense than a table of conflicting evidence from different trials and of the extent of the difference. The fact that screening mammography in women less than 50 years of age is without value can be seen at a glance in Figure 5.3. Not one of the trials demonstrates a relative risk that is significantly less than one and three of them show a relative risk greater than one, although once again the confidence intervals are wide indicating a result without statistical significance. Screening mammography in women under age 50 merits little further discussion, but it is remarkable that there are still enthusiastic advocates for the procedure in this age group.[15,16] Some have gone so far as to deliberately exclude from consideration the trial results that do not fit with the preconception that mammography should work at all ages.[15,17] It is noteworthy that in an objective analysis of the quality of all randomized trials of mammographic screening that included women under 50 years of age,[18] the highest quality score was assigned to the Canadian study that was so viciously attacked on multiple spurious grounds and deliberately excluded from some meta-analyses.[17,19,20] The Canadian study has been well defended against the criticisms[18,21,22]

Table 5.3. Results of randomized, controlled trials

| | | Relative Risk (95% CI) | |
	Entry Years	Women 40-49 years	Women 50-74 years
HIP	1963-66	0.77 (0.5-1.16)	0.68 (0.49-0.96)
Kopparberg	1977-80	0.75 (0.41-1.36)	0.67 (0.5-0.9)
Ostergotland	1978-81	1.28 (0.76-2.33)	0.75 (0.57-0.99)
Malmo	1976-78	0.51 (0.22-1.17)	0.86 (0.64-1.16)
Edinburgh	1979-81	0.78 (0.46-1.51)	0.85 (0.63-1.14)
Stockholm	1981-85	1.04 (0.53-2.05)	0.65 (0.4-1.08)
Canadian	1980-85	1.36 (0.84-2.21)	0.97 (0.62-1.52)
Gothenburg	1982-84	0.73 (0.27-1.97)	0.91 (0.53-1.55)

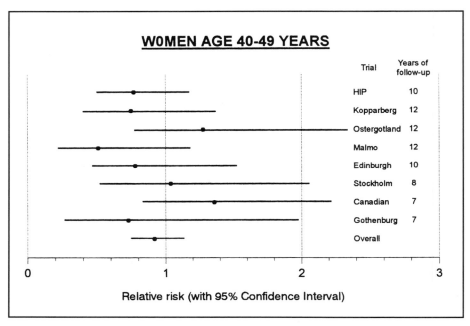

Fig. 5.3. Women age 40-49 years. Relative risk and 95% confidence interval for breast cancer in a screened population. Historical sequence of trials from top to bottom.

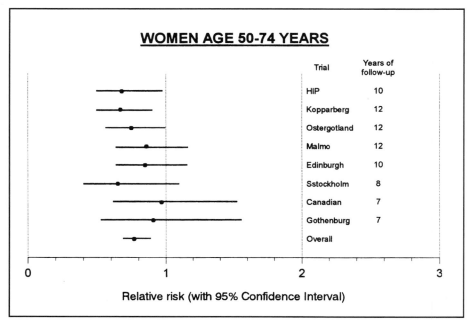

Fig. 5.4. Women age 50-74 years. Relative risk and 95% confidence interval for breast cancer in a screened population. Historical sequence of trials from top to bottom.

and fortunately a more objective, balanced view has prevailed.[23,24] Concerning younger women, therefore, screening mammography must be rejected as being of no value even before bringing considerations of harm and cost into the debate.

For women over 50 years of age the results are more encouraging, but Table 5.3 and Figure 5.4 demonstrate how tenuous the claim of benefit is even in this age group. The trials are listed in historical sequence and it is interesting to note that only the first two (HIP and SNBH) demonstrated a statistically significant mortality reduction from screening. Meta-analyses have shown a statistically significant reduction of breast cancer deaths in older women[9,23] but if this result is valid it is certainly difficult to explain the trend towards less and less effect when the trial results are viewed in historical sequence. How can this apparently diminishing return be explained? The increasing use of adjuvant chemotherapy may have been a factor, but is unlikely to be a confounder since this would appear in both arms of the trials. It is also noted that mortality falls sequentially even in the control groups in the separate trials, but once again the confounding factors that may be responsible for this would act in both experimental and control groups. In view of the vast and progressive improvement in the quality of mammography over the last 30 years and the increasing rigor of trial design and execution, it is truly bizarre that more attention should be paid to the older studies than those more recent, yet the oft-quoted figure of 30% for the mortality reduction is based only on these older studies. It is understandable that researchers should present data in the way that best illustrates the claim of benefit for an intervention under study, but the public have uncritically accepted it, causing increasing demand for mammography among women of all ages. Pleas for a more cautious approach based on comprehensive statistical and epidemiological analyses[25-30] have had little effect on the enthusiasm of radiologists and the clamor for mass screening mammography programs.

THE BENEFIT IN PERSPECTIVE

As discussed above, the publicity for screening mammography emphasizes the *relative* mortality reduction in mortality of 20-30%. It is equally important to consider the *absolute* mortality reduction, that is the difference between the proportion of women dying of breast cancer in the entire screened and unscreened populations. A 20-30% relative mortality reduction after 10 years represents an absolute mortality reduction of 0.04-0.14 depending on the prevalence of breast cancer. The difference between *relative* and *absolute* reductions is best understood by taking an actual example. The HIP Study at 10 years[5] reported 46 deaths per 10,000 women in the screened group and 60 in the control group. This can be accurately portrayed as a 23% reduction in relative mortality from breast cancer. Calculating the absolute mortality reduction, it is seen that the death rate in the screened group at 10 years was 0.46% and in the control group 0.6%, giving an absolute mortality reduction of 0.14%.

It is the importance of considering the absolute mortality reduction that has led to the "number to treat" concept that is now increasingly used in evaluating interventions. Simply stated, the "number to treat" is the total number of persons that must be subjected to an intervention in order to achieve benefit for one. Mathematically, it is the reciprocal of the difference between the event rates in the two groups. Again using the above example from the HIP Study, the "number to treat" is 714, that is 714 women must be screened over 10 years to yield one death prevented. Figure 5.5 (reproduced by courtesy of the Lancet)[30] illustrates a similar analysis of the results of screening mammography over 7 years based on data from the SNBH Study. For 10,000 women screened, 137 (1.37%) had breast cancer diagnosed and there were 11 (0.11%) deaths from breast cancer compared with 15 (0.15%) among 10,000 unscreened controls. Once again this represents a 30% reduction in mortality (relative reduction), but the end result is that 4 women out of 10,000 screened

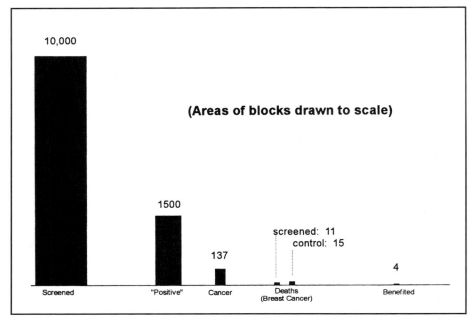

Fig. 5.5. Screening mammography: results per 10,000 women after 7 years based on SNBH data. Reproduced by permission of the Lancet Limited, Wright, CJ, Mueller, CB. Screening mammography and public health policy; the need for perspective. Lancet 1995; 346:29-32.

have benefited. In this example the absolute mortality reduction was 0.04% and the "number to treat" was 2,500, that is, 2,500 women were screened for one to benefit over 7 years.

In the Canadian Study, there was actually a small increase in breast cancer mortality in the screened population, mainly due to the results in the younger women. Deaths from colon cancer were reduced in the Canadian screened group by almost the same number as the breast cancer deaths were increased.[12,13] As in all the studies on screening mammography, there was no difference in all-cause mortality between the screened and unscreened groups. This may be inevitable because of the much larger proportion of deaths from causes other than breast cancer, but it is noteworthy that from this perspective ultimately not a single life is "saved." If, as many health economists now claim,[31] the effect to be measured for a cost-effectiveness analysis should be all-cause mortality rather than disease-specific mortality,

then the cost per life saved in the case of screening mammography would not be calculable at all (at infinity) as the denominator would be zero. The trial results also demonstrate that the eventual outcome of death due to breast cancer for the large majority of women is unaffected by screening mammography.

The fact that mammography ultimately benefits only such a small proportion of women screened is not surprising in view of what is known about the cytokinetics of breast cancer. The growth rate is very variable,[32] but in the majority of cases it is much slower than popularly imagined. Models of cancer growth rates in humans can only be speculative, but with a tumor volume doubling time in the range of 100-200 days, most cancers will have been present for several years before detection by any method. It should not be surprising that screening mammography is usually ineffective in altering the course of the disease, as mammography cannot detect a mass until 25-30 doublings have already occurred, representing already two-thirds of the interval between the cancer's inception and a lethal tumor burden.[33,34] In addition, there is evidence that huge numbers of cancer cells are shed into the circulation daily from an early stage,[35] and indeed there would be no reason to expect any fundamental change in the capacity of cancers to metastasize in the interval, for example, between 25-30 doublings. This is illustrated in a very simplified form in Figure 5.6 derived from Spratt's data.[33] The time interval between the cancer becoming detectable by mammography and then clinically is approximately the time it takes for the cancer to grow from a few millimeters in diameter to one centimeter or more. This in turn represents six or seven further doublings of the tumor. The actual time scale in this model would be very dependent on the aggressiveness of the tumor and the growth rate is not constant throughout, but Figure 5.6 serves to illustrate the point that the interval between mammographic and clinical detection represents a small proportion of the tumor's life span.

THE HARM CAUSED BY MAMMOGRAPHY

The evidence on mortality reduction is controversial and conflicting, but the harm caused by mammography has been well recognized and described. False-positive mammograms cause unnecessary intervention, false-negative mammograms cause inappropriate reassurance, false hopes of cure of breast cancer are generated, breast cancer is being overdiagnosed as a result of screening programs, there is increased fear and anxiety about breast cancer and there is the radiation risk.

The major problem that first drew the author's attention to the harm caused by breast cancer screening was the procession of women referred to a surgical clinic because of a mammographic abnormality. This inevitably sets in motion a train of events that is difficult to stop before a definitive tissue diagnosis is made. Approximately 6% of screening mammograms are assessed as being abnormal, that is either "positive" or "suspicious." The rate at which screening mammograms are labeled abnormal and the subsequent follow up

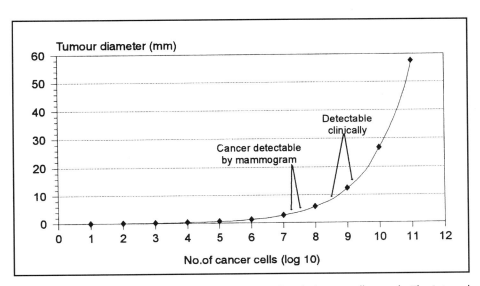

Fig. 5.6. Representation of breast cancer tumor size in relation to cell growth. The interval between detectability by mammography and by palpation is equivalent to about 5-6 doublings of tumor volume.

procedures generated are displayed in Table 5.4. These data are derived from an analysis of over 30,000 women referred for mammography to the University of California, San Francisco mobile mammography screening program between 1985-1992[36] and may not represent the full extent of the problem throughout community radiology practice. The breast cancer detection rate of 0.54% of women screened is within the range found in all studies for first screen mammography. The positive predictive value of 8.5% is at the lower end of the range from different studies of 4-20%,[36-39] that is only between 1:5 and 1:25 women with a positive screen is found to have cancer. The better results for positive predictive value are often claimed by the highly specialized centers for mammography, but there is little doubt that in the real world of community practice the results are usually at the other end of the scale; that is, the positive predictive value is very low. In fact, a recent large study of screening mammography in community practice found the extraordinarily high rate of abnormal screening mammograms of 11%, with a positive predictive value of only 4%.[39] As with so many other interventions in medical practice requiring great skill, care and attention, it is not possible to generalize the ideal findings of highly specialized practice to the community at large.

The most serious of the consequences of false positive mammography in the short term is the unnecessary surgery that is caused. As seen in Table 5.4, the newer less invasive diagnostic techniques are useful, but many women still come to open surgical biopsy. The general public and even many physicians who do not have a surgical background, may not realize that operations for nonpalpable mammographic "disease" are often more difficult and traumatic than operations for a palpable lesion. Once again, in expert hands the trauma can be minimized, but breast surgery is still being performed by a large number of general surgeons with many other interests. Life threatening complications of breast surgery are fortunately rare but hemorrhage and infections do occur and the results of open biopsy, especially if repeated frequently due to recurrent suspicious lesions on annual mammography, can be very unsightly.

Using the overall results from the recent meta-analyses of the trial results in older women[9,11,23] together with a current analysis of the consequences of false positives,[36-39] Figure 5.7 illustrates the fate of 10,000 women over 10 years in a typical community screening program in North America. For the 14 deaths avoided, more than 2,500 women have had multiple investigations and 700 have had surgical procedures. The calculation of harm caused must at least include those subjected to unnecessary interventions and those who died in any case, whose only "advantage" of screening was to be given more years of living with the knowledge of their cancer (see Fig. 5.2). The adverse effects of this have yet to be

Table 5.4. Follow up procedures from screening mammography

	% of Abnormal Screens	% of all Screens
Abnormal screening result	100	5.8
Additional mammography	>100*	6.2
Ultrasound of breast	20.1	1.2
Needle aspiration and/or biopsy	8.4	0.5
Open surgical biopsy	27.7	1.6
Breast cancer found	8.5	0.54

* This exceeds 100% because of multiple procedures in same cases

measured in terms of patient-assessed quality of life. Whereas cost-effectiveness analysis is increasingly used as a means of evaluating interventions, we still do not have any widely accepted means of objectively or quantitatively analyzing harm in relation to benefit. Any attempt to perform a formal "harm-effectiveness analysis" would founder on the seeming impossibility of finding units for harm and effectiveness that

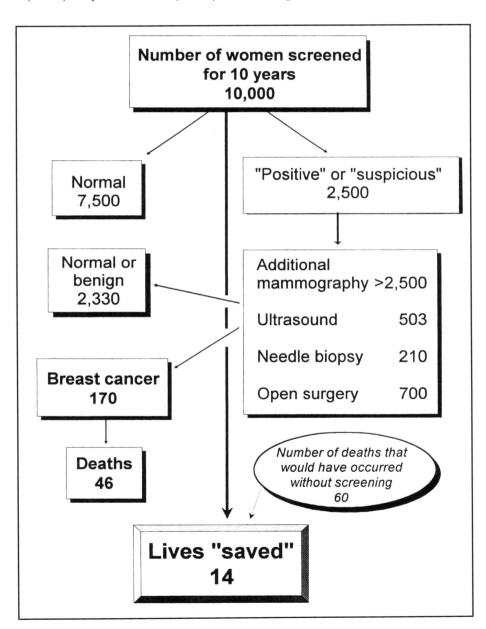

Fig. 5.7. Demonstration of the sequential outcomes from screening mammography in 10,000 women.

make sense with each other. However, cost-effectiveness analysis basically assesses the cost per unit of effect and if one assesses the harm per unit of effect as a ratio of the number of women harmed (regardless of degree) to the number saved from death due to breast cancer, it is 2376/14, that is 170:1. The problem with this type of analysis is, obviously, the difficulty in equating the 170 units of harm with the 1 life saved, but the issue merits careful consideration and research. It must be emphasized again that this calculation is derived from the most hopeful trial results rather than those published more recently showing no statistically significant benefit. It could also be argued that all women screened are harmed to some degree (see below) but those with a false positive screen and those who died despite screening are most important.

Mammography screening programs are causing another significant problem in over diagnosing cancer of the breast. Most reported results include cases of carcinoma in situ which is still a poorly understood disease whether of the ductal or lobular variety. It is certainly not, by definition, an invasive cancer but rather a high risk marker,[40,41] and its ultimate behavior is still subject to speculation. The incidence of in situ carcinoma (stage 0) among screen-detected "cancers" ranges from 10-23%.[8,10]

The level of anxiety about breast cancer among women is very high in our society partly because there is currently a serious misperception about the level of risk.[42-44] The bald statement that one in ten women will develop breast cancer and all the publicity surrounding screening have contributed to the gross overestimate of the risk perceived by women. This misperception is greatest in younger women who perceive their risk of developing breast cancer to be up to 40 times as high as it actually is.[44] The fear and anxiety caused by this misperception and by false positive mammograms is a serious burden for women today. The negative emotional impact of screening is extremely difficult to quantify, but it has probably been seriously underestimated.[26,45-47] Dr. Maureen Roberts, who was the Director of the Edinburgh Breast Screening Trial, wrote a very poignant article about this only months before her own unfortunate and untimely death from breast cancer.[26] It is customary in the evaluation of breast cancer screening programs to consider mortality or "life years saved" as the only important outcome. In spite of the methodological difficulties, a study needs to be done to measure these negative effects and factor them into the calculation to arrive at quality adjusted life years (QALYs) rather than life years alone.

The false reassurance of a negative mammogram is another serious issue, as 10-15% of early breast cancers are missed by mammography, that is for every 10 cancers found at mammography, one or two more will become apparent between annual screens. There is therefore no justification for the argument that one of the advantages of screening mammography is the comfort and reassurance that cancer is not present.

Death from breast cancer following screen detection of an early lesion is a cruel disappointment. Even if the highest claimed level of mortality reduction is accepted, namely 30%, this means that the natural history of the disease progressing to death is not changed in 70% of cases. Some radiologists would like to do everything possible to increase the sensitivity of mammography[16] without apparently realizing that in a screening situation like this with low prevalence of the target disease, this would inevitably lead to even worse positive predictive value and an even higher false positive rate with all the attendant complications. The radiation hazard in screening mammography is very low and can only be assessed by mathematical models, but it is not entirely negligible and may be significant in specific circumstances.[48,49]

Lastly, mammography for many women is uncomfortable and may be frankly painful. Approximately half of women screened report that the procedure causes discomfort or pain and 4% would never return for a further screen for this reason.[50,51]

THE COST OF SCREENING PROGRAMS

Any cost-effectiveness analysis requires a number of assumptions and decisions to be made including the boundaries of the study, the extent of the claimed benefit, the perspective to be considered and the method of cost determination. Several cost-effectiveness analyses of screening mammography have been performed.[52-55] The outcome of interest is usually taken as the number of "life years saved" or the number of "lives saved" at 10 years. The estimates of cost per life year saved range from $9,000 to $145,000 and for cost per "life saved" at 10 years all the way up to $1.5 million. The overwhelming proportion of the cost involved in screening programs is the cost of the actual mammography, but few studies adequately take into account all of the costs that spin out from the investigation of false positives and even fewer deal with the issue of utility which would attempt to measure the negative impact of the lead time in diagnosis, the false positive screens and all the other undesirable consequences of the program. As discussed earlier, these economic analytic techniques have limited application at present because of the serious difficulty in achieving objectivity in the prevailing political climate surrounding breast cancer. A detailed cost-effectiveness analysis is outside the scope of this chapter, but simple arithmetic from Table 5.4 and Figure 5.7 supports the upper range of reported cost per life saved. A recent detailed national survey of the cost of mammography[56] suggests a mean of around $100 (US). Annual mammography for 10,000 women for 10 years would, therefore, cost $10m. In view of the very small number of deaths avoided the treatment costs avoided are relatively inconsequential. Without even including the costs of all the additional investigations and surgery following the screening episode, the cost-effectiveness ratio is 10,000 x 100 x 10/14, that is $714,000 per death avoided.

PUBLIC INFORMATION OR INTEMPERATE PROPAGANDA?

On reviewing all the outcomes of screening mammography trials, it is seen that there is a modest mortality reduction confined to women over the age of 50 in exchange for a significant toll of undesirable effects. The extent of the benefit has been translated into remarkably optimistic messages to the public. The researchers involved in the HIP Study state that "most women with breast cancer could be saved by detection... with mammography."[57] The American Cancer Society has issued public education pamphlets stating "mammography helps your doctor see breast cancer before there is a lump when the cure rates are near 100%."[58] There are billboards in the USA suggesting that for Mother's Day you should give her the gift of life—a mammogram and the television and magazine advertisements attempt to convince women that "if you are over 35 and haven't had a mammogram, you need more than your breasts examined." This kind of grossly inaccurate overstatement is in itself a major contributing factor to the unrealistic expectations and subsequent inevitable disappointment. The statements quoted above by researchers themselves and by the American Cancer Society are particularly reprehensible and it can only be hoped that there was no deliberate intention to misrepresent the facts. To speak of "most women" being saved by early detection with cure rates of "near 100%" is to ignore completely the results even of the most promising studies in the literature showing at best that the outcome of breast cancer for 70% of screened women is unchanged. However, statements such as these have raised public awareness and have increased the clamor for screening programs. Mammography has spawned a major industry and is responsible for a large proportion of the income of many radiologists. In the formulation of public health policy, it is important that vested interests not be permitted to distort the truth in this manner.

THE NEED FOR A BALANCED PERSPECTIVE

What should women do in the light of all this information and what would constitute healthy public policy in view of the conflicting evidence. It is clear that we do not have any good answers to the terrible problem of breast cancer but we need to consider carefully whether the net result of all the current screening efforts is to increase rather than decrease the net burden caused by the disease. For women under the age of 50, the answer is clear, namely women should be actively discouraged from having screening mammograms. No other conclusion can be reached if the major consideration is the best interests of patients rather than those of radiologists and the screening mammography industry that has developed in the western world.

The summary of the evidence in women over 50 years of age is that there is potential benefit, but only for a tiny proportion of those screened and in exchange for significant harm caused to a large proportion at enormous cost. A balanced assessment of all these factors suggests that healthy public policy should stop promoting mass population screening even of older women in favor of more selective targeted application. For example, screening women with known high risk factors such as family history of premenopausal breast cancer and those actually carrying the breast cancer gene would by definition raise the prevalence of breast cancer in the screened population and thereby improve the positive predictive value of the test. In other words, there would be a higher yield with fewer false positives. The contrary argument that this policy would deny screening to the majority of women who will indeed develop breast cancer in the absence of these high risk factors, would only be cogent if the poor positive predictive value and all the resulting problems in this group could be justified by the size of the benefit. Unfortunately, this is not the case. The massive resources currently consumed by unselective screening mammography would be better channeled into more realistic and more extensive public education and into research. Questions about the allocation of limited resources among competing demands are very uncomfortable, but public health policy, especially on proposed mass population inter-

ventions, must be based on an unequivocal case for benefit in the absence of significant harm and at acceptable cost. Mammography as a screening procedure for breast cancer does not meet these criteria.

REFERENCES

1. Mueller CB, Jeffries W. Cancer of the breast: its outcome as measured by the rate of dying and causes of death. Ann Surg 1975; 182:334-340.
2. Baker L. Breast cancer detection demonstration project: 5-year summary report. Cancer J Clin 1982; 32:194-225.
3. Miller AB. The costs and benefits of breast cancer screening. Am J Prev Med 1993; 9:175-180.
4. Shapiro S. Determining the efficacy of breast cancer screening. Cancer 1989; 63:1873-1880.
5. Shapiro S, Venet W, Strax P et al. Ten to fourteen year effects of breast cancer screening on mortality. J Natl Cancer Inst 1982; 69:349-355.
6. Tabar L, Fagerberg CJ, Gad A et al. Reduction in mortality from breast cancer after mass screening with mammography. Lancet 1985; i:829-832.
7. Tabar L, Fagerberg G, Duffy SW et al. Update of the Swedish two-county program of mammographic screening for breast cancer. Radiol Clinics of North America 1992; 30:187-210.
8. Andersson I, Aspegren K, Janzon L et al. Mammographic screening and mortality from breast cancer: the Malmo mammographic screening trial. BMJ 1988; 297:943-948.
9. Nystrom L, Rutqvist LE, Wall S et al. Breast cancer screening with mammography: overview of Swedish randomized trials. Lancet 1993; 341:973-978.
10. Roberts MM, Alexander FE anderson TJ et al. Edinburgh trial of screening for breast cancer: mortality at 7 years. Lancet 1990; 335:241-246.
11. Fletcher SW, Black W, Harris R et al. Report of the international workshop on screening for breast cancer. J Natl Cancer Inst 1993; 85:1644-1656.
12. Miller AB, Baines CJ, To T et al. Cana-

dian national breast screening study: 1. Breast cancer detection and death rates among women aged 40 to 49 years. Can Med Assoc J 1992; 147:1459-1476.

13. Miller AB, Baines CJ, To T et al. Canadian national breast screening study: 2. Breast cancer detection and death rates among women aged 50 to 59 years. Can Med Assoc J 1992; 147:1477-1488.

14. Frisell J, Eklund G, Hellstrom L et al. Randomized study of mammography screening—preliminary report on mortality in the Stockholm trial. Breast Cancer Res Treat 1991; 18:49-56.

15. Kopans DB. Mammography screening and the controversy concerning women aged 40 to 49. Radiol Clinics of North America 1995; 33:1273-1290.

16. Feig, SA. Strategies for improving sensitivity of screening mammography for women aged 40 to 49 years. JAMA 1996; 276:73-74.

17. Smart CR, Hendrick RE, Rutledge JH et al. Benefit of mammography screening in women ages 40 to 49 years. Cancer 1995; 75:1619-1626.

18. Glasziou PP, Woodward AJ, Mahon CM. Mammographic screening trials for women aged under 50. A quality assessment and meta-analysis. Med J of Australia 1995; 162:625-629.

19. Kopans DB, Feig SA. The Canadian national breast screening study: a critical review. AJR 1993; 161:755-760.

20. Warren Burhenne LJ, Burhenne HJ. The Canadian national breast screening study: a Canadian critique. AJR 1993; 161: 761-763.

21. Basinski ASH. The Canadian national breast screening study: opportunity for a rethink. Can Med Assoc J 1992; 147: 1431-1434.

22. Baines CJ. The Canadian national breast screening study: a perspective on criticisms. Ann Int Med 1994; 120:326-334.

23. Kerlikowske K, Grady D, Rubin SM et al. Efficacy of screening mammography: a meta-analysis. JAMA 1995; 273: 149-154.

24. Fletcher SW. Why question screening mammography for women in their forties? Radiol Clinics of North America 1995; 33:1259-1271.

25. Wright CJ. Breast cancer screening: a different look at the evidence. Surgery 1986; 100:594-598.

26. Roberts MM. Breast screening: time for a rethink? BMJ 1989; 299:1153-1155.

27. Skrabanek P. Mass mammography. The time for reappraisal. Intl J of Technology Assessment in Health Care 1989; 5:423-430.

28. Schmidt JG. The epidemiology of mass breast cancer screening—a plea for a valid measure of benefit. J Clin Epidemiol 1990; 43:215-225.

29. Mueller CB. Breast cancer: reporting results with inflationary arithmetic. Am J Clin Oncol 1994; 17:86-92.

30. Wright CJ, Mueller CB. Screening mammography and public health policy: the need for perspective. Lancet 1995; 346: 29-32.

31. Mandelblatt JS, Fryback DG, Weinstein MC, Russell LB, Gold MR, Hadorn DC. Assessing the effectiveness of health interventions. In: Gold MR, Siegel JE, Russell LB, Weinstein MC, eds. Cost-effectiveness in health and medicine. Oxford University Press, 1996:158-159.

32. Spratt JS, Greenberg RA, Heuser LS. Geometry, growth rates and duration of cancer and carcinoma-in-situ of the breast before detection by screening. Cancer Res 1986; 46:970-974.

33. Spratt JS, Spratt JA. What is breast cancer doing before we can detect it? J Surg Oncol 1985; 30:156-160.

34. Spratt JA, Von Fournier D, Spratt JS et al. Mammographic assessment of human breast cancer growth and duration. Cancer 1993; 71:2020-2026.

35. Butler TP, Gullino PM. Quantitation of cell shedding into efferent blood of mammary adenocarcinoma. Cancer Res 1975; 35:512-516.

36. Kerlikowske K, Grady D, Barclay J et al. Positive predictive value of screening mammography by age and family history of breast cancer. JAMA 1993; 270: 2444-2450.

37. Norton LW, Zeligman BE, Pearlman NW. Accuracy and cost of needle localization breast biopsy. Arch Surg 1988; 123:947-950.

38. Baines CJ, McFarlane DV, Miller AB.

Sensitivity and specificity of first screen mammography in 15 NBSS centres. J Can Assoc Radiol 1988; 39:273-276.

39. Rosenberg RD, Lando JF, Hunt WC et al. The New Mexico mammography project—screening mammography performance in Albuquerque, New Mexico, 1991 to 1993. Cancer 1996; 78: 1731-1739.

40. Page DL, Dupont WD, Rogers LW et al. Intraductal carcinoma of the breast: follow up after biopsy only. Cancer 1982; 49:751-758.

41. Rosen PP, Kosloff C, Lieberman PH et al. Lobular carcinoma in situ of the breast: detailed analysis of 99 patients with average follow up of 24 years. Am J Surg Pathol 1978; 2:225-251.

42. Eddy DM. Screening for breast cancer. Ann Int Med 1989; 111:389-399

43. Baines CJ. Breast cancer: can good news be news? Can Med Assoc J 1994; 150: 139-140.

44. Smith BL, Gadd MA, Lawler C et al. Perception of breast cancer risk among women in breast center and primary care settings: correlation with age and family history of breast cancer. Surgery 1996; 120:297-303.

45. Marteau T. Psychological costs of screening. BMJ 1989; 299:527.

46. Jatoi I, Baum M. American and European recommendations for screening mammography in younger women: a cultural divide? BMJ 1993; 307: 1481-1483.

47. Lidbrink E, Elfving J, Frisell J et al. Neglected aspects of false positive findings of mammography in breast cancer screening: analysis of false positive cases from the Stockholm trial. BMJ 1996; 312:273-276.

48. Howe GR, Sherman GJ, Semenciw RM et al. Estimated benefits and risks of screening for breast cancer. Can Med Assoc J 1981; 124:399-403.

49. Swift M, Morrell D, Massey RB et al. Incidence of cancer in 161 families affected by ataxia-telangiectasia. N Eng J Med 1991; 325:1831-1836.

50. Jackson VP, Lex AM, Smith DJ. Patient discomfort during screen-film mammography. Radiology 1988; 168:421-423.

51. Nielsen BB, Miaskowski C, Dibble SL et al. Pain and discomfort associated with filmscreen mammography. J Natl Cancer Inst 1991; 83:1754-1756.

52. De Koning HJ, Van Ineveld BM, Van Oortmarssen GJ et al. Breast cancer screening and cost-effectiveness; policy alternatives, quality of life considerations and the possible impact of uncertain factors. Int J Cancer 1991; 49:531-537.

53. Brown ML. Sensitivity analysis in the cost-effectiveness of breast cancer screening. Cancer suppl 1992; 69:1963-1967.

54. Brown ML, Fintor L. Cost-effectiveness of breast cancer screening: preliminary results of a systematic review of the literature. Breast Cancer Research and Treatment 1993; 25:113-118.

55. Kattlove H, Liberati A, Keeler E et al. Benefits and costs of screening and treatment for early breast cancer. Development of a basic benefit package. JAMA 1995; 273:142-148.

56. Brown ML, Fintor L. U.S. screening mammography services with mobile units: results from the national survey of mammography facilities. Radiology 1995; 195:529-532.

57. Strax P. Control of breast cancer through mass screening: from research to action. Cancer 1989; 63:1881-1887.

58. American Cancer Society. Pamphlet 86-(30mm); no 2077-LE. Washington: ACS, 1986.

CHAPTER 6

Screening by Breast Self Examination

Anthony B. Miller, Cornelia J. Baines and Bart J. Harvey

INTRODUCTION

B reast self examination (BSE) is a widely promoted breast cancer screening method. Few methods of breast cancer detection have the appeal of BSE, being self-generated, nonintrusive, inexpensive and avoiding radiation risk. However, BSE is not without risks.[1-6] It can generate considerable anxiety in women. In addition, both false positive and false negative detections carry costs and risks. Further if BSE leads to an earlier detection without affecting breast cancer mortality, it just extends the period of time a woman is aware of her diagnosis. For these reasons it is important to ensure that the benefits of BSE practice outweigh its costs and risks.[7,8]

In this chapter we first review the evidence available from others on the efficacy of BSE in reducing mortality from breast cancer. We then consider in more detail our own studies of BSE, those based on the Canadian National Breast Screening Study (CNBSS) and that based on a special cohort of women in Finland. We then attempt to draw a practical conclusion on the role of BSE in screening.

STUDIES ON THE EFFECTIVENESS OF BSE

While BSE has been advocated for more than 60 years,[9,10] the first studies to provide evidence of BSE's effectiveness were only published in 1978.[11,12] Both were correlational studies. Despite Moore's[8] plea for more rigorous studies of BSE the investigations that followed were largely similar. Only recently have more rigorous studies been reported.

CORRELATIONAL STUDIES

Following the initial studies[11,12] ten other correlational studies[13-22] found a relationship between reported BSE practice and the diagnosis of earlier, more favorably staged breast cancer.

Foster et al[11] studied the relationship between BSE practice and the clinical stage of histologically diagnosed invasive breast cancer. The study subjects were 335 of the earliest registrants in the Vermont Breast Cancer Network Demonstration Project. Each woman's physician was asked to report whether the patient performed BSE monthly, less than monthly or never. Information regarding BSE practice was obtained for 246 (73%) of the women. There was a significant relationship between more frequent BSE practice and more favorable clinical stage, especially evidenced as smaller tumors and fewer instances of cancerous axillary lymph nodes. The results were unaffected by adjusting for age. The authors estimated that monthly BSE might result in a 27% improved survival compared to nonpractice.

Greenwald et al[12] examined the effects of BSE and clinical breast examination (CBE) on the clinical and pathologic stages of diagnosed breast cancer. The 293 women studied were those identified in the Regional Breast Cancer Program for Northeastern New York and Western Massachusetts who agreed to be interviewed. Results from the study showed that a higher proportion of late stage cancers were discovered by accident rather than by BSE or CBE. This result persisted even after controlling for age, education, a history of previous benign breast disease, religion, marital status and menstrual status. The study found no significant difference in the stages of BSE and CBE detected cancers. Using stage-specific 5-year survival rates, the authors estimated that BSE might result in a 10-20% improvement in 5-year survival.

Huguley and Brown[13] examined the relationship between reported BSE practice and the clinical and pathologic stages of breast cancer at diagnosis. The study included 2,092 women diagnosed with breast cancer in the Georgia Cancer Management Network who agreed to be interviewed. Competency of BSE practice was assessed by oncology nurses. After adjusting for race, age, education and economic levels, the study found that smaller, earlier staged tumors were diagnosed more frequently among BSE practitioners, especially those practicing competent BSE. Women practicing BSE were found to seek medical attention for their tumors more promptly than did nonpractitioners.

Feldman et al[14] used information collected from 996 newly diagnosed breast cancer patients entered in the Brooklyn Breast Cancer Demonstration Network to study the relationship between BSE practice and the pathologic stage of breast cancer. The investigators found a significant association between practicing BSE at least three times per year and the diagnosis of smaller, early staged tumors. This relationship was unchanged by adjustments for age, marital status, education level, economic status, menopausal status and oral contraceptive use. The authors estimated this benefit of BSE might increase 5-year survival up to 20%.

Tamburini et al[15] studied the relationship of BSE practice and clinical and pathologic stage among a group of 500 unselected women diagnosed with breast cancer at an outpatient department in Milan Italy. BSE practitioners were more frequently diagnosed with earlier stage cancers, both a higher proportion of smaller tumors and a lower proportion involving axillary lymph nodes.

Owen et al[16] examined the relationship between the method of breast cancer detection and cancer stage at diagnosis among 2,063 women with newly diagnosed breast cancer. A multivariate analysis, adjusted for age, marital status, race and quadrant of cancer location, showed that tumors detected by BSE were at a significantly earlier stage than those detected by accident.

Mant et al[17] examined the relationship between BSE and clinical and pathological stage at diagnosis in 616 women who had discovered their own tumor. History of BSE was categorized as taught and done at least monthly, taught and done less frequently than monthly, not taught but done and not done. Those taught and practicing any frequency of BSE had the most favorably staged cancers at diagnosis, with a higher proportion of smaller tumors and a lower proportion involving axillary lymph nodes. These findings persisted after adjusting for the confounding effects of age, oral contraceptive use and social class.

Ogawa et al[18] compared the clinical and pathologic stage of tumors diagnosed in 150 women: 30 who reported monthly BSE practice, 60 reporting less frequent BSE practice and 60 reporting infrequent or no previous BSE practice. The proportion of tumors found by "accident" were 30%, 60% and 97% for the monthly, less than monthly and rarely/never groups, respectively. Women practicing monthly BSE were more frequently diagnosed with smaller tumors without axillary lymph node involvement than women in either of the other two groups.

Dowle et al[19] examined the characteristics of the first 319 breast cancers diagnosed in the Nottingham Center of the United Kingdom (UK) Trial of Early Detection of Breast Cancer. All women living in the Nottingham area were invited to attend BSE educational sessions. The invasive tumors diagnosed among study woman were found to be significantly smaller than the 319 breast cancers diagnosed in Nottingham women immediately prior to the trial. There was, however, no difference in the proportion of tumors involving axillary lymph nodes while the two groups had similar proportions of advanced cancers diagnosed (19.7% and 16.9%, respectively). Nevertheless women with cancer who had attended the BSE educational sessions had significantly better 5-year survival than those with cancer who did not attend the sessions.

To examine the relationship between stage at diagnosis and reported BSE practice, Shugg et al[20] studied 117 women diagnosed with breast cancer in Tasmania. Compared to less frequent practitioners, women who reported practicing BSE at least every 3 months had a higher proportion of tumors that were < 2 cm in diameter (39% vs. 21%) and no axillary lymph node involvement (77% vs. 56%).

Bonett et al[21] used South Australian Central Cancer Registry data concerning breast cancers diagnosed between 1980-1986 to investigate the effects of a state-wide BSE campaign on tumor diameter, axillary lymph node status and case survival. The campaign began on October 1, 1982 and concluded January 31, 1983. Compared to tumors diagnosed during other time periods, a higher proportion of tumors diagnosed during the campaign had uninvolved axillary lymph nodes (60% vs. 52%). However, the higher proportion with tumors smaller than 2 cm in diameter (33% vs. 28%) did not achieve statistical significance and the 5-year survival for the 146 cases, diagnosed during the campaign (78%) was similar to that of the other cases (76%).

The Interdisciplinary Group for Cancer Care Evaluation (GIVIO)[22] examined the relationship of BSE practice and stage of disease among 1,315 women with newly diagnosed nonmetastatic breast cancer enrolled in a clinical trial of breast cancer treatment. Their BSE practice was assessed and classified into one of three categories. Women practicing BSE correctly and at least monthly had significantly more early stage tumors (59% < 2 cm and 52% stage I); the proportions for women practicing incorrect or less frequent BSE were 54% < 2 cm and 48% stage I; while for women not practicing BSE the proportions were 46% and 41%, respectively.

During the same period seven additional correlational studies[28-34] were published which did not demonstrate a beneficial effect associated with BSE practice.

Smith, Francis and Polissar[28] assessed the relationship between the mode of breast cancer detection and the stage at diagnosis in a group of 230 women identified through the Washington state population based cancer registry. They found that the pathologic stage, extent of nodal involvement and sizes of tumors detected by BSE did not differ from those discovered accidentally. This lack of relationship persisted after adjustment for factors such as histologic type, menopausal status, age, race, marital status, occupation and level of education.

Senie et al[29] examined the relationship of BSE practice and physician evaluations of the breast to stage of breast cancer among 1,216 breast cancer patients consecutively admitted to the Memorial Sloan Kettering Cancer Center. After adjusting for factors, such as family history of breast cancer, history of benign breast disease, education level and relative body weight, BSE practice was found to be unrelated to both tumor size and positive axillary lymph nodes. However, there was a significant relationship between the frequency of physical breast examinations by physicians and the diagnosis of more favorably staged disease.

Gould-Martin et al[30] studied 274 women with local or regional breast cancer diagnosed at one of 11 Los Angeles hospitals. Women with distant metastases were excluded because 45% of them had died before they could be reached for interview. They found no evidence linking BSE practice with the diagnosis of more favorably staged tumors. Localized disease was diagnosed in 64% of the women reporting no BSE practice and in 59% of BSE practitioners. In addition, 59% of the tumors discovered by accident and 52% of those identified during BSE were diagnosed at a localized stage. Even among the 31% of women judged to be performing 'adequate' routine self examination, BSE practice appeared to provide no advantage.

Philip et al[31] studied the first 153 breast cancers diagnosed at the Huddersfield Center of the UK Trial of Early Detection of Breast Cancer. While a larger proportion of the women who had attended the educational sessions were diagnosed with tumors < 2 cm in diameter (45% vs. 31%), a similar proportion of attenders and nonattenders had no axillary lymph node involvement (53% vs. 54%). However, a larger proportion of tumors detected by BSE were < 2 cm in diameter (40% vs. 31%) and had no axillary nodal involvement (59% vs. 52%).

Philip et al[32] subsequently studied 304 consecutive patients diagnosed during the Huddersfield center's second, third and fourth years. They found a larger proportion of BSE practitioners to have clinically early cancers (48% vs. 35%). However, there was no association between BSE practice and either tumor size or pathologic evidence of axillary lymph node involvement.

Hislop, Coldman and Skippen[33] interviewed 416 women with breast cancer listed in the British Columbia cancer registry. They found that twice as many women who inspected their breasts thoroughly had tumors smaller than 2 cm (P = 0.05) and that those who did not palpate their breasts were twice as likely to have involved axillary

lymph nodes (P = 0.05). Nevertheless, the probability of a tumor being self-detected was not affected by BSE practice.

Smith and Burns[34] studied 365 cases of newly diagnosed breast cancer between the ages of 20-54 years at diagnosis identified through the Iowa cancer registry. They found 20.8% of BSE detected tumors and 18.5% of those discovered accidentally were < 2 cm in diameter while 59.4% and 50.0% were early stage (in situ or local). However, there was a significant relationship between physician detected tumors and diameter < 2 cm (42.3%) and early stage (65.8%) at diagnosis.

More recently four additional correlational studies[23-27] were carried out to examine the relationship between BSE practice and survival of women diagnosed with breast cancer. Each found better survival among those reporting BSE practice.

Foster and Costanza[23,24] studied the 1,004 invasive breast cancer cases identified through the Vermont state wide registry between July 1, 1975 and December 31, 1982. Each woman's physician was asked whether the patient performed BSE monthly, less than monthly or never. Follow up and BSE information was obtained on 835 (83%) of the patients. The median period of follow up for surviving patients was 52 months with a maximum follow up of 92 months. Consistent with the results of an earlier study[11] they found that the 5-year survival for BSE performers was 75% but only 57% for the nonperformers (P < 0.001). This result remained unchanged after adjusting for age, family history of breast cancer, method of detection and delay in treatment. The authors assert that at least a 3-year lead time would be needed to negate a survival benefit of this magnitude.

Huguley et al[25] determined the survival of 2,079 women from a previously studied cohort of breast cancer patients[13] with follow up and BSE information available. They found that BSE performers had significantly better 5-year survival than the nonperformers; 77% vs. 61% respectively (P < 0.0001). The investigators estimated that only 25% of the survival benefit was due to factors such as age, race, education, marital status, menstrual status, family history of breast cancer, patient delay and treatment. They also suggested that a lead time of 3 years would be required to explain the observed survival difference.

Kuroishi et al[26] compared the survival of 347 women with BSE detected breast cancer with that of 1,322 patients with accidentally discovered breast cancer. The 5-year survival for patients with BSE detected breast cancers was 94% but only 86% for those with chance discovered tumors (P < 0.001). The beneficial effect of detection by BSE remained after adjusting for patient age, year of diagnosis and histologic type.

Le Geyte et al[27] followed a previously identified cohort of 616 women diagnosed with breast cancer[17] whose tumor was discovered by themselves. During the 6 years of follow up, 190 (31%) of the women died: 60 of the 226 (27%) who had been taught and practiced BSE prior to their diagnosis and 130 of the 390 (33%) patients who had never been taught BSE (P = 0.07). The survival benefit was largely limited to those diagnosed with Stage I disease.

The correlational studies published prior to 1986[11-14,23-24,28-31,33-34] were included in the 1987 critical review of BSE completed by O'Malley and Fletcher[3] for the US Preventive Services Task Force. The authors found that 'descriptive' studies were the predominant source of evidence concerning BSE's effectiveness and concluded "these studies demonstrated either no or small, nonsignificant associations of BSE to tumor size/ stage." O'Malley and Fletcher suggested that "the problem with BSE is not evidence of a lack of effect, but lack of evidence."[3]

In 1988 Hill et al[35] published the results of a meta-analysis which included results from the descriptive studies published before 1987.[11-16,23,28-30,32-34] Based on their analysis the authors drew conclusions somewhat divergent from those of O'Malley and Fletcher:[3]

1. results among the examined studies were generally consistent with one another;

2. a significantly lower proportion of women who had practiced BSE prior to their diagnosis had tumors of 2 cm or more in diameter (56% vs. 66%) and evidence of cancerous axillary lymph node involvement (39% vs. 50%) compared to women never having practiced BSE;

3. no difference in the extent of disease was found between those tumors detected by BSE and those found accidentally;

4. because of the misclassification that results from using method of tumor detection, reported past history of BSE practice is a more appropriate classification to assess BSE's effectiveness;

5. the data reviewed provide good grounds to encourage women to practice breast self examination regularly.

However, Hill et al[35] in agreement with O'Malley and Fletcher[3] and others[1,2,6,8,36-42] highlighted the methodologic limitations inherent in correlational studies of BSE. Thus the findings of these studies have been questioned because of the inherent potential of post disease reporting (recall), loss to follow up, nonresponse and self-selection biases and because of the screening specific lead time and length biases.

To eliminate or at least minimize these potential biases, studies using more rigorous methodologies are required to evaluate the effectiveness of BSE.[43,44] These include randomized and nonrandomized, controlled trials, cohort studies and case-control studies. The potential effects of lead time and length biases are eliminated if, rather than stage of disease or survival since diagnosis, disease-specific mortality rates are used to estimate the effect of screening.

CONTROLLED TRIALS

The strongest evidence comes from controlled trials which can eliminate all of the methodologic shortcomings described above. However, the two randomized, controlled trials currently in progress, one in St. Petersburg and Moscow, Russia[45-47] and the other in Shanghai, China underway in an occupational setting (Thomas D, personal communication April 1995) are not yet able to provide results. The Russian trial used BSE in conjunction with physical examination of the breasts by medical care practitioners and the controls received physical examination without the teaching of BSE in the largest component (St. Petersburg).[47] The nonrandomized UK trial found divergent results from the two BSE centers during the period 6-10 years from entry, the relative risk being 1.13 (95% confidence interval (CI) 0.95-1.35) for Nottingham and 0.78 (95% CI 0.61-1.00) for Huddersfield.[48]

COHORT STUDIES

Well-conducted cohort studies provide an intermediate level of evidence. While results may be affected by self-selection bias, cohort studies can eliminate the effect of the other potential biases described above. There has been one such study reported which examined the experience of 29,000 women enrolled in the BSE-containing Mama Program in Finland.[49-51] This is described in a later section of this chapter.

CASE CONTROL STUDIES

Case control studies also provide intermediate level evidence. Application of case control methodology to the evaluation of screening has received a great deal of attention.[1,2,6,52-73]

The case control design may be used in a population if screening has been available for some time. If BSE is effective a history of BSE practice will be found significantly less often in cases than controls. In etiologic case control studies of breast cancer, cases are women diagnosed with histologically proven breast cancer. In contrast cases in case control studies of breast cancer screening are women who have had the adverse consequences, particularly death and distant metastases, that screening is intended to avoid. Thus they are failures of the screening process. The control group is selected to estimate the exposure to BSE in the population from which the cases arose. It is as-

sembled by randomly selecting women who do not meet the case definition from the same population from which the cases came. In this design cases and controls have comparable BSE opportunities. The control group may include women with less advanced stages of the disease as well as those not diagnosed with breast cancer but the cases of breast cancer will not occur with greater frequency than they do in the general population. A control group drawn exclusively from cases with early breast cancer is biased. By employing the case control methodology, any possible effects of length or lead time biases are eliminated.

Three case control studies of BSE have been reported. Newcomb et al[74] carried out a population based case control study to examine the relationship between BSE and the occurrence of advanced breast cancer. They found no beneficial effect associated with either the practice of BSE or its frequency. However, the small proportion of women who reported more thorough BSE had a significantly decreased occurrence of advanced disease relative to those who either did not perform BSE or performed it less proficiently.

In a case control study of 435 women with advanced breast cancer identified through the Connecticut Tumor Registry and 887 matched neighborhood controls, Muscat and Huncharek[75] found that 57.7% and 27.4% of the cases and only 48.5% and 20.5% of the disease-free controls reported practicing BSE at least twice yearly and monthly, respectively. Stepwise multiple regression, controlling for a family history of breast cancer, age at first birth, race and frequency of mammography found an odds ratio associated with BSE frequency of 1.27 (95% CI 0.77-2.07).

In contrast, a case control study nested within the Nottingham BSE Center of the UK Trial of Early Detection of Breast Cancer conducted by Locker et al[76,77] found attendance for BSE education to be protective of breast cancer death (odds ratio = 0.70; 95% CI 0.50-0.97). However, because the breast cancer mortality rate of the Nottingham nonattenders was higher than in the comparison districts, Moss[62] suggests the demonstrated benefit is the result of selection bias.

STUDIES OF BSE BASED ON THE CANADIAN NATIONAL BREAST SCREENING STUDY

THE CANADIAN NATIONAL BREAST SCREENING STUDY (CNBSS)

The CNBSS was designed primarily to determine the efficacy of mammography plus physical examination of the breasts in reducing mortality from breast cancer in women age 40-49 on entry and the benefit of mammography over and above physical examination in women age 50-59 on entry.[78] An individually randomized, controlled trial with informed consent, 50% of the participants were randomly allocated to receive mammography and physical examination (PE) annually and another 50% were allocated to receive PE alone. Of those allocated to PE alone women age 40-49 received only one screening examination and were subsequently followed by mailed annual questionnaires, while women age 50-59 received PE annually. PE was performed by nurse examiners in 12 screening centers across Canada and by physicians in three centers located in the Province of Quebec. All participants were taught BSE by the nurse or physician examiners at their first attendance and their technique was reinforced at their subsequent screening visits. The CNBSS began in 1980 and screening ceased in May 1988. A total of 89,835 participants were recruited and were eligible to receive up to five annual screens.

The role of the practitioner

Integrated with PE the nurse or physician taught BSE and in all examinations subsequent to the initial screen BSE evaluation accompanied BSE instruction. Even though screening associated anxiety may have made it difficult for women to learn a complex skill the participants' BSE performance improved consistently each year of their screen-

ing schedule. In each succeeding year of the screen schedule more women reported doing BSE 12/yr, 19% at screen 1 increasing up to 61% at screen 5.[79] BSE instruction and evaluation caused some problems and the examiners varied in their motivation and ability to teach BSE. However, less than 2% of the participants reported they were not interested in BSE.[80]

The CNBSS has shown that instruction by health care practitioners is critical to ensure that women gain sufficient expertise to practice BSE well and to allow them to achieve maximum benefit from the practice. With the increasing recognition of the role of nurses in various health care delivery roles it is possible that nurses will take over some of the roles that physicians are not inclined to provide, especially many male physicians.

The study from Finland (see below) emphasizes an additional role for physicians, that of giving an informed opinion on the nature of any abnormality discovered by the BSE practitioner. It is critical that women are able to obtain such informed advice. Physicians must acquire the necessary skills in the detection of early breast cancer (with visual inspection for subtle signs of breast cancer an important component) recognizing that the physical signs taught in medical school are of advanced breast cancer. They should also be prepared on the basis of the woman's testimony to refer her to a specialist with the necessary skills.

Compliance with BSE

The CNBSS provided an opportunity to evaluate not only women's attitudes and intentions with respect to BSE[80] but also their actual BSE performance.[79] In the first instance, understanding can be gained from factors associated with compliance and in the second, compliance as reflected by actual performance is measured.

Women's attitudes to BSE

A self-administered, mailed questionnaire was sent to 2,800 CNBSS participants who had been enrolled at two CNBSS centers and had completed their screening protocol. The sample was stratified according to age, study arm (mammography containing vs. other), compliance with the annual screening schedule and the consequences of screening (referral to a surgeon with or without a subsequent biopsy). An 82% response rate was achieved.

Responders who had been good compliers with the screening schedule (n = 1,612) were more likely to be "very interested" in BSE than less good compliers (n = 548), 81% and 73%, respectively (p = 0.0004). Good compliers were also more likely to express an intention to perform BSE in the future—91% vs. 84%, respectively (P<0.0001). Of 1,061 reasons offered why it was difficult to do BSE, the most frequent was forgetfulness (32%), followed by laziness (15%), "difficult" (11%), time restrictions (9.2%), fear and anxiety (8%) and lumpy or scarred breasts (7%). The arm of the study to which respondents had been randomized did not affect attitudes to BSE.

Some inferences about compliance can be drawn from these observations.

- Women who are motivated to accept routine breast screening appear to be most positively motivated to perform BSE. Paradoxically, women who avoid routine screening may be most able to profit from BSE.
- In women who are favorably disposed to do BSE for whom forgetfulness is a major problem it may be helpful to offer aides memoirs.
- If "difficulty" is associated with insufficient BSE instruction and a consequent lack of self confidence the importance of effective BSE instruction is reinforced.
- Given that "time restrictions" affect the majority in our society it would be helpful to streamline the recommended components of BSE. Women who cannot find the time to examine themselves lying down (with pillows or folded towels) and standing up and who may well dislike pinching their nipples, might be more compliant if only one position were recommended

and the nipple squeeze were deleted.

- "Fear and anxiety" about breast cancer is prevalent in our society. It has been observed that women severely overestimate their risk of getting and dying of breast cancer.[81]

BSE performance in the CNBSS

Participants were instructed in BSE on each and every annual visit. After the first screening visit, the participants' BSE technique was also evaluated although the method for this varied according to circumstance. Ideally the participant demonstrated her technique to the screen examiner. However, in order not to threaten or antagonize, the examiners sometimes would depend on the participant's verbal report of her BSE technique.

The specific BSE components evaluated were: visual examination performed; three digits used; finger pads applied in palpation; a systematic search pattern (spoke or concentric circles); most of the breast examined; axillae examined; and a frequency of 12 times a year.

The results revealed that compliance with each BSE component increased from year to year. The improvement occurred whether women were perfect attenders (attending all screening visits) or less perfect attenders, although the improvement was greatest in the perfect attenders. For example among perfect attenders compliance with the visual examination of the breasts was 69% at the second screening visit and 84% at the fifth, while for less perfect attenders the compliance was 63% and 74%, respectively. In both groups of attenders and for all BSE components the trend for improvement over screens was highly significant.

With respect to BSE frequency, younger (age 40-49 on entry) and older (age 50-59 on entry) women were similar at the first screening examination with 19% reporting BSE frequency of 12 or more times annually. By the fifth screen significantly more older women reported this frequency (64%) than younger (57%). Significantly associated with BSE scores (based on all BSE components with the exception of frequency) was a family history of breast cancer. Better scores were observed in women with two or more relatives with breast cancer compared to women with one affected relative who in turn had better scores than women with no affected relatives. Women with higher educational experience had higher BSE scores than those reporting only public school education, but by the final screens those with public school education showed a greater improvement from baseline than those with higher education.

The inferences which can be drawn from these observations are:

- women's BSE competence can improve over time in the context of a large screening program and with a relatively brief intervention from health professionals;
- annual feedback on BSE leads not only to a higher prevalence of BSE performance but also to improved compliance with the various components of BSE technique;
- improvements over time can be achieved in spite of education level;
- women with a family history of breast cancer appear to be motivated to perform BSE well;
- for women aged from 40-64 years, age is not a barrier to performing BSE.

THE CASE CONTROL STUDY

To measure the effect of BSE practice on breast cancer mortality, we conducted a case control study nested within the CNBSS. Eligible subjects for the case control study were all CNBSS participants except those diagnosed with breast cancer prior to their second year in the CNBSS who were excluded to eliminate the influence of prevalent cancers.

Cases were women who had either died of breast cancer or who had been reported as developing distant metastatic disease during follow up. Study cases were identified by the ongoing annual CNBSS follow up for all women diagnosed with breast cancer and by record linkages with Statistics Canada's National Mortality Database and the cancer registries of the six provinces where the CNBSS operated. There were 220 cases in all, 153 women dead due to breast cancer and 67 with distant metastases.

For each case ten controls were randomly selected from the remaining eligible women. All who were alive at the time the case either died or was determined to have distant metastatic disease were eligible. Therefore the controls could include women with diagnosed breast cancer. However, if they subsequently developed distant metastases or died of breast cancer they were eligible to become a case. The controls were matched by age group (40-44, 45-49, 50-54 and 55-59 years) screening center, enrollment year and CNBSS randomization group.

During the CNBSS prospectively collected BSE data included: self-reported BSE frequency prior to CNBSS enrollment; annual self reports of BSE frequency during the screening program; and annual assessments of BSE proficiency by the CNBSS examiners. Because objective, structured assessment of BSE proficiency by the examiners was instituted after the CNBSS started, approximately 15% of the participants did not have their BSE assessed at their year 2 screening visit. Women aged 40-49 years randomly allocated to the comparison (usual care) group were not eligible for re-screening so their BSE proficiency was not assessed.

The examiners conducted their assessments of BSE proficiency prior to performing physical examination of the breasts. The assessment of BSE proficiency was based on eight factors (the practices considered proficient are noted within parentheses): visual examination (included); fingers used for examination (middle three); surfaces used for examination (finger pads); search pattern used (not random); palpation technique used (small circles); coverage of the examination (all/most); axillae examination (included); and BSE frequency (12 or more times/year). BSE practice was evaluated up to the time of diagnosis. For each case control set assessment of BSE and other screening practices was limited to the time of breast cancer diagnosis within the set.

Cases and controls were compared for self-reported BSE frequency prior to CNBSS enrollment, annual self reports of BSE frequency during the program and principally the annual objective assessments of BSE proficiency. The effect of covariates such as age, family history of breast cancer, age at menarche, past history of breast problems, parity, age of first live birth, age of menopause, marital status, smoking history, education and occupation were examined.

Self-reported information about BSE practice was available for over 85% of the eligible cases and controls. Failure to return follow up questionnaires (8%) and questionnaires returned without specifying BSE practice (6%) were responsible for the missing responses. Screen examiner assessment information was available for over 80% of eligible cases and controls. When not available the reasons were: failure to attend the rescreening visit (11%); the rescreening visit occurred before the structured assessment of BSE proficiency was implemented (6%); and the assessment was not completed during the rescreening visit (1%).

Fewer cases than controls reported having practiced BSE before study entry, 44% vs. 50%, respectively. However, this difference did not attain statistical significance (P = 0.10).

Self-reported BSE frequency post entry was not found to be associated with an increased risk of dying of breast cancer or developing advanced metastatic disease. However, the odds ratios associated with failure to perform three of the eight assessed BSE characteristics: a visual examination, palpation with the three middle fingers and examination with the finger pads were found to be greatest for the assessment 2 years prior to diagnosis. Relative to women who visually examined their breasts, used their finger pads for palpation and examined with their three middle fingers, the odds ratio for breast cancer death or distant metastatic disease for women omitting at least one factor was 2.20 (95% CI 1.30-3.71; P = 0.003).

The odds ratio for those omitting one factor was 1.82 (95% CI 1.00-3.29; P = 0.05), omitting two factors 2.84 (95% CI 1.44-5.59; P = 0.003) and omitting all three factors 2.95 (95% CI 1.19-7.30; P = 0.02). The results remained unchanged after adjustment for potential confounders.

Although the effect of BSE practice was found to be evident only when assessed 2 years prior to breast cancer diagnosis, this appears consistent with Weiss et al[54] who pointed out that effective screening must focus on the period of time when the tumor is both detectable and curable. Our results suggest that BSE practice 1 year prior to diagnosis was too late to have an effect, while practice 2 years earlier provided an effect. This seems reasonable because the cases in this study are, by definition, women in whom screening failed because they either died of breast cancer or developed distant metastatic disease.

We conclude that this study, using prospectively collected data, provides strong evidence of BSE's effectiveness in reducing breast cancer mortality.

THE FINNISH COHORT STUDY

The Mama Program in Finland provided an opportunity to evaluate by a historical cohort design the impact of a specially designed and comprehensive BSE containing program on mortality from breast cancer in a group of women who were exposed to the program and subsequently returned calendars detailing their BSE practice over a 2-year period.[82]

The Mama Program strategy was based on the experience that women were able to detect changes in their breasts indicative of early breast cancer if they had first learned the normal appearance and structure of their breasts.[51] Two nationwide Finnish women's organizations that work for home care and home economics planned a "health project year" in 1972 and chose to concentrate on the early detection of breast cancer through the Mama Program.

The Mama Program strategy consisted of three elements. The initial element was information provided by health professionals in two way communications face to face in groups or sometimes individually. The women were usually initially exposed to the program in groups of 20-50 persons. The message included information on the Mama screening program, healthy and changed breasts at different ages, breast cancer symptoms, the BSE technique and frequency, the monthly use of the calendar for recording the date and findings from BSE and the self referral system. Opportunity for discussion was provided during the information sessions.

The second element in the strategy was continuous interaction between key volunteer lay people and the women enrolled in the program including reminders to continue BSE with specially designed Mama calendars acting as prompts. For the woman the calendar served as a reminder of the date BSE was due by writing it down every month in the appropriate space. The name of the local breast specialist (usually a radiologist) who agreed to examine women who discovered breast abnormalities was written down in a space on the calendar. For the health personnel in charge of the initial communication and the key persons in charge of the follow up communication, the calendar provided basic information while encouraging individual women to continue with the program. The material for this study consists of the first calendar which was returned after the first 2 years of follow up.

The third element in the strategy was provision of diagnostic mammography for those women who reported discovering changes in their breasts through BSE. Women could self refer directly for a mammography examination or may have been referred by other physicians.

The population in the study was based on women who belonged to selected clubs from the two organizations from urban and rural areas across Finland, who were included in the Mama Program and who returned the calendars. The membership of the selected clubs was 56,177 women aged 20 years or more. Calendars were returned by 29,018 women. Since the vast majority of the women had recorded dates of BSE

performance once a month on the calendar they were regarded as BSE compliers. The data were entered on tape and the tape linked the Finnish Cancer Registry through the unique ID number. Information on all breast cancers diagnosed in the study population, time of all deaths and the cause of death was extracted. Stage was available for the majority of the cancers, coded localized, metastases only in regional node(s) and distant metastases. This categorization was routinely applied within the cancer registry for all cancers without knowledge of BSE practice. Data for the year 1980 (the mid-year of observation of the study cohort) was extracted from the cancer registry files for comparison purposes.

Those women who were symptomatic at the time they attended the initial information session (and were therefore in part attending for this reason) and those with prevalent detectable breast cancer at the time they started practicing BSE were excluded from the study cohort. As the women who returned their calendars did so only after the end of the second year of keeping calendars the first 2 years of observation were also excluded from the analysis. The study findings therefore relate to women in whom breast cancer had not been found before the first 2 years of the program had elapsed.

The reference population in this study constituted the general female population of Finland, with observed rates of incidence of breast cancer and mortality available on an age, sex, and calendar time-specific basis. The general female population was not exposed to the Mama screening program, though it was exposed to general publicity concerning BSE outside the Mama program.

Of the 28,785 women followed from the beginning of the third year since enrollment, 2,658 (9%) were known to have died by the end of 1986. This compared with 125 (28.9%) of the 432 with breast cancer. The observed and expected numbers of breast cancers diagnosed among the 28,785 women by year from enrollment and age at enrollment compared to the numbers expected from Finnish national rates were similar. The cumulative rates over years 3-13 were greater than expected and for all ages combined the rate ratio was 1.2. The stage distribution for the cancers observed compared to the distribution from the Finnish Cancer Registry for 1980 were very similar.

The difference between the observed total of 95 breast cancer deaths and the expected number of 133.9 is statistically significant (P < 0.001) for a ratio of 0.71 (95% CI 0.57-0.87). Half of the deficit in breast cancer deaths occurred in the period between 3-6 years after enrollment (11 observed compared to 32 expected). When the study population was subdivided into those under the age of 50 and above, the observed to expected ratio of deaths was 0.64 for those under the age of 50 and 0.74 for those 50 or older on entry to the study, and a formal test of homogeneity indicated no significant difference in the degree of effect by age group (chi-square 1.95, P > 0.75). The mortality from all causes was lower than in the general population, an effect seen in previous studies of compliers with breast screening.

The fact that there was no indication that the stage distribution of breast cancers in the study population was affected by the Mama program in comparison with the expected distribution from the Finnish population has to be reconciled with the lower breast cancer mortality in the study population than that expected from Finnish national rates. Change in stage distribution as an effect of screening has been regarded as a necessary component of reduced breast cancer mortality in screening programs.[83] However, in this study the information on stage was relatively crude because it originated from routine notifications to the cancer registry. This crude classification does not exclude the possibility of a difference within the localized or within the nonlocalized cases in favor of the BSE group. Earlier detection of advanced disease has been suggested as one of the means benefit was derived in the first trial of breast cancer screening.[84] Further on the basis of a mathematical model improved survival within stage has been regarded as one of the mechanisms for reduced breast cancer mortality in that study.[85]

In a population invited to be screened, those with previously diagnosed breast cancers are excluded and therefore a simple comparison of observed numbers of breast cancer deaths with that expected from the person years experience of a cohort of women drawn from the general population will be biased to showing lower breast cancer deaths than expected. In the Finnish study this bias was avoided as national survival rates were applied to the expected number of incident breast cancer cases to compute the expected breast cancer mortality. This method corrects for the selection of healthy screenees, i.e., for the exclusion of women with previously diagnosed breast cancer at the beginning of follow up. The study population was of slightly higher socio-economic status than the Finnish population at large as indicated by the greater proportion of women with college education. Although survival from breast cancer is somewhat related to socio-economic status, any bias arising from the use of national survival rates was probably compensated by the use of expected rather than observed breast cancer incidence in computing the expected number of breast cancer deaths. However, while the incidence of breast cancer was higher the total all cause mortality was lower than the general Finnish population. The deficit of such deaths in the early period of follow up is analogous to the healthy screenee effect in that only the relatively healthy are likely to attend for screening.

In conclusion, although this study could not avoid the major disadvantage of most observational studies of screening compliers as distinct from invitees, namely selection bias, the findings are consistent with an effect of a comprehensive BSE program in reducing mortality from breast cancer, which appears to be independent of age.

CONCLUSION

The evidence on the effectiveness of BSE as reviewed in this chapter clearly does not reach the level of certainty that we would normally expect before sanctioning the introduction of a screening test as public health policy.[64] The absence of randomized, controlled trial data confirming efficacy in reducing breast cancer mortality is particularly troubling. However, given the importance of breast cancer and the fact that the Cancer Societies of many countries usually advocate BSE, we believe that lesser degrees of evidence must be used to guide policy decisions on BSE as we simply cannot afford to wait until the necessary controlled trials are designed and performed.

It is our view that BSE should be adopted as an important contributor to breast cancer control for the following reasons:

- it is an approach to early detection that women can perform themselves and it contributes to their empowerment in relation to breast cancer;
- its teaching and reinforcement in the context of a breast screening program helps to avoid false reassurance from a false negative screening test (both mammography and physical examination);
- the evidence that is available from our studies suggests that it is equally effective in women under and over the age of 50;
- our studies suggest that good BSE practitioners have a 20-30% lower risk of death from breast cancer than poor or nonpractitioners.

In this chapter we have avoided discussing the age at which BSE instruction should commence. We are not convinced that teaching BSE to women younger than 40 (unless they are at especially high risk) is likely to be beneficial. Indeed there is some evidence that it is likely to lead to an unacceptable frequency of false positive surgery. However, we believe that BSE should be taught by health professionals and therefore its use should begin at the same time as annual physical breast examinations are recommended, i.e., from the age of 40. There is no upper age limit for its use. BSE and physical examinations of the breast are complementary and unless there is a major cultural barrier that can not be overcome by properly directed education, both should be an important element of cancer control

in any country where breast cancer is deemed a sufficiently high priority to justify investment in its early detection.

REFERENCES

1. Prorok PC. Epidemiologic approach for cancer screening: Problems in design and analysis of trials. Am J Pediatr Hematol Oncol 1992; 14:117-28.
2. Hurley SF, Kaldor JM. The benefits and risks of mammographic screening for breast cancer. Epidemiol Rev 1992; 14: 101-30.
3. O'Malley MS, Fletcher SW. Screening for breast cancer with breast self-examination: A critical review. J Am Med Assoc 1987; 257:2197-2203.
4. Frank JW, Mai V. Breast self-examination in young women: More harm than good? Lancet 1985; ii: 654-7.
5. Cole P, Austin H. Breast self-examination: An adjunct to early cancer detection. Am J Public Health 1981; 71:572-4.
6. Cole P, Morrison AS. Basic issues in population screening for cancer. J Natl Cancer Inst 1980; 64:1263-72.
7. Sox HC, Woolf SH. Evidence-based practice guidelines from the US Preventive Services Task Force. J Am Med Assoc 1993; 269:2678.
8. Moore FD. Breast self-examination. N Engl J Med 1978; 299:304-5.
9. Adair FE. Clinical manifestations of early cancer of the breast—with a discussion on the subject of biopsy. N Engl J Med 1933; 208:1250-5.
10. Haagensen CD. Self-examination of the breasts. J Am Med Assoc 1952; 149: 356-60.
11. Foster RS Jr, Lang SP, Costanza MC et al. Breast self-examination practices and breast cancer stage. N Engl J Med 1978; 299:265-70.
12. Greenwald P, Nasca PC, Lawrence CE et al. Estimated effect of breast self-examination and routine physician examinations on breast cancer mortality. N Engl J Med 1978; 299:271-3.
13. Huguley CM Jr, Brown RL. The value of breast self-examination. Cancer 1981; 47:989-95.
14. Feldman JG, Carter AC, Nicastri AD et al. Breast self-examination, relationship

to stage of breast cancer at diagnosis. Cancer 1981; 47:2740-5.

15. Tamburini M, Massara G, Bertario L et al. Usefulness of breast self-examination for an early detection of breast cancer. Results of a study on 500 breast cancer patients and 652 controls. Tumori 1981; 67:219-24.

16. Owen WL, Hoge AF, Asal NR et al. Self-examination of the breast: Use and effectiveness. South Med J 1985; 78:1170-3.

17. Mant D, Vessey MP, Neil A et al. Breast self examination and breast cancer stage at diagnosis. Br J Cancer 1987; 55:207-11.

18. Ogawa H, Tominaga S, Yoshida M et al. Breast self-examination practice and clinical stage of breast cancer. Jpn J Cancer Res 1987; 78:447-52.

19. Dowle CS, Mitchell A, Elston CW et al. Preliminary results of the Nottingham breast self-examination education programme. Br J Surg 1987; 74:217-9.

20. Shugg D, Hill D, Cooper D et al. Practice of breast self-examination and the treatment of primary breast cancer. Aust NZ J Surg 1990; 60:455-62.

21. Bonett A, Dorsch M, Roder D et al. Infiltrating ductal carcinoma of the breast in South Australia: Implications of trends in tumor diameter, nodal status and case-survival rates for cancer control. Med J Aust 1990; 152:19-23.

22. GIVIO (Interdisciplinary Group for Cancer Care Evaluation). Practice of breast self examination: Disease extent at diagnosis and patterns of surgical care. A report from an Italian study. J Epidemiol Community Health 1991; 45:112-6.

23. Foster RS Jr, Costanza MC. Breast self-examination practices and breast cancer survival. Cancer 1984; 53:999-1005.

24. Costanza MC, Foster RS Jr. Relationship between breast self-examination and death from breast cancer by age groups. Cancer Detect Prev 1984; 7:103-8.

25. Huguley CM Jr, Brown RL, Greenberg RS et al. Breast self-examination and survival from breast cancer. Cancer 1988; 62:1389-96.

26. Kuroishi T, Tominaga S, Ota J et al. The effect of breast self-examination on early detection and survival. Jpn J Cancer Res 1992; 83:344-50.

27. Le Geyte M, Mant D, Vessey MP et al. Breast self-examination and survival from breast cancer. Br J Cancer 1992; 66:917-8.

28. Smith EM, Francis AM, Polissar L. The effect of breast self-exam practices and physician examinations on extent of disease at diagnosis. Prev Med 1980; 9: 409-17.

29. Senie RT, Rosen PP, Lesser ML et al. Breast self-examination and medical examination related to breast cancer stage. Am J Public Health 1981; 71:583-90.

30. Gould-Martin K, Paganini-Hill A, Casagrande C et al. Behavioral and biological determinants of surgical stage of breast cancer. Prev Med 1982; 11:429-40.

31. Philip J, Harris WG, Flaherty C et al. Breast self-examination: Clinical results from a population-based prospective study. Br J Cancer 1984; 50:7-12.

32. Philip J, Harris WG, Flaherty C et al. Clinical measures to assess the practice and efficiency of breast self-examination. Cancer 1986; 58:973-7.

33. Hislop TG, Coldman AJ, Skippen DH. Breast self-examination: Importance of technique in early diagnosis. Can Med Assoc J 1984; 131:1349-52.

34. Smith EM, Burns TL. The effects of breast self-examination in a population-based cancer registry: A report of differences in extent of disease. Cancer 1985; 55:432-7.

35. Hill D, White V, Jolley D et al. Self examination of the breast: is it beneficial? Meta-analysis of studies investigating breast self examination and extent of disease in patients with breast cancer. Br Med J 1988; 297:271-5.

36. Venet L. Self-examination and clinical examination of the breast. Cancer 1980; 46(4 Suppl):930-2.

37. Early diagnosis and survival in breast cancer (editorial). Lancet 1981; 2:785-6.

38. Del Greco L, Spitzer WO. Breast self-examination: A call for scientific answers. Can J Public Health 1984; 75:425-8.

39. Diem G, Rose DP. Has breast self-examination had a fair trial? NY State J Med 1985; 85:479-80.

40. Feldman J. Breast self-examination—a practice whose time has come? NY State

J Med 1985; 85:482-3.

41. Morrison B. The periodic health examination: 3. Breast cancer. Can Med Assoc J 1986; 134:727-9.

42. Screening for Breast Cancer. In: US Preventive Services Task Force. Guide to Clinical Preventive Services Task Force: An Assessment of the Effectiveness of 169 Interventions. Baltimore, Md: Williams & Wilkins, 1989:39-46.

43. Goldbloom R, Battista RN. The periodic health examination: 1. Introduction. Can Med Assoc J 1986; 134:721-723.

44. Methodology. In: US Preventive Services Task Force. Guide to Clinical Preventive Services Task Force: An Assessment of the Effectiveness of 169 Interventions. Baltimore, Md: Williams & Wilkins, 1989: xxvii-xxxviii.

45. Semiglazov VF, Sagaidak VN, Moiseyenko VM et al. Study of the role of breast self-examination in the reduction of mortality from breast cancer: The Russian Federation/World Health Organization Study. Eur J Cancer 1993; 29A: 2039-46.

46. Semiglazov VF, Moiseyenko VM. Current evaluation of the contribution of self-examination to secondary prevention of breast cancer. Eur J Epidemiol 1987; 3:78-83.

47. Semiglazov VF, Moiseyenko VM. Breast self-examination for the early detection of breast cancer: A USSR/WHO controlled trial in Leningrad. Bull WHO 1987; 65:391-6.

48. UK Trial of Early Detection of Breast Cancer Group. Breast cancer mortality after 10 years in the UK trial of early detection of breast cancer. Breast 1993; 2:13-20.

49. Gastrin G. Self-examination in early detection of breast cancer: Is it effective? Recent Res Cancer Res 1987; 105: 106-110.

50. Gastrin G. Programme to encourage self-examination for breast cancer. Br Med J 1980; 281:193.

51. Gastrin G. New technique for increasing the efficiency of self-examination in early diagnosis of breast cancer. Br Med J 1976; ii: 745-6.

52. Weiss NS. Application of the case-control method in the evaluation of screening. Epidemiol Rev 1994; 16:102-8.

53. Gefeller O, Windeler J. The misuse of attributable and prevented fractions in the evaluation of screening in case-control studies. Cancer Det Prev 1993; 17:591-9.

54. Weiss NS, McKnight B, Stevens NG. Approaches to the analysis of case-control studies of the efficacy of screening for cancer. Am J Epidemiol 1992; 135: 817-23.

55. Morrison AS. Screening in Chronic Disease. 2nd Edition. New York, Oxford University Press Inc., 1992:104-28.

56. Knox G. Case-control studies of screening (response). Public Health 1992; 106:130.

57. Weiss NS. Case-control studies of screening: A response to George Knox. Public Health 1992; 106:127-29.

58. Knox G. Case-control studies of screening procedures. Public Health 1991; 105:55-61.

59. Friedman DR, Dubin N. Case-control evaluation of breast cancer screening efficacy. Am J Epidemiol 1991; 133:974-84.

60. Connor RJ, Prorok PC, Weed DL. The case-control design and assessment of the efficacy of cancer screening. J Clin Epidemiol 1991; 44:1215-21.

61. Sasco AJ. Validity of case-control studies and randomized controlled trials of screening (letter). Int J Epidemiol 1991; 20:1143-4.

62. Moss SM. Case-control studies of screening. Int J Epidemiol 1991; 20:1-6.

63. Sobue T, Suzuki T, Fujimoto I et al. Population-based case-control study on cancer screening. Environ Health Persp 1990; 87:57-62.

64. Miller AB, Chamberlain J, Day NE et al. Report on a workshop of the UICC project on evaluation of screening for cancer. Int J Cancer 1990; 46:761-9.

65. Dubin N, Friedman DR, Toniolo PG et al. Breast cancer detection centers and case-control studies of the efficacy of screening. J Chron Dis 1987; 40:1041-50.

66. Sasco AJ, Day NE, Walter SD. Case-control studies for the evaluation of screening. J Chron Dis 1986; 39:399-405.

67. Morrison AS. Screening in Chronic Dis-

ease. New York, Oxford University Press Inc., 1985:100-17.

68. Baum M, MacRae KD. Screening for breast cancer (letter). Lancet 1984; 2:462.

69. Breast screening: New evidence (editorial). Lancet 1984; 1:1217-8.

70. Prorok PC, Miller AB. Discussion of methodology of evaluation. In: Prorok PC, Miller AB, eds. Screening for Cancer. UICC Technical Report Series, Vol. 78. Geneva: International Union Against Cancer; 1984:94-105.

71. Berrino F, Gatta G, D'Alto M et al. Use of case-control studies in the evaluation of screening programmes. In: Prorok PC, Miller AB, eds. Screening for Cancer. UICC Technical Report Series, Vol. 78. Geneva: International Union Against Cancer; 1984:29-43.

72. Weiss NS. Control Definition in case-control studies of the efficacy of screening and diagnostic testing. Am J Epidemiol 1983; 118:457-60.

73. Morrison AS. Case definition in case-control studies of the efficacy of screening. Am J Epidemiol 1982; 115:6-8.

74. Newcomb PA, Weiss NS, Storer BE et al. Breast self-examination in relation to the occurrence of advanced breast cancer. J Natl Cancer Inst 1991; 83:260-5.

75. Muscat JE, Huncharek MS. Breast self-examination and extent of disease: A population-based study. Cancer Det Prev 1991; 15:155-9.

76. Locker AP, Caseldine J, Mitchell AK et al. Results from a seven-year programme of breast self-examination in 89,010 women. Br J Cancer 1989; 60:401-5.

77. Blamey RW, Locker AP, Mitchell AK et al. The Nottingham breast self-examination project. Acta Oncol 1989; 28:869-71.

78. Miller AB, Howe GR, Wall C. The national study of breast cancer screening. Clin Invest Med 1981; 4:227-58.

79. Baines CJ, To T. Changes in breast self-examination behaviour achieved by 89,835 participants in the Canadian National Breast Screening Study. Cancer 1990; 66:570-6.

80. Baines CJ, To T, Wall C. Women's Attitudes to screening after participation in the National Breast Screening Study. Cancer 1990; 65:1663-9.

81. Black WC, Welch HG. Advances in diagnostic imaging and over-estimations of disease prevalence and the benefits of therapy. New Engl J Med 1993; 328: 1237-43.

82. Gastrin G, Miller AB, To T et al. Incidence and mortality from breast cancer in the Mama Program for breast screening in Finland, 1973-1986. Cancer 1994; 73:2168-74.

83. Day NE, Williams DRR, Khaw KT. Breast cancer screening programmes: the development of a monitoring and evaluation system. Br J Cancer 1989; 59:954-8.

84. Miller AB. Screening for cancer: issues and future directions. J Chron Dis 1986; 39:1067-77.

85. Chu KC, Connor RJ. Analysis of the temporal patterns of benefits in the Health Insurance Plan of Greater New York trial by stage and age. Am J Epidemiol 1991; 133:1039-49.

CHAPTER 7

BREAST CANCER SCREENING BY PHYSICAL EXAMINATION

Indraneel Mittra

INTRODUCTION

In a clinical setting, breast cancer has traditionally been detected by physical examination (PE). However, in the setting of breast cancer screening, of the various modalities, PE is the least researched. While there have been seven randomized trials of mammography (for a review see ref. 1) and two of breast self examination (BSE),[2,3] there has been no trial to compare PE with no screening. When PE has been employed, it has been used in conjunction with mammography in some randomized trials or in other nonrandomized screening programs. Nevertheless, these studies provide information regarding the tumor detection potential of PE and its sensitivity and specificity as a screening procedure, in comparison to mammography. They also allow us to draw inferences regarding the potential that PE alone might have, relative to mammography, in reducing mortality from breast cancer. This chapter is intended to be a discussion on the potential effectiveness of PE in relation to mammography, in terms of tumor detection, mortality reduction and cost and benefit. After reviewing the evidence, PE appears to be as effective as mammography in reducing mortality from breast cancer while being far more cost-effective in both human and economic terms.

THE TECHNIQUE OF PHYSICAL EXAMINATION OF THE BREAST

In the same way that it has been urged that screening mammography must be of the highest technical standard, so too must it be urged that PE should be done well. PE of the breast in the setting of breast cancer screening demands greater care and attention than is normally paid in a clinical setting. In the latter circumstance, a suspicion has already been aroused, but in the former no abnormality has been perceived and examination must be more thorough and exhaustive to exclude any abnormality. Readers interested in a detailed description of the technique of PE as a screening test for breast cancer are referred to an article by Bassett.[4]

The extent of PE should include the entire mammary area bounded by the second and the sixth ribs and the lateral border of the sternum and the mid-axillary line. It should also

Breast Cancer Screening, edited by Ismail Jatoi. © 1997 Landes Biosience.

include the axillae and supraclavicular fossae. According to Bassett,[4] the breast should be divided into imaginary radial sectors. The flat surfaces of the middle three fingers should be used applying pressure firmly but gently against the chest wall. The fingers should be rotated in small circular movements from the periphery to the nipple within each sector to detect an abnormality in texture or a lump. Pinching of the breast tissue should be avoided as this is likely to give false impression of the presence of a tumor. The nipples should be gently squeezed to express any discharge.

The breast is examined in three positions: upright, supine and oblique. With the subject in the upright position the breasts are carefully inspected for any differences in size or contour. The nipples are examined for retraction or inversion. The aerolae and nipples are examined for skin changes. Presence of edema, redness or any ulceration of the skin if any are noted. The subject is then asked to raise both her arms above her head and any skin dimpling or localized fullness in the breasts is noted. She is then asked to put her hands on her waist and to press firmly, causing the pectoral muscles to contract thereby accentuating any previously noted abnormality. Although a thorough palpation of the breast is conducted when the subject is supine, a small percentage of lumps are best felt with the subject sitting in the upright position. To palpate the breast in this position, the woman is asked to place her hands behind her head with elbows outwards. To examine the axillae the subject is asked to put her arms, one at a time, on the examiner's shoulder and each axilla is examined with the opposite hand. This is followed by an examination of the supraclavicullar fossae.

With the subject now in the supine position the breasts are examined as described earlier using rotatory finger movements.[4] The axillae are examined again with the opposite hand. The woman is now asked to rotate by about 15° away from the examiner with her forearm resting on the pillow and lateral half of each breast is re-examined with special reference to the axillary tail.

The entire procedure of PE of the breast should take approximately 10 minutes.

Observer variability with respect to breast physical examination was investigated by Boyd et al.[5] The authors found that variability was restricted largely to patients who did not have breast cancer. Where breast cancer was confirmed by biopsy, there was little variation with respect to the recommendation as to which tumor should be biopsied.

BREAST CANCER DETECTION BY PHYSICAL EXAMINATION

Published results are available from four studies that have combined mammography with PE, on the relative contribution of the two modalities with respect to tumor detection (Table 7.1). The Health Insurance Plan (HIP) Study of Greater New York was conducted in the 1960s in which 62,000 women aged 40-64 were randomized to receive either annual PE plus mammography or no screening.[6] The study was conducted in the early stages of development of mammography, and a disproportionately large number of tumors in that study were detected by PE. Although in the 50-59 age group the proportion of tumors detected by PE alone and mammography alone were almost equal (40% vs. 42%), in the 40-49 age group PE was vastly superior to mammography in terms of tumor detection (61% vs. 19%). It has been calculated that, overall, as much as 70% of the mortality reduction in the HIP study might have been derived from PE.[7]

The Breast Cancer Detection Demonstration Project (BCDDP) conducted in the United States in the 1970s used modern mammography machines and is the largest screening study conducted to date.[8] The BCDDP was an uncontrolled study in which women aged 35 years or more were screened annually with mammography and PE. The study was carried out in 29 centers in 27 locations throughout the United States. Many of the centers concentrated largely on mammography and it is possible that some of the apparently increased sensitivity of mammography compared with PE may have resulted from relatively less efficient PE.

Table 7.1. Detection rates of breast cancer in different studies by mammography and PE

Method	HIP Study		BCDDP		Edinburg*	NBSS		Average
	40-49 Yrs.	50-59 Yrs.	40-49 Yrs.	50-59 Yrs.	45-64 Yrs.	40-59 Yrs.	50-59 Yrs.	All Ages
Mammography alone	19%	42%	35%	42%		41%	56%	39%
Mammography & PE	19%	18%	50%	50%		27%	26%	32%
PE alone	61%	40%	13%	7%		32%	18%	29%
Total detected by mammography	38%	60%	85%	92%	96%	68%	82%	74%
Total detected by PE	80%	58%	63%	57%	74%	59%	44%	62%

* Results for first year of screening.
The method of detection was unknown for a small fraction of tumors in the BCDDP. Adapted from refs. 6,8-11.

That this may indeed be so is suggested by the fact that while detection rate by mammography only in the 50-59 year age group was 42% for both the BCDDP and the HIP study, detection rate by PE alone was only 7% for the former compared to 40% for the latter. A similar trend was observed in the 40-49 year age group in which PE alone detected 13% of the tumors in the BCDDP compared to 61% in the HIP study.

The Edinburgh study was a randomized trial started in 1979 in which 45,130 women aged 45-64 were randomized.[9] A combination of PE and two-view mammography was given in the first year followed by PE alone in years 2, 4 and 6 and a combination of the two modalities in years 3, 5 and 7. In the first year of the study, 96% of cancers were detected by mammography compared to 74% by PE.

The National Breast Screening Study (NBSS) was conducted in Canada in the early 1980s and had two components. Women between the ages of 40-49 were randomized to receive annual mammography plus PE or no screening (after an initial PE).[10] Women aged of 50-59 were randomized to receive either annual PE plus mammography or annual PE alone.[11]

The quality of mammograms in the Canadian NBSS has been much criticized.[12,13] It was claimed that over 50% of the mammograms were technically suboptimal in the first 2 years of the study and that only in the last 2 years was satisfactory image quality achieved in 70% of the films.[12] It was also reported that in several sites the mammography equipment were suboptimal and radiologists and technicians had not received adequate training.[12,13] The suggestion was made that in the 40-49 year age group, more advanced cancers were allocated to the screened arm than the control arm.[14,15]

The organizers of the NBSS have, however, refuted these charges. Only 5.1% of the mammograms, which were alleged to have been of suboptimal quality, had been taken in the first 2 years of the study,[16] and no direct evidence of improper randomization was found.[17] They also reported that the sensitivity of mammography in the NBSS was

not inferior to data published from other trials.[18,19] Most importantly, the breast cancer detection rates and incidence of interval cancers per 1000 women in the NBSS was virtually identical to that observed in the BCDDP.[20]

An examination of Table 7.1 suggests that tumor detection by mammography in the NBSS was, if anything, superior than that in the BCDDP; mammography alone detected more cancers in both age groups in the former than in the latter (41% vs. 35% and 56% vs. 42% in the 40-49 year and 50-59 year age groups, respectively). The higher detection rate by mammography alone in the NBSS could, however, have been due to a relatively poor quality of PE. But this was not the case, since the detection rate by PE alone was also higher in the NBSS for both the age groups compared to the BCDDP. In conclusion, regardless of whether or not the quality of mammograms in the Canadian NBSS was suboptimal, the tumor detection rate in that study was, if anything, superior than that in the most classical screening study of that era.

Overall, Table 7.1 shows that there are considerable variations in the relative proportions of cancers detected by PE and mammography in the different studies. These variations may have been due as much to the quality of mammography as to that of PE. Table 7.1 also shows clearly that a large proportion of tumors detected at mammographic screening are palpable. When the figures for all ages in the four studies averaged, 62% of all cancers are detectable by PE compared to 74% by mammography. If data from only those studies that used modern mammography machines are included (excluding the HIP study), 59% of cancers were detected by PE compared to 85% by mammography (not shown in Table 7.1). It is also noteworthy that a substantial proportion of cancers that are missed by mammography are detectable by PE. These figures are 13% and 32% in the 40-49 year age group and 7% and 18% in the 50-59 year age group in the BCDDP and NBSS, respectively.

Finally, it should be pointed out that the figures given in Table 7.1 include both invasive and noninvasive cancers. Since the latter are much more frequently detected by mammography than by PE, differences in cancer detection rates between the two modalities are likely to become less pronounced if in situ cancers were to be excluded from analysis (see later). The detection of non-invasive in situ cancers is generally not considered to be a primary goal of screening.[21]

SENSITIVITY AND SPECIFICITY OF PHYSICAL EXAMINATION

Two studies have estimated the sensitivity and specificity of PE. These are the Canadian NBSS[22] and the UK Trial of Early Detection of Breast Cancer.[23] In the Canadian study, PE was conducted by trained nurses. Interval cancers were used as an index of a false negative examination while the proportion of normal women (false positives) referred to review clinic (conducted by a study surgeon) was used as an index of specificity. The specificity of examinations conducted by the nurses in the NBSS was uniformly high and improved with time with an average which was well over 90%. The sensitivity was nearly 74.4% for the study as a whole for the 50-59 age group and was 70.8% for the single examination in the 40-49 age group. The Canadian study emphasizes that PE conducted by trained nurses can achieve a high degree of sensitivity and specificity with respect to breast cancer detection and suggests that PE may be a useful yet simple screening procedure. The use of nurse examiners rather than clinicians reduces the cost of examinations to a considerable extent and also helps to improve coverage.

The sensitivity of PE obtained in the Canadian NBSS cannot be directly compared with that achieved with mammography in other studies. With mammography it is possible to retrospectively review films and decide whether a false negative interpretation occurred at the previous film. Nevertheless, a sensitivity of 86% was reported for the Swedish two county study[24] of mammography in the 50-59 year age

group compared to an average of 74.4% for PE for the same age group of women in the Canadian study.

In the UK Trial of Early Detection of Breast Cancer, PE plus mammography was given in the first year and PE alone in years 2, 4 and 6, and a combination in the intervening years.[23] Since PE followed screening in which mammography had been performed a year earlier in rounds 1, 3 and 5, sensitivity calculation for the year following combined screening with mammography and PE does not apply to our current discussion. In rounds 2, 4 and 6 in which PE was used on its own, an average sensitivity of 65% was obtained.

TUMOR SIZE AND NODAL STATUS OF INVASIVE CANCERS DETECTED BY PHYSICAL EXAMINATION

The size of invasive tumors is an important indicator of the effectiveness of screening. In the BCDDP, when all women were considered, 45% of infiltrating cancers < 1 cm were detected by PE (alone or in combination with mammography) and 53% by mammography alone (Table 7.2). On the other hand, 64% of cancers >1 cm in size were detected by PE and 34% by mammography. When all tumors are considered, 61% were detected by PE and 37% by mammography alone. The important message from this table, therefore, is that a large majority of invasive breast cancers detected at screening are palpable.

Axillary nodal status is an intermediate end-point of a screening study the ultimate goal of which is mortality reduction. Comparative data on nodal status with respect to the method of detection (mammography or PE) for invasive cancers have been reported by the authors of the Canadian study and these are given in Table 7.3. It is noteworthy that when invasive cancers alone were considered, twice as many tumors were detected by PE (or PE and mammography) compared to mammography alone in the 40-49 year age group (138 vs. 67 out of a total of 205). Nevertheless, of the cancers detected, more tumors detected by

Table 7.2. Size of infiltrating tumors according to method of detection in the BCDDP

Method of Detection	< 1 cm	> 1 cm	All Tumors
Mammography alone	195 (53%)	631 (34%)	826 (37%)
PE *	166 (45%)	1199 (64%)	1365 (61%)
Unknown	10 (3%)	41 (2%)	51 (2%)
Total	371 (100%)	1871 (100%)	2242 (100%)

* Tumors detected by PE alone or by PE and mammography

mammography had negative nodes compared to those detected by PE (79% vs. 59%). The PE group also had more tumors with greater than four positive nodes (18% vs. 4%).

In the 50-59 year age group, PE (or PE and mammography) again detected more invasive cancers than did mammography alone in the intervention arm (141 vs. 127 out of a total of 268). In this age group, both modalities detected similar proportion of tumors that were node negative (67% and 62%) although somewhat more of the PE detected cancers had more than four involved nodes compared to the mammography group (11% vs. 4%). The nodal status of tumors detected in the control arm, which received PE only, is comparable to those in the intervention arm detected by PE alone.

DOES THE DETECTION OF NONPALPABLE CANCERS CONTRIBUTE TO MORTALITY REDUCTION?

The ultimate goal of screening is to reduce death rate from cancer and early detection is a necessary prerequisite for achieving this goal. The question is how early in its natural history do we need to detect breast cancer to achieve a reduction in mortality? Is it necessary to detect cancers as early as possible or only as early as needed to produce an improvement in outcome? Mammography detects many occult cancers, both invasive or noninvasive, but we do not know whether these lesions would ever cause

symptoms or pose a threat to woman's life? Are these nonpalpable cancers worth detecting?

A study was carried out by Neilsen et al[25] in Denmark to determine the incidence of occult cancers that occur in ostensibly healthy women. They identified 110 women aged 20-54 with a median age of 39 who had died of medico-legal causes such as suicide, road traffic accident, etc. They simulated bilateral modified mastectomies on these women and undertook an extensive histopathological examination of their mammary glands. They observed that 20% of women harbored occult cancers, and that this figure increased to 33% when women between the ages of 50-54 were considered. Multicentric lesions in their study were 40% and 41% were bilateral. Since these figures are much higher than the actual incidence of breast cancer in the population, many women apparently live through life carrying multiple occult cancers in their breasts which never pose a threat to them; and the incidence of these cancers rises with increasing age. The study raises the question as to how many of these occult and apparently biologically "benign" cancers are detected by mammography and whether their detection makes any contribution to reduction in mortality from breast cancer?

It has, indeed, been reported that mammographically detected cancers are biologically less aggressive than clinically detected ones.[26-28] One such study was carried out by Klemi et al[26] in Finland between 1987-1990 during which period

Table 7.3. Nodal status of all invasive tumors according to method of detection in the Canadian NBSS

| | 40 - 49 Yrs. | | | | 50 - 59 Yrs. | | | |
| | | Mammo. + PE | | | | Mammo. + PE | | |
	All	Mammo. alone	PE *	NS **	All	Mammo. alone	PE *	PE only
None	134 (65%)	53 (79%)	81 (59%)	34 (57%)	173 (65%)	85 (67%)	88 (62%)	86 (58%)
1 - 3	38 (19%)	8 (12%)	30 (22%)	16 (27%)	50 (19%)	20 (16%)	30 (21%)	32 (22%)
> 4	28 (14%)	3 (4%)	25 (18%)	5 (8%)	21 (8%)	5 (4%)	16 (11%)	22 (15%)
Unknown	5 (2%)	3 (4%)	2 (1%)	5 (8%)	24 (9%)	17 (13%)	7 (5%)	8 (5%)
Total	205 (100%)	67 (100%)	138 (100%)	60 (100%)	268 (100%)	127 (100%)	141 (100%)	148 (100%)

* Tumors detected by PE alone or by PE and mammography
** No screening after an initial PE.
Adapted from refs. 10,11.

mammography was introduced for population screening in a gradual manner. The authors compared the biological properties of 125 mammographically detected cancers matched for tumor size with a similar number of cancers detected clinically. The biological parameters studied included: histological differentiation, tumor necrosis, mitotic counts, estrogen and progesterone receptors, histological type, invasion of lymphatic vessels, DNA ploidy and S-phase fraction. When compared, each of these biological parameters was significantly less aggressive in case of mammographically detected cancers than those that were detected clinically. The study supports the argument that many cancers detected mammographically are indolent which may never surface during the lifetime of a women or be the cause of her death.

It is agreed that the detection of non-infiltrating in situ cancers is unlikely to contribute substantially to mortality reduction.[21] However, what about occult invasive cancers that are potentially lethal? How early do we need to detect these to make an impact on mortality reduction? It is calculated that a single transformed cell undergoes 30 doublings to reach a size of 1 cm (1 billion cells) when it has a good chance of being detected clinically. If we consider the average diameter of a nonpalpable mammographically detected cancer to be 0.5 cm, the lead time gained by mammographic over PE detection is equivalent to only one doubling (from 0.5-1 cm) (Fig. 7.1). Is this gain in lead time of one doubling in the long natural history of 30 doublings likely to impact significantly on mortality reduction?

It should be remembered that when invasive cancers alone are considered, more cancers are detected by PE than by mammography alone (61% vs. 37% in the BCDDP—Table 7.2). In women aged 40-49, twice as many invasive cancers are detected by PE than purely by mammography (138 vs. 67 in the Canadian NBSS—Table 7.3). What is the contribution of these small invasive, nonpalpable cancers that are detected purely by mammography in terms of mortality reduction? Presumably, some of these are bio-

logically so indolent as to never pose a threat to life, and for the others, the lead time gained by mammographic detection over PE detection is so small as to make little difference to mortality reduction. Is the detection of nonpalpable cancers worth the effort, cost, anxiety and trauma involved?[29]

The only trial that has addressed this issue is the Canadian NBSS.[11] The study was designed to answer the question as to whether mammography adds anything to mortality reduction over an above that achieved by PE. Women aged 50-59 were randomly allocated to receive either annual mammography plus PE conducted by trained nurses or annual PE alone. Since PE was present in both arms of trial, the study had the potential to answer the question as to whether the detection of nonpalpable cancers in the mammography arm had any bearing on mortality reduction. At the end of 7 years, the number of breast cancer deaths in the two arms of the study have been found to be identical.[11] No evidence of mortality reduction has emerged in the mammography arm even after 10 years of follow up (Miller, personal communication). Although longer follow up may reveal a benefit, currently there is no evidence to suggest that the detection of nonpalpable cancers by mammography has any impact on mortality reduction.

The controversy over the quality of mammography in the Canadian NBSS has been alluded to earlier. Even if we were to accept that the quality of mammograms was indeed a weakness of the study, the Canadian NBSS also had certain strengths. First, mammography was given annually as opposed biennially as was done in other modern breast cancer screening trials. But in spite of this, no added benefit of mammography was seen. Second, unlike the other screening trials, the Canadian NBSS tested the efficacy (rather than effectiveness) of screening. Only those women who agreed to participate in the study were randomized. Consequently, any benefit of mammography should have been magnified as there was no dilution effect due to noncompliance in the intervention arm (usually around 30%).

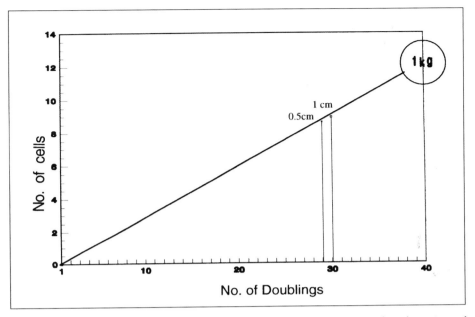

Fig. 7.1. Schematic representation of lead-time gained by mammographic detection of nonpalpable cancers over PE detection.

It can be concluded from the above discussion that although the real usefulness of mammography lies in the detection of nonpalpable cancers, the majority of invasive cancers detected at mammographic screening are palpable and that there is no evidence that the detection of nonpalpable cancers has any impact on mortality reduction.

COST AND BENEFIT OF SCREENING BY PHYSICAL EXAMINATION

An ideal screening test should be simple, inexpensive and effective. Mammography is complex, expensive and only partially effective (say in comparison with the PAP smear test). Yet to attain this partial effectiveness is required a very high degree of expertise at every level of mammographic screening which is achieved at a huge cost.[29] PE, on the other hand, is simple, inexpensive and apparently as effective as mammography.[29]

Like in mammography, staff training and quality control of screening by PE must also be of the highest standard.[22] But, com-pared to mammography, the scale and cost of achieving this goal is likely to be a great deal smaller. In the Canadian NBSS,[22] for example, the nurse examiners were only given 2-4 weeks of out patient training by study surgeons with further reinforcement at the screening centers. Screening with PE would require little additional training for surgeons and pathologists, since they are well accustomed to dealing with palpable lesions in the breast.

The human cost of mammography has not been fully emphasized.[30] The anxious waiting period after mammography (of a week to ten days) until the test results are known can itself be a traumatic experience. Since many thousands of women are being (repeatedly) screened, this human cost of screening mammography is actually enormous. Screening by PE would eliminate the anxious waiting period for the vast majority who have no breast abnormality and can be reassured on the spot.[29]

Localization of nonpalpable mammographically detected lesions is another source of considerable anxiety[31] and this would be eliminated if PE is used as a screening test. A recent paper has analyzed the anxiety and cost related to false positive mammography in the Stockholm trial of mammographic screening.[32] The authors report that 352 women who had a false positive screen in the first round made 1112 visits to the physician, had 397 fine needle aspiration biopsies, 180 mammograms and 90 surgical biopsies, all of which, of course, to no avail, before being declared free of cancer. For two-thirds of the women it took 6 months for them to be declared cancer free and some were not declared free of cancer until 2 years.

Although it might be expected that reassurance after a false positive biopsy would be a source of relief, this supposition is not supported by reported studies. A false positive diagnosis of hypertension led to more symptoms of depression and a lower state of general health in spite of reassurance, than a matched group who were initially found to be normotensive at screening.[33] Similar findings have been reported in pregnant woman who had a false positive alpha-fetoprotein result.[34]

Compared to mammography, screening by PE would lead to fewer benign biopsies to detect a cancer. Rates of biopsy detection for benign lesions per 1000 women has been reported for the Canadian NBSS with respect to the method of detection (Table 7.4).

The proportion of benign biopsies was greater in case of mammography detected lesions compared to those detected by PE. The difference was more pronounced in the 50-59 year age group in which twice as many benign biopsies were performed for mammography detected lesions.

Mammography would detect many more in situ cancers than would PE.[8] The malignant potential of these cancers is unknown, and for most women, their detection would lead to unnecessary treatment with all the attendant anxiety and financial cost. Above all, women will be wrongly labeled for life as having "cancer."[35]

The economic cost of mammographic screening has been reported by several authors, and this varies with the age group of women screened. Kattlove et al[36] calculated that the cost to save one life at 10 years works out to $1.48 million—$0.18 million and $0.15 million for age groups 40-49, 50-59 and 60-69, respectively. Similar figures have been reported by others.[37,38]

The economic cost of screening by PE has not been accurately calculated. However, Miller reported that the comparative economic cost of PE and mammography in the Canadian NBSS was of the order of 1:3.[39] This calculation, however, did not take into account the cost of equipment, buildings, mobile vans, etc. Nor did it include the huge cost of mammographic screening related to

---

Table 7.4. Rates of biopsy detected benign lesions per 1000 women according to method of detection in the intervention arms in the Canadian NBSS

| Year | Mammo. + PE (40 - 49 Yrs.) | | Mammo. + PE (50 - 59 Yrs.) | |
	Mammo.*	PE**	Mammo.*	PE**
1	18.1	15.5	24.3	10.5
2	10.2	7.4	8.9	5.0
3	7.9	5.3	6.7	3.5
4	7.6	4.4	5.7	2.7
5	8.8	4.4	7.1	1.7
TOTAL	52.6	37.0	52.7	24.4

* Detected by Mammography
** Detected by PE alone or by Mammography + PE
Adapted from refs. 10, 11.

programs of staff training and quality control and of professional accreditation. When these are taken into account the economic cost of PE may be 5- to 10-fold lower than that of mammography.

Finally, 50% of the world's breast cancer load is in the developing world.[40] The advocacy for mammographic screening ignores the fact that this modality of early detection is utterly beyond the reach of three-fourths of the world's population. Yet opportunistic screening with mammography is on the increase in poorer countries as a result of motivated publicity without the necessary expertise, infrastructure or attention to perfection, and is probably doing more harm to their women than good. Since BSE is unlikely to be very effective,[41] PE would appear to be the ideal screening test for countries with limited resources.[42] Two randomized trials to compare PE (plus BSE) with no screening are about to commence in Manila (Parkin, personal communication) and in Mumbai.

SHOULD PHYSICAL EXAMINATION REPLACE MAMMOGRAPHY?

It is agreed that in most countries in which mammography is a part of a public health-care program financed by the state, yearly mammography will not be affordable. The U.K., for example, has opted for a single-view mammography given triennially to women between the ages of 50-64.[43] PE, being relatively inexpensive, on the other hand, can be given annually. The question, therefore, is whether annual PE can replace biennial (or triennial) mammography? The results of the Canadian study of the 50-59 year age group,[11] which showed no added benefit of (even) yearly mammography over yearly PE, would suggest that the answer to this question may be in the affirmative. If PE were to replace triennial mammography in the NHS Breast Screening Program, it could certainly prevent the unacceptably high rate of interval cancers (31%, 52% and 82% at 12, 24 and 36 months, respectively) that is now obtained in the U.K.[44] Clearly, what we need is a randomized trial to compare annual screening by PE with bi- or triennial mammography in women above the age of 50.

In the 40-49 year age group, both the HIP and the Canadian studies compared annual mammography plus PE with no screening. But the effects of screening on mortality reduction in these two studies have been in opposite directions.[6,10] The HIP study[6] showed a nonsignificant 25% benefit in the screened arm in spite of the fact that the standard of mammography in this study was poor by modern standards. Only 19% of cancers were detected by mammography alone while 61% of cancers were detected by PE alone (Table 7.1). Consequently, PE must have played a major role in mortality reduction seen in that study.

The Canadian study,[10] on the other hand, showed a 36% nonsignificant excess mortality in the screened arm in this age group. Compared to the HIP study, more than twice as many cancers (41% vs. 19%) in the NBSS were detected by mammography alone and fewer cancers by PE alone (32% vs. 61%).

Why then was there an adverse effect of screening in the intervention arm in spite of relatively superior mammography in the Canadian NBSS? In fact, why has, in every other modern trial of mammographic screening, there been an excess mortality (albeit to a lesser extent) in the screened arm in the first few years in younger women? (for a review see ref. 1). One explanation for this counterintuitive finding is that women with screen-detected cancers may not have been given adjuvant systemic therapy while women in the control arm who developed cancer were treated by this modality since their tumors were more advanced.[17]

But, an entirely different issue has also been raised: does mammography itself have a detrimental effect?[45] In keeping with this conjecture is the suggestion that breast compression during mammography might cause dissemination of cancer cells.[46] Is it possible that the discrepancy between the HIP and the Canadian studies can be attributed to the fact that the former used equipment of an older generation that caused less compression of the breast[6] compared to modern mammography machines that were used in the latter study (and other modern randomized trials)? Can the relatively greater detrimental effect in the screened group in the Canadian study compared to other randomized trials be due to the fact that mammography was given annually, rather than biennially, in that study?[10] Is it possible that the positive finding in the HIP study in the 40-49 year age group was due to a combination of a relatively large proportion of tumors being detected by PE and to the use of older mammography equipment that produced less compression of the breasts?

There is much current debate on whether younger women should be given mammography every year rather than every 2 years.[47,48] But when there is evidence that PE detects twice as many invasive cancers (and far fewer in situ cancers) in this age group than does mammography alone (Table 7.3), and the possibility that yearly mammography might have an even greater detrimental effect than two-yearly mammography, should the debate not focus on whether PE should replace mammography in the 40-49 year age group as the preferred screening test?

CONCLUSIONS

The natural clinical intuition is that the earlier the stage at which breast cancer is detected the greater is the benefit. Mammography is driven by the instinct that "earliest is best." But this intuitive clinical belief is not in accord with the epidemiological view. The latter suggests, instead, that we need to detect breast cancer only as early (or as late) as is necessary to produce an improvement in outcome. PE as a screening test derives its support from this epidemiological view. PE may well detect breast cancer at a relatively later stage, but this is still early enough to make it as effective as mammography in reducing mortality from breast cancer. Although the real usefulness of mammography lies in the detection of nonpalpable tumors, the majority of invasive cancers detected at mammographic

screening are palpable, and there is no evidence to suggest that the detection of nonpalpable cancers has any impact on mortality reduction. PE should, therefore, be the logical alternative to mammographic screening. Yet mammography has come to be accepted as the standard screening test in spite of the enormous complexities related to optimization and huge financial and human costs. The simple, inexpensive and humane alternative that exists in screening by PE is ignored. The time has come for serious soul-searching and to ask the question as to whether we have not gone too far down the wrong road? It may still not be too late to make a retreat and pursue the alternative course.

REFERENCES

1. Elwood JM, Cox B, Richardson AK. The effectiveness of breast cancer screening by mammography in younger women (article). Online J Curr Clin Trials (serial online) 25 Feb. 1994 (Doc. No. 32).

2. Semiglazov VF, Moiseenko VM. Breast self-examination for the early detection of breast cancer: a USSR/WHO controlled trial in Leningrad. Bulletin of the World Health Organization 1987; 65: 391-396.

3. Thomas DB, Gao D, Self S et al. A randomized trial of breast self examination in Shanghai. 20th Annual Meeting of American Society of Preventive Oncology, Bethesda, Maryland (Abstract), 1996.

4. Bassett AA. Physical Examination of the Breast and Breast Self-Examination. In: Miller AB, ed. Screening for Cancer. Orlando: Academic Press, 1985:271-291.

5. Boyd NF, Sutherland HJ, Fish EB, Hiraki GY, Lickley HL, Maurer VE. Prospective evaluation of physical examination of the breast. Am J Surg 1981; 142:331-334.

6. Shapiro S, Venet W, Strax P, Venet L. Periodic Screening for Breast Cancer: the Health Insurance Plan Project and its Sequelae 1963-1986. Baltimore: Johns Hopkins University Press, 1988.

7. Bailar JC. Mammography: a contrary view. Ann Intern Med 1976; 84:77-84.

8. Baker LH. Breast cancer detection dem-

onstration project: 5-year summary report. CA 1992; 32:194-225.

9. Roberts MM, Alexander FE, Anderson TJ et al. Edinburgh trial of screening for breast cancer: mortality at seven years. Lancet 1990; 335:241-246.

10. Miller AB, Baines CJ, To T, Wall C. Canadian National Breast Screening Study: Breast cancer detection and death rates among women aged 40 to 49 years. Can Med Assoc J 1992; 147:1459-1476.

11. Miller AB, Baines CJ, To T, Wall C. Canadian National Breast Screening Study: Breast cancer detection and death rates among women aged 50 to 59 years. Can Med Assoc J 1992; 147:1477-1488.

12. Kopans D. The Canadian screening program: a different perspective. Am J Radiol 1990; 155:748-750.

13. (Anonymous). Canadian study of breast screening under 50. Lancet 1992; 339: 1473-1474.

14. Day NE, Duffy SW. Breast screening in women under 50. Lancet 1991; 338: 113-114.

15. Kopans DB. Breast screening in women under 50. Lancet 1991; 338:447.

16. Miller AB. Breast screening in women under 50. Lancet 1991; 338:113-114.

17. (Anonymous). Breast cancer screening in women under 50. Lancet 1991; 337: 1575-1576.

18. Baines CJ, Miller AB, Wall C et al. Sensitivity and specificity of first screen mammography in the Canadian National Breast Screening Study: A preliminary report from five centers. Radiology 1986; 160:295-298.

19. Baines CJ, McFarlane DV, Miller AB et al. Sensitivity and specificity of first screen mammography in 15 NBSS centers. J Can Assoc Radiol 1988; 39: 273-276.

20. Miller AB, Baines CJ, Sickles EA. Canadian National Breast Screening Study. Am J Radiol 1990; 155:1134-1135.

21. Lidbrink E. Mammographic Screening for Breast Cancer: Aspects on Benefits and Risks. Doctoral thesis. Stockholm: Karolinska Institute, 1995.

22. Baines CJ, Miller AB, Bassett AA. Physical examination: Its role as a single screening modality in the Canadian National Breast Screening Study. Cancer 1989; 63:1816-1822.

23. UK Trial of Early Detection of Breast Cancer Group. First results on mortality reduction in the UK Trial of early detection of breast cancer. Lancet 1988; ii:411-416.

24. Tabar L, Fagerberg G, Duffy SW, Day NE, Gad A, Grontoft O. Update of the Swedish two-county program of mammographic screening for breast cancer. Radiol Clin North Am 1992; 301: 187-210.

25. Nielsen M, Thomsen JL, Primadahl S, Dyreborg U, Andersen JA. Breast cancer and atypia among young and middle-aged women: A study of 110 medicolegal autopsies. Br J Cancer 1987; 56:814-819.

26. Klemi PJ, Joensuu H, Toikkanen S et al. Aggressiveness of breast cancers found with and without screening. Br Med J 1992; 304:467-469.

27. Kallioniemi OP, Karkkainen A, Auvinen O, Mattila J, Koivula T, Hakama M. DNA flow cytometric analysis indicates that many breast cancers detected in the first round of mammographic screening have a low malignant potential. Int J Cancer 1988; 42:697-702.

28. Hakama M, Holli K, Isola J et al. Aggressiveness of screen-detected breast cancers. Lancet 1995; 345:221-224.

29. Mittra I. Breast screening: the case for physical examination without mammography. Lancet 1994; 343:342-344.

30. Fentiman IS. Pensive women, painful vigils: consequences of delay in assessment of mammographic abnormalities. Lancet 1988; i:1041-1042.

31. Marteau TM. Psychological costs of screening. BMJ 1989; 299:527.

32. Lidbrink E, Elfving J, Frisell J, Jonsson E. Neglected aspects of false positive findings of mammography in breast cancer screening: analysis of false positive cases from the Stockholm Trial. Br Med J 1996; 312:273-276.

33. Bloom JR, Monterossa S. Hypertension labelling and sense of well-being. Am J Public Health 1981; 71:1228-1232.

34. Marteau TM, Kidd J, Cook R et al. Screening for Down's syndrome. BMJ 1988; 297:1469.

35. Foucar E. Carcinoma in situ of the breast. Have pathologists run amok? Lancet 1996; 347:707-708.

36. Kattlove H, Liberati A, Keeler E, Brook RH. Benefits and costs of screening and treatment for early breast cancer. JAMA 1995; 273:142-148.

37. Eddy DM, Hasselblad V, McGivney W, Hendee W. The value of mammography screening in women under age 50 years. JAMA 1988; 259:1512-1519.

38. Wright CJ, Mueller CB. Screening mammography and public health policy: the need for perspective. Lancet 1995; 346: 29-32.

39. Miller AB. The role of screening in the fight against breast cancer. World Health Forum 1992; 13:277-285.

40. Parkin DM, Pisani P, Ferlay J. Estimates of the worldwide incidence of eighteen major cancers in 1985. Int J Cancer 1993; 54:594-606.

41. Morrison AS. Is self-examination effective in screening for breast cancer? J Natl Cancer Inst 1991; 83:226-227.

42. Mittra I. The role of screening in the fight against breast cancer. World Health Forum 1992; 13:287-289.

43. Breast Cancer Screening: report to the Health Ministers of England, Wales, Scotland and Northern Ireland by a working group chaired by Sir Patrick Forrest. London; HM Stationery Office, 1987.

44. Woodman CBJ, Threlfall Ag, Boggis CRM, Prior P. Is the three year breast screening interval too long? Occurrence of interval cancers in NHS breast screening programm's north western region. Br Med J 1995; 310:224-226.

45. Stacey-Clear A, McCarthy KA, Hall DA et al. Breast cancer survival among women under age 50: is mammography detrimental? Lancet 1992; 340:991-994.

46. Watmough DJ, Quan KM. X-ray mammography and breast compression. Lancet 1992; 340:122.

47. Kerlikowske K, Grady D, Barclay J, Sickles EA, Ernster V. Effect of age, breast density, and family history on the sensitivity of first screening mammography. JAMA 1996; 276:33-43.

48. Feig SA. Strategies for improving sensitivity of screening mammography for women aged 40 to 49 years (Editorial). JAMA 1996; 276:73-74.

CHAPTER 8

THE MEDICO-LEGAL IMPLICATIONS OF BREAST CANCER SCREENING

David Plotkin

INTRODUCTION

In order to focus on the medico-legal aspects of breast cancer screening, the definition of screening must be scrutinized. The implication of benefit from screening requires that we study how benefit is measured. This leads us to examine the definition of cure as the prime determinant of benefit.

All of these generic considerations must then be applied to the specifics of breast cancer screening. By rational estimation of the preclinical life of a cancer in the breast and its metastases will the role of screening be fully realized. Moreover, this insight into the biology of breast cancer will reveal the relationship between screening and the extraordinary prevalence of malpractice suits brought about because of the alleged failure to diagnose breast cancer in a timely manner.

GENERIC SCREENING

Screening seeks to identify a symptomless disease (or a state of relatively high risk for the disease) by some fairly simple means. Taking a bit of history, doing a partial physical examination, running a test on a readily available body fluid, or examining cells scraped from a surface organ or exfoliated from an "internal" organ that communicates to the "outside", are all usable in screening. More troublesome is the need to image an organ. Tedious, labor-intensive imaging procedures that require highly-trained professional administration do not satisfy the requirement of relative simplicity. Indeed, chest x-rays and mammograms have proven to be the only imaging procedures uncomplicated enough to apply on a large scale. The waned interest in the former (screening chest x-rays in lung cancer detection) with the continued enthusiasm for mammography for breast cancer detection carries a message to be elaborated on in due course. The continued use of Pap smears in controlling uterine cervical cancer is essentially unchallenged.

A second axiom of screening is that detection of the disorder prior to the time of routine clinical diagnosis leads to an intervention that produces benefit. There are few arguments that earlier detection by screening of an untreatable illness has a rational basis. Insurers may have a vested interest in this type of discovery. An afflicted individual may need to settle affairs but usually even the most grim prognosis allows sufficient time for this. Without evidence that screening benefits at least a significant proportion of patients harboring the disease or its immediate precursor, while routine diagnosis does not, the widespread application of health resources in such endeavors makes no sense. Benefit is held out as the carrot to justify the stick of screening expense, inconvenience and even modest discomfort.

How to Measure Benefit From Screening

Benefit is not, as a rule, all or nothing. It must be carefully measured to permit comparison of studies. Demonstrating that benefit is derived from a particular medical intervention would seem at first blush to be easy. Simply obtain an answer to the question, does the test group do better than the control group? It is in the term "better" that we find the rub. "Better," it turns out, is many things to many people and is not precise enough to use as a measurement without very careful definition. And the possibility that the test and control group are not equivalent must also be considered.

Decrease in Morbidity

The quest for benefit, at times owing to the intrinsic difficulty in controlling a disease, may have a modest goal that is nevertheless worthwhile. One wholly acceptable means of measuring benefit, is to document significantly less morbidity in a test group compared to a control group. Of many possible examples, the use of a less drastic surgical procedure in a test group that preserves the survival rate seen in a control group is straightforward.

Improvement in Disease Free Survival

A goal that may evoke minimal celebration is the documentation of substantial delay to time of first recurrence in a test intervention group as compared to a control group. If time to death from diagnosis,

however, is the same in the two groups, the benefit has a shadow cast over it unless time intervals of difference are striking. See Figure 8.1, Example A. A relatively unimportant distinction between test and control group can also be seen in Figure 8.1, Example B. If the intervention only minimally delays first recurrence, does not postpone death and is at all costly (physically or economically) the benefit is probably not worth it.

Improvement in Crude Survival

Survival percentage is the most commonly used clinical yardstick in oncology. When it does not take into account deaths from causes other than the specific cancer under consideration, the term crude survival is often used. It typically records the number of patients of the original cohort that are alive 5 years after diagnosis as the numerator. The original starting number is the denominator. A comparison of a test and control group produces two sets of numerators and denominators from which percentage is computed. Does the test group have a "better," i.e., larger percentage of surviving patients than the control group? If so, and underwritten statistically whenever possible, a conclusion with 95% confidence, i.e., $P = .05$, is reached.

Improvement in Timed Survival Rates

There are problems with heavy reliance on timed survival data because of the influence of biases, i.e., selection, lead time and length bias. Selection bias occurs when the control group and test group are not comparable. The biologic deck is unknowingly stacked, e.g., one group has an undue prevalence of bad-acting cancers. Unless a treatment is dramatically or universally effective, the conclusion that the group with the less malevolent constituency has done better will be reached erroneously. Another pitfall of timed survival, lead time bias, occurs when there is an introduction of a diagnostic modality that drops the threshold for detection resulting in an "earlier" sampling of tissue leading to diagnosis that starts the

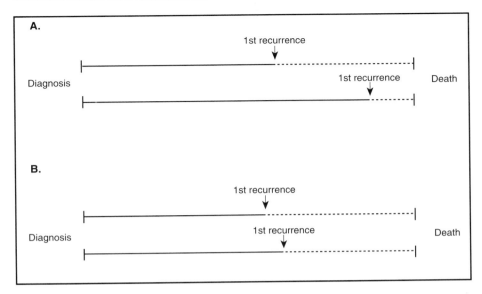

Fig. 8.1. Difference in time to first recurrence.

survival meter running sooner. Higher resolution imaging detecting smaller lesions, with no added benefit of treatment, will provide the basis for improved specific timed survival rate with no alteration in true curability.[1]

Length bias occurs when slower-growing cancers are picked up disproportionately by screening. More dangerous cancers appearing between screens, so called interval cancers, are not attributed to the effect of screening.

CONCEPT OF CURE

The goal most commonly sought is of course either significant postponement of death, e.g., from middle to very old age, or cure, i.e., the total eradication of the disease in question as a threat to life. Although the term cure has a remarkably uniform meaning to epidemiologists and biostatisticians, it is more complicated than it may seem when first considered. To clinicians, a less than rigorous definition may suffice, e.g., 5-year survival rate. To the scientifically unsophisticated public the term is more an emotional wish than a carefully defined statement. Regardless of how many defini-

tions of cure are used in society, the definition for our purpose must be free of any ambiguity.

The dictionary defines cure as a remedy that restores one to health[2] with no comment as to the permanence of health. Unstated but acknowledged is ultimate mortality of any cohort for some reason. Implicit, and probably the crucial element in the definition, is freedom from recurrence of the treated disease that is total and for the individual's lifetime. Death due to the disease under consideration is eliminated. It is this permanent eradication of a disease that most pristinely defines cure and it is termed actuarial cure.[3,4] Simple examples of this precise definition of cure includes appendectomy for appendicitis, antibiotics for many infections, etc. In oncology, the successful use of chemotherapy in childhood acute leukemia, the use of radiation therapy in eliminating some cancers of the uterine cervix, the surgical removal of a low grade sarcoma lead to unqualified cures. A less clear, widely used expression is 5-year cure—a potentially oxymoronic term that means "alive" 5 years after diagnosis of a cancer. The irony of death due to the cancer sometime in the 5 years following the first 5-year mark is therefore probably made especially bitter. Five-year cure is then indeed an oxymoron. A better and totally accurate expression is simply 5-year survival. Accurate notation of survival for any length of time after primary diagnosis and treatment, e.g., 1, 3, 5, 10, 15, 20, 30, etc. is above any reproach.

An expression, "personal cure," has appeared over the years in the United Kingdom oncology literature.[5] It is defined as death following treatment for cancer that is totally unrelated to the cancer. Implicit in this definition is the fact that many patients with malignancy, especially the elderly, have other illnesses competing for their mortality. The avoidance of cancer death by demise earlier owing to cardiovascular disease is actually fairly common.

The term statistical cure provides no clarification. All definitions of cure, even those lacking precision, are statistical, i.e., the assembly and classification of numeric data so as to present significant information. The problem we have, therefore, is to select or develop a commonly accepted definition of cure that is accurate. If all patients treated for a particular cancer are totally and forever free of recurrence after a 5-year free interval, the term 5-year cure is not only not oxymoronic, it is quite accurate. Sadly, in the zeal to display good results, many authors and spokesmen, fail to acknowledge the limited value in our struggle with cancer by reporting the timed survival data that unfortunately represent a comical (but not so funny in this instance) metaphorical "partial score."

FLATTENING OF RELATIVE (DISEASE-SPECIFIC) SURVIVAL CURVE

The shape of a survival curve carries a powerful visual message. A shallow descending slope, reflecting relatively few deaths over 20 years, is generally viewed with favor. Such a disease is not severely malevolent. Conversely, a rapidly descending survival curve communicates the ominous information that a highly lethal disease is at work. An important means of measuring

benefit from new diagnostic or therapeutic interventions therefore is the application of the relative or disease-specific survival method. It is computed by dividing the crude survival rate by the expected survival rate of a gender and age equivalent but "normal" population multiplied by 100% (see Fig. 8.2). This small mathematical maneuver excludes deaths in the observed cohort that are due to illnesses other than the one under consideration. If the relative survival curve becomes horizontal, one can conclude that the remainder of the original intervention group has a hazard for death that is precisely the same as the normal, noncancer afflicted population. Conversely, the persistence of a negative slope of the relative survival curve can only be interpreted as a failure to restore usual mortality expectation to the original group. Until such time as survival reaches zero, the hope can be held that some of the remaining subset may yet prove to be cured by prior treatment. In most visceral cancers, the vast majority of studies reveal a persistent negative slope of the relative survival curve.

DECREASED MORTALITY (FEWER DISEASE-SPECIFIC DEATHS/100,000)

Another telling measure of how a particular cancer is being combated is the determination of the number of deaths per unit population, usually per 100,000. The age spectrum of the U.S. population has changed in this century due to the small baby boom of the 1920s and the better known, large baby boom of the 1950s. The latter requires adjusting late 20th century data to the age spectrum of 1970 to eliminate the extra deaths attributable to the temporally advancing population bulge. In this manner, the true mortality impact of a particular cancer is seen (see Table 8.1).

BREAST CANCER SCREENING

INTRODUCTION

The definition, goal and implementation of breast cancer screening are issues well documented in other chapters of this text. The preceding largely epidemiologic

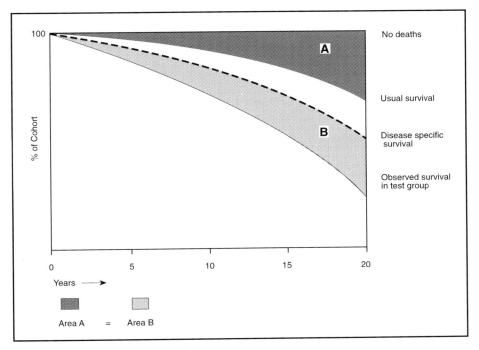

Fig. 8.2. Disease-specific survival.

discussion within this chapter has set the stage for a more focused view of breast cancer screening and its medico-legal aspects. The extraordinary direct relationship between the advent of screening and the rise in malpractice actions based on failure to diagnose breast cancer in a timely manner is by now generally well known, especially to radiologists, malpractice attorneys and underwriters. Breast is the organ site that is the most common basis of litigation in cancer. This phenomenon, quite aside from the costs of screening, warrants careful appraisal of screening's purported benefits. Unfortunately, expressing skepticism about the public health value of screening is akin to questioning the value of mom, apple pie and the flag.

SPECIFIC FEATURES OF BREAST CANCER SCREENING

There is nothing particularly unique about *breast* cancer screening from a technical standpoint. The definition and goals are the same as they are for the successful screening seen with uterine cervical cancer. Both mammography and Pap smear are screening tests that are considered part of a general check up for female patients. There may well be an emotional overtone to breast cancer screening because of its politicization and demographics. The demand by the white female upper middle class for an "appropriate" response to the perceived epidemic of breast cancer and its essentially unchanged mortality (age adjusted number of deaths/100,000) gets disproportionately more attention than the uterine cervical malignancy. Although conclusive proof of benefit is required before routine application of most medical procedures, screening included, the circumstances with breast cancer screening seem almost to disregard this axiom. The burden of proof appears to be shifted to those who question the value of mammography. Assuming this perhaps unfair burden but with the goal of pursuing logical discourse on the subject, the theories

Table 8.1. Breast cancer demographics

Year	1970	1995
USA Female Population	104,300,000	134,000,000
Number of 100,000 units of USA FP	1,043	1,340
Incidence of Breast Cancer		
Absolute total	76,500	185,000
Absolute total/100,000	73.3	138
Age adjusted to 1970/100,000*	–	107.4
Noninvasive total	1,000	37,600
Noninvasive total/100,000	0.96	28
Age adjusted to 1970/100,000*	–	21.9
Invasive total	75,500	147,400
Invasive total/100,000	72.3	110
Age adjusted to 1970/100,000*	–	85.6
Mortality of Breast Cancer		
Absolute number of deaths	27,000	46,000
Not age adjusted deaths/100,000	25.8	34.3
Age adjusted deaths/100,000*	25.8	26.7

*age adjustment based on 1043 ÷ 1340 = .778

and evidence supporting the use of screening mammography and the countervailing positions will be reviewed. But first, definitions of medical negligence and related terms, i.e., causation and damages, are required.

MEDICAL LEGAL ISSUES

STANDARD OF CARE

Standard of care is defined as the general duty of a physician to maintain a level of competence that a reasonably capable and prudent physician practicing under similar circumstances exercises. It is not practical in advance to set forth guidelines that separate acceptable vs. unacceptable behavior in *all* of the myriad possibilities posed by medical practice. Expert witnesses are required to review the specifics of a case and offer opinions as to adherence to standard of care. Both plaintiff and defense attorneys are able

to hire respectable-appearing, appropriately credentialed experts to solemnly express their views that are predictably diametrically opposed. The issue is often over the management of either a questionable lump or a mammographic abnormality in the breast. Polemics from both sides ensue about whether the area was "suspicious enough" to warrant biopsy or was watchful waiting for a benign tissue change to resolve on its own a reasonable approach. Why not biopsy any suspicious focus—no matter how seemingly innocent? What is there to lose? A lot in my view. When a woman has a biopsy of the breast, waiting for the result is agonizing. The ratio of biopsies to cancer diagnoses in competent hands is in the range of three to five to one. About three out of four women will therefore be subjected to the anxiety and physical discomfort of a biopsy so that one of them will know she absolutely had to have a biopsy that discovered breast cancer. Most regard this as a reasonable price to pay. But some take the quixotic view that ratios of 10 or greater are justified in avoiding a missed diagnosis of breast cancer. About 210,000 breast cancers are currently diagnosed yearly, 180,000 invasive and 30,000 CIS. The ratio of patients referred for biopsy to diagnosis of cancer is approximately 4:1. Therefore, 800,000 breast biopsies are done annually. If the ratio is increased to 10:1, in the neighborhood of 2,000,000 biopsies per year would be required. Since there are about 60 to 70 million women in the age groups in which possible breast malignancy is an issue, nearly one woman in 33 would be biopsied yearly.

The shades of gray, the vague densities, the question of fine or coarse calcifications bedevil radiologists in a manner quite analogous to the tactile difficulties primary care physicians have in the interpretation of palpable breast cancers. In either case, whether a questionably palpable breast mass or an uncertain mammographic density is ignored or unduly watched, an ultimate diagnosis of cancer may lead to a charge of negligence.

There are many instances when the doctor's care, although perceived by the patient as substandard, is actually adequate. The expectation that all doctors must perform at an exemplary level is neither realistic nor fair. As much as we would like to think that radiologists make no mistakes, it must be acknowledged that competence, approximately measured, is portrayed as a range by the same bell-shaped frequency distribution curve that produces student grades. Not everyone is going to deserve an A or a B grade. (We won't even get into the "off day" that even the A performer has now and then.) Where does a C grade or radiologist of average competence fit into this picture? If you get your television set or auto repaired, most of the time are the technicians or mechanics notably good to outstanding? A rhetorical joke of course. Average is acceptable and you routinely pay people to perform at that level. D, meaning poor, is lumped with F for failure and in health care delivery probably deservedly so.

The education parallel permits a course to be taken again without great prejudice while the errant physician does not get a second chance to read the films properly. Acknowledging human (yes, doctors do qualify) imperfection, the reason a physician should carry malpractice insurance is to protect himself or herself financially for the time the *inevitable* error with *serious consequence* occurs and is *discovered*.

The theoretical ideal application of mammography occurs when there is no unusual lumpiness to the breasts but the films reveal an abnormality. Even when technical factors permit detection of suspicious findings, there are occasions when an abnormal mammogram, although read properly, is not reported to the responsible attending physician. The radiology office may not have mailed the report or it was mailed but never received by the referring physician's office. Or it did get there but it was filed without the doctor seeing it or it was inadvertently discarded. And so on. In any case the "missed report" is negligence that borders on *res ipsa loquitor*. The basis for this, despite its relative infrequency, is that the occurrence is in a zero tolerance situation. No one can claim that failure to follow up on an acknowledged abnormal mammogram is within the standard of care.

Most commonly the failure to diagnose breast cancer is due to a doctor relying too heavily on a mammogram that misses a cancer. This problem is seriously aggravated if there is a dominant breast mass. Not adhering to the dictum that a dominant breast mass requires biopsy, irrespective of mammographic findings, puts a defendant doctor into a legally dangerous position. From the radiologist's perspective he can't report a finding that he doesn't see. At times, even the radiologist who is being sued for malpractice agrees that a lesion suspicious enough to warrant follow up was discernible but simply not seen at the time. This is a form of negligence that almost matches the un- or misfiled report, circumstances that contribute to the frequency of missed diagnosis.

No matter how the charge of failure to diagnose in a timely manner originates following a surgical pathologic diagnosis of breast cancer, especially stage 2 cancer, a review of previous "unremarkable" mammograms is prompted. Unremarkable is a "waste basket" term that communicates to the attending physician that only routine follow up is needed. With the benefit of an expert's hindsight the films reveal an "obvious" abnormality that would have prompted further action immediately in the wake of the procedure. I have been struck that these retrospectoscope experts are made into uniformly brilliant diagnosticians when a lawyer walks into their offices with a set of mammogram films to "review." Why in the world would this attorney ask a radiologist to review a set of mammograms unless he had a client interested in suing a doctor because of a missed diagnosis? Despite this painfully obvious algorithm, I have yet to see the only counterplay that puts the onerous task of reading mammographic films into the real world of a busy radiologist. Ask the plaintiff's expert to identify truly worrisome sets of mammographic films out of 20 cases shown to him, allowing the amount of time he routinely spends on such a number of films. Two abnormal cases should be included in the mix along with the one forming the basis for the lawsuit, all suitably disguised as to origin. And don't tell him how many cancer cases there are in the batch. This challenge ought to lower the pontification level of some plaintiff's radiology experts on standard of care.

Causation

The failure to diagnose in a timely manner is virtually always described by the plaintiff's attorney to have harmed the patient. Either more treatment was required—surgical, radiation or chemotherapy—because of the delay in diagnosis or the patient's stage of disease was worsened or life expectancy was adversely affected. Usually the malpractice action stakes out all of these claims. The key task of the defendant's attorney then is to show that there was no damage to the patient that would not have

taken place even with timely diagnosis. This requires resorting to the principle of causation. This less than self-explanatory legal doctrine, put indelicately but more to the point, asks "so what if the miss occurred?!" Acknowledging that the patient's clinically problematic cancer was due to the negligence of the doctor, did the negligence make any difference in the patient's morbidity (disease or treatment-related) or mortality?

Plaintiff's attorney invariably attempts to document injury to his client caused by the delay in diagnosis. The typical circumstance that has the potential to lead to a malpractice suit occurs when there is a real of perceived failure to diagnose cancer. From the point in time when the diagnosis could have been made until the time of actual diagnosis is alleged to be inappropriate delay. During this interval, with the benefit of hindsight, the primary is invariably seen as growing. With this primary tumor enlargement depending on what staging method is being used, there will be a worsening of the stage (so-called stage creep).[6] In addition, it is usual for the allegation of harm done to the patient to include the involvement of regional axillary lymph nodes. At the least, the nodes harboring metastatic deposits at time of diagnosis are recognized to have progressed with the delay in diagnosis. Commonly, it is alleged that nodes went from negative to positive during the delay in diagnosis. Degree of nodal involvement is regularly expressed as a fraction with the number of metastatic nodes as numerator and the number of total nodes examined as the denominator. Predictably, plaintiff's counsel will argue that the number of involved nodes increased. Rarely are the actual size of the metastatic deposits reported although retrieval of archival slides permits this with considerable accuracy even many years later.

Two very important observations about nodal status must be made. Assuming that the primary and the nodal metastases are clonal, their relationship in size is meaningful. Although a primary may be 30 mm in diameter and a metastatic deposit in an axillary lymph node be 10 mm in diameter the spawning of the latter by the former occurred typically within a year or so. Unless a significant difference in growth rate is supportable by clinical, pathological or molecular biological data, the interval of time between the origin of the metastases and the primary is regularly remarkably brief. Further discussion of when metastases occur will soon follow.

The other key issue in this context is the comparability of growth rates of primary vs. metastases. It is a startling irony that critics of using tumor growth rate as a means of determining when a primary cancer and its metastases began will invoke extraordinarily fast growth rates to account for metastases that began only after the opportunity to diagnose the primary was missed by the defendant. Typically, plaintiff's expert will attribute the worsening of stage by lymph node involvement without realizing what is cell kinetically involved.

With the demonstration of enlargement of the primary by palpation or mammography and/or worsening of the degree of lymph node involvement by surgical pathology, the upstaging of the cancer may reduce the *timed*, i.e., 5-year survival rate from above 50% to below. Generally, a lower stage, e.g., stage 1, with a near 80-90% 5-year survival is alleged to have been squandered by delay in diagnosis with a loss of chance of (*5 year*) survival, specifically to less than 50%.

Rarely, delay in diagnosis permits an in situ breast cancer to become invasive. An example of this would be the demonstration of axillary node deposits of only a very few cells by monoclonal antibody-aided immunohistochemistry. The time of origin of such tiny clumps of metastases could well post-date the opportunity to diagnose a primary that was unusually large relative to the size of the metastases. In this infrequent circumstance the loss of chance for the patient goes well beyond a decreased likelihood of 5-year survival. Loss of life expectancy of several to many years is then probable. If the malignancy that went from in situ to microinvasive is very slow-growing and the patient is elderly with significant compet-

ing illness then even this type of delay is of no consequence. The patient will not die of breast cancer.

A frequently invoked consequence of delay, especially in the context of explaining the presence of sizable lymph node metastases, is to allege a genetic transformation within the primary that spawned metastases of much faster growth rate. This departure from the concept of the clonality of cancer (or lack of it) is more ascertainable than commonly realized. Molecular biological profiles of the primary and metastases demonstrating their similarity or difference are infrequently offered as evidence. Defense experts may well use the comparability of primary and metastatic breast profiles to support the contention of at least similar growth rates.

Although genetic transformation in cancer in general and breast cancer in particular is not debatable, the imputed change in growth is. Two lines of evidence support the conclusion that acceleration of tumor growth rate is uncommon. If the vertical coordinate for the surviving fraction of an original cohort of cancer patients is changed from linear to log scale, the characteristic reverse sigmoid curve describing survival is converted to a straight line (see Fig. 8.3). If acceleration of tumor growth rate within any of the surviving cohort regularly occurred, then the straight, negatively sloped line would at some point become more steeply sloped, i.e., acquire a downward bend. This would reflect the extra thrust of mortality owing to the genetically transformed, faster growth rate group. It can be argued that this may occur so early in the preclinical life of a cancer that this actuarial observation will be missed. Demonstration of this in human clinical oncology is thus far virtually impossible. In experimental animal models, supporting examples of this concept are not known to me.

Lastly, the review of Figure 8.4 permits the relatively straight forward conclusion that effective treatment of metastatic disease selects out the clone of resistant cells whose original numbers are quite small compared to the dominant cell type of the untreated

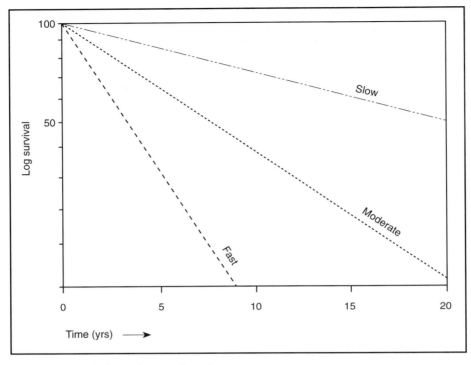

Fig. 8.3. Survival shown by semi-log plot.

clone. Differences in growth rates of dominant vs. nondominant fractions of the cellular population of the original tumor would require ratios of 100:1 or 1000:1 to account for the manifestly slower growth rate for the surviving clone.

IMPACT OF SCREENING BY OTHER THAN MAMMOGRAPHY

Only to quickly dismiss means of breast cancer screening other than mammography, should breast self-examination (BSE), thermography, ultrasound and magnetic resonance imaging (MRI) be mentioned. As an adjunct to palpation, fine needle aspiration and/or breast ultrasonography are useful in separating fluid filled from solid breast lesions. MRI in women with implants may become standard of care because of purported greater accuracy and the means of avoiding compression views. A measure of the level of uncritical acceptance of any

screening is the widespread recommendation to women to do breast self-examination. The logic that a breast cancer might be discovered earlier with self palpation seems compelling. More important is the fact that only infrequently is there a claim of reduction in breast cancer mortality owing to BSE. Most breast cancers are still discovered by the patient.

MAMMOGRAPHY DECREASES BREAST CANCER MORBIDITY AND MORTALITY: SUPPORTING AND COUNTERVAILING THEORIES AND EVIDENCE

The laudable goal of breast cancer screening is reduction of morbidity and mortality attributable to the malignancy.

There is no question that mammography has permitted the diagnosis of many cancers when they are small enough to be

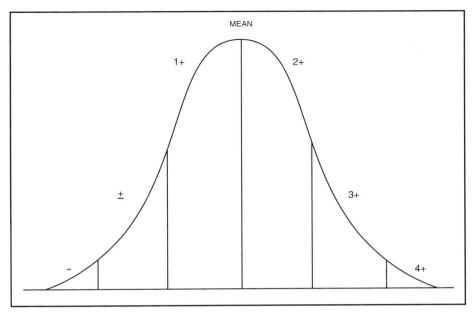

Fig. 8.4. Selection of resistant clone by effective treatment. Legend: 4+: subpopulation very highly sensitive to treatment; 3+: subpopulation highly sensitive to treatment; 2+: subpopulation moderately sensitive to treatment; 1+: subpopulation somewhat sensitive to treatment; ±: subpopulation slightly sensitive to treatment; –: subpopulation resistant to treatment.

treated by lumpectomy. The average size of a breast cancer diagnosed mammographically is probably near or even less than a centimeter while diagnosis by palpation remains near 3 cm. With the 4 cm upper limit for lumpectomy usually applied by surgeons, the margin for lumpectomy is clearly increased by mammographic diagnosis.

Were reduction in surgical morbidity to be the sole impact of mammography in breast cancer morbidity there could be no question of its value in this regard. There are, however, some probable negatives to the use of mammography that affect public health. The well-documented spurt in incidence from 1980 (probably about 4% increase per year annually compounded) through the early 1990s, is largely due to the discovery of many more carcinoma in situ and minimally invasive cancers. The proportion of all breast cancers diagnosed as in situ 50-25 years ago was 1-2%. In screening studies such as the Breast Cancer Detection and Demonstration Project (BCDDP) done in the 1980s, it was 20%. Routine community incidence is probably near 10%. This 5- to 10-fold increase in relative occurrence should be further amplified by comparing the absolute USA incidence of about 70,000 cases of breast cancer in 1970 against 185,000 per year in the mid-1990s. But why would the value of diagnosing at least 20 times more carcinoma in situ (CIS) currently than a generation ago be questioned? If a high proportion of such cases progress to invasive cancer, and this can be avoided, why not promote such intervention? On the other hand, if only a small proportion of CIS progresses to a dangerous stage, then recognition and intervention is a two-edged sword. Without much exception, women diagnosed with any kind of breast cancer are initially shocked. No matter how we emphasize the distinction between in situ and invasive, the word cancer seems gets most of the attention. Moreover, we often suggest treatments for CIS that not only sound like but are identical to the treatments used for invasive cancer. If we were so sure that noninvasive cancer was not such a threat, why the magnitude of treatment? The reason of course is that about 20-25% of the in situ patients go on to develop invasive breast cancer over the ensuing 10-15 years with an attendant risk, albeit small, in absolute terms, for mortality. With upwards of 40,000 women per year currently dying of breast cancer, words of reassurance based on a diagnosis of CIS are therefore probably not fully, if at all, heeded. But what of the 75-80% of women with CIS, an absolute number per year in the range of 30,000, who will never hear from the breast cancer again. If their disease had never been discovered would their subsequent lives have been affected? Are not the postmortem studies of remarkably high incidence of atypical hyperplasia and CIS in asymptomatic and undiagnosed women not a clue that there is a wide range of biologic malevolence posed by the pathologic diagnosis of breast cancer and its precursor lesions?[7]

In the meantime, the current practice is the almost invariable use of radiation therapy to the remaining breast after lumpectomy, certainly for invasive cancer and often for even CIS. This is based on a substantial reduction in local recurrence in the group receiving radiation therapy as compared to a control group treated without radiation therapy although these data have been largely accumulated for less than 15 years. Assuming that there is no biologic downside to this treatment, the economic cost still ought to be considered and not regarded dismissively. Moreover, the consequences of radiation injury to the breast and immediately contiguous tissues may well loom larger as many more cases are treated that enter their second decade of survival and beyond. Acknowledging that improved local control if sustainable is worthwhile, the argument that radiation therapy as a supplement to lumpectomy with and without adjuvant systemic treatment actuarially "cures"

breast cancer, i.e., impacts mortality, has never been convincingly made.

CURE OF BREAST CANCER

Actuarial cure of invasive breast cancer is probably not possible with our current therapeutic armamentarium. Of the lines of evidence supporting this view an analysis of relative or disease-specific survival in measuring the impact of medical/surgical intervention in breast cancer is required. As with most cancers a negative slope of the disease-specific survival curve is seen with breast cancer. In a few long-term follow up studies, however, even when the breast cancer cohort death rate due to all causes approached the control group's death rate at 20-30 years, there was persistent excess breast cancer mortality, 15 times the rate of the general population.[5,8] Late excess mortality due to breast cancer has been observed even up to 40 years after diagnosis.[9]

The role of cardiovascular and other causes of death in a cohort of breast cancer patients becomes increasingly important as one looks at survival potential of progressively older groups of women.[10,11] In a number of very large premammography registry-based studies it has been shown that, if a woman was diagnosed as having breast cancer, there was an approximately 80% chance of dying of it.[10-12] Reciprocally, the 20% of women who did not die of breast cancer died of other causes that in a real sense competed with breast cancer. It is of course theoretically possible that all of the women who die of other causes might never die of breast cancer. This possibility is not at all likely, when the observation of Mueller et al in a study of 3,558 women with breast cancer are considered. They noted that breast cancer was the cause of death in 96.5% of women in the age group 21-50, 90% in the 51-70 age group, and 77.5% in the group older than 70.[10] Following the diagnosis of breast cancer at a relatively young age, survival of 30-40 years is rarely seen. Indeed, such an occurrence warrants a careful reexamination of the original tissue for accuracy.

But the studies showing a relative survival rate of only 20% in 20 years are old, i.e., they took place in the premammography era. Indeed, proponents of mammography point to the BCDDP data collected during the 1980s that show a much shallower slope of mortality and by all estimates will at least double the percentage of 20 year survivors of breast cancer. As an aside there is irony in the fact that the oft claimed 91% cure rate (a euphemism for 5-year survival) is followed by the death of another 11% of the original cohort so that the 10 year survival is 80%. Since the curve is probably descending further (we await 15 year data), it is likely that more 5 and even 10 year "cures" will die. It is also true that any reasonable projection of these curves to 20 years will produce a disease-specific survival rate in the 50% range.

Another type of database that those alleging cure of breast cancer find difficult to explain is the age-adjusted incidence and disease-specific mortality/100,000 female population tracked for the last 60 years. Following the publicity of breast cancer diagnosed in the wives of well-known political figures in the late 1970s, mammography promotion began in earnest. The approximately 1% rise in incidence per year from the mid-1930s through the 1970s was increased four-fold from 1980 until the mid 1990s. In the Health Insurance Plan of New York (HIP) study (to be further discussed) breast cancer mortality was purportedly reduced in the test group beginning 7 years after entry. One would expect a similar impact nationwide from the widespread use of mammography. No decline was seen in the late 1980s. Indeed, despite the much greater use of mammography in breast cancer screening, the *absolute* mortality rate for breast cancer rose about 25% between 1985-1992. Eliminating the baby boomer effect in producing a bulge in the at risk population by *age-adjusting* back to 1970, the mortality rate remains about as flat as it had been since the mid 1930s, i.e., 26-27 deaths/100,000 female population, until quite recently. Over the 5 year span of 1991-1995 a probably unsustainable *relative* 6.3% decline in mortality has been attributed to "advances," e.g., early detection and treatment. No apportioning of the decline between detection and treatment is made; both efforts are assumed to be working. This relative decline from 1991-1995 is probably temporally related to the widespread use of tamoxifen and other systemic therapies. Many patients with clinically occult and hormone and/or chemotherapy responsive metastatic disease would have had deaths postponed by such intervention. Destined to die in the last decade of this century, some patients were given a pharmacologic stay of demise.

With no authority contending responsibly that *metastatic* breast cancer is actuarially curable, the patients with at least initially responsive breast cancers will eventually relapse and die of it. When that happens the mortality rate rolling along behind and numerically lower than the usual incidence burden, will have the delayed deaths added. This will probably increase the mortality rate in the next few years and will be commensurate with the transient drop of the 1990s. It should last as long and be seen to the same but opposite degree as when it was suppressed.

Of course, another major advance in systemic treatment might produce another transient dip in mortality. With nothing dramatically new and effective in the treatment pipeline a second dip seems unlikely. Eventually, though, when there is enough therapeutic impact on metastatic disease, the median duration of survival (MDS) of breast cancer patients will exceed the MDS for cardiovascular diseases in the same age groups and the mortality rate for breast cancer will drop more meaningfully.

Just as was described in the general epidemiologic discussion earlier in this chapter, bestowing definitive credence to timed survival is a mistake. Selection, lead time and length biases in the BCDDP are strongly suggested from the remarkably shallow slope of the mortality curve attributed to this study. The argument that this experience with its extraordinarily high survival should be the "gold standard" in our management of breast cancer ignores the marked difference in the intrinsic biology of mammographically diagnosed breast cancer against cancers that are diagnosed by palpation. The average doubling time (DT) measured at one BCDDP site was nearly three-fold slower than the generally observed DTs seen with metastatic disease.[13]

The belief that breast cancer mortality can be reduced rests heavily on the observations made in the HIP and the Swedish Two County (WE) trials. It is remarkable that authorities cite seven references in support of mammography's role with only two (HIP and WE trials) having statistical significance.[14] The other five, especially the Canadian trial, where the results are "counterintuitive," are apparently given little weight. The allegation that radiologic competence and equipment involved in the USA's HIP study of the 1960s was superior to the Canadian trial of the early 1980s is curious if not provincial.

A letter to the editor of the New England Journal of Medicine criticizing the HIP and WE trials was sent in the wake of the medical progress series of articles on breast cancer in July and August of 1992. Although it was never published, the key points remain germane to the issue. The letter is excerpted here:

"We have focused on the 10 year follow up data of the HIP study since it seems to be the point of maximum benefit of the screening. The difference in size of the study (30,239) vs. the control (30,756) group was 517 and has been attributed to a greater number of exclusions in the study group owing to pregnant women and women with prior mastectomies, a difference considered to be slight by Shapiro et al.[15] However, if a large contribution to the excluded women was because of mastectomy for breast cancer, the number of exclusions in the screened group in relationship to the total number of breast cancers diagnosed in the entire group: 1234 (study: 617, control: 617), has potential significance. It seems unlikely that pregnancy could have made much of a contribution to exclusion of women aged 40-64. The authors of the study noted that the status of control group women for pregnancy and mastectomy were "most completely ascertained." But how precise was the ascertaining of... prior mastectomy in the control women when that determination was made years later?" The following is a modification of the 1992 letter: Suppose only 10% of the approximately 500 women who should have been excluded from the control group were included by misplacing the date of their mastectomies to *after* 1963 instead of *before* (the time of initiation of the trial) because of faulty patient memory being the only source of history. With 50 such patients slipping through the ascertaining process and experiencing an approximately 50% 10-year mortality rate, the number of deaths in the control group would be reduced to a number insignificantly different from the test group.

The Swedish Two County study showed one-third the effect on breast cancer mortality as that purportedly shown by the HIP study.[16] The same problem that possibly occurred in the HIP study might have taken place in Sweden as well. Perhaps a totally different confounding factor, e.g., the use of tamoxifen in stage 2 breast cancer in Sweden during those years, would have delayed mortality in the screened group. Lastly, Skrabanek[17] has observed that although breast cancer specific mortality was reduced over the observation interval, overall mortality in the Swedish test group was slightly higher than the control group.

In the context of examining large breast cancer survival databases it is intriguing to look at the 10-year follow up data of the National Surgical Adjuvant Breast Project (NSABP) and Breast Cancer Trialists Organization (BCTO). These survival curves wend their way between the old tumor registry data and BCDDP observations. It is plausible that the NSABP and BCTO data is a blend of the obvious selection, lead time and length-biased statistics of the BCDDP with the mammographically uninfluenced observations of three to five decades ago. But there is of course no argument that the survival curves of breast cancer patients tabulated in the last 15-20 years are less ominous than those seen in the old breast cancer survival data. The explanation for this must in major part be related to the use of mammography over the same interval of time. This effect of mammography appears to be grafted onto the one percent rise in incidence beginning in the mid-1930s. The evidence that mammography picks up biologically more indolent cancers is irrefutable. Mammographically detected cancers are better differentiated, are disproportionately diploid with low S-phase fractions, are disproportionately more hormonally dependent and have actually been measured to be slower growing, i.e., have longer doubling times.[13] With this in mind it is likely that the NSABP and BCTO disease-specific survival at 15 years will probably be in the 40-50% range.

BREAST CANCER SCREENING AND BIOLOGY

THE THEORETICAL BASIS OF SCREENING

For screening to be effective it must make diagnosis possible before metastases begin. Figure 8.5 graphically addresses the theory of effective screening. Average detection for the diagnosis of breast cancer by palpation is generally accepted as a 30 mm diameter mass that corresponds with 35 doubling times. Average detection for diagnosis of breast cancer by mammography has also been approximated at about a 7 mm diameter, reflecting 27 doublings to reach that point. The detection *thresholds* for diagnosis by palpation vs. mammography are 10 and 2 mm, respectively, with corresponding diminution in the number of DTs required to reach those points. A comparison of the two average and two threshold sizes, when viewed on a semi-log plot, reveals the modest difference between them. If the metastatic process begins before the primary is clinically detectable with mammography then the rationale for this procedure is lost.

WHEN DO METASTASES OCCUR?

The growth of a primary malignancy in the breast need almost never be the cause of death as it was 100 years ago (before Halsted's operation). If after detection by any means, screening or routine clinical, the primary is surgically removed, the mortal threat that it specifically posed goes with it. But what of its metastatic potential? When metastases are encountered after appropriate intervention in operable breast cancer no conclusion can be reached other than that the spread of the cancer had to occur before the mastectomy. When metastatic disease is never diagnosed in a patient with primary breast cancer, i.e., there is long term (20+ year) survival, there are three possible explanations. There may be no metastases to diagnose because the primary was removed before it embolized tumor cells capable of generating viable clones elsewhere in the body. This hypothesis seems very unlikely. Over the last half century our ability to detect metastatic breast cancer has continuously improved. With each advance, from clinical estimates to surgical pathology, to extra sections taken of axillary lymph node dissections, and finally with immunocytochemical assay using monoclonal antibodies, we see no threshold for metastatic potential of invasive breast cancer. But we also have to consider the possibility that metastases were eradicated with systemic treatment. The evidence supporting our ability to do this is nonexistent.

In either of the two above circumstances, actuarial cure could theoretically result. Were actuarial cure of metastatic breast cancer more than a theoretical possibility, there would be cause for rejoicing in the community of people interested in breast cancer and there would almost certainly follow a substantial reduction of malpractice actions.

Personal cure, an ever more frequent phenomenon, occurs when there are metastases that are growing so slowly that they never reach the threshold for clinical diagnosis, even to the point of a patient's death from a cause other than breast cancer. It is in particular in the circumstances of personal cure that we erroneously take undue credit for systemic intervention.

If it is assumed that the metastases occur before the primary is removed, the next question is specifically *when* did the metastases occur? My best estimate of when the

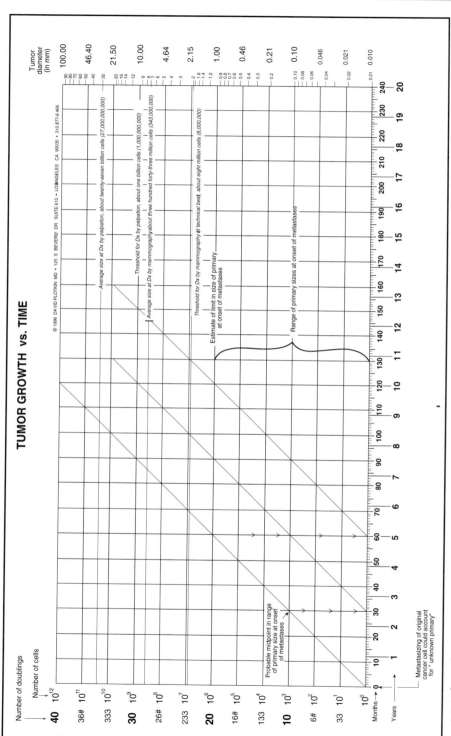

Fig. 8.5. Where do metastases occur?

metastatic process begins is portrayed in Figure 8.5. A wide range of primary sizes up to one million cells with a midpoint of an assumed bell-shaped frequency curve at 1,000 cells, or 0.1 mm in diameter, consistent with 20 doubling times seems plausible. The justification for this estimate is based on two lines of evidence. The first of these is the mathematics of survival curve analysis. The relationship between doubling time and survival has been pointed out in a number of publications.[18-25] This information is graphically summarized in Figure 8.6. The shape of breast cancer survival curves appears to be dictated by the frequency distribution of the doubling times of metastases, the acceptance of an average lethal tumor burden at 10^{12} (1 kg of tumor), and the onset of metastatic disease as suggested above. These factors seem to provide the best fit of the observed survival curves. The variation in the slope of the curves appears to be pri-

marily a function of the frequency distribution of the cancers within each cohort. Premammography breast cancer as reflected by curves A and B in Figure 8.7, diagnosed by palpation, had a range of DT from about 30-300 days with a mean of 90 days. Breast cancer as encountered in the NSABP and BCTO trials are reflected by curves C and D; they have about the same limit on the fast side but extends into the several thousands on the slow side. The fact that breast cancer diagnosed by palpation has relatively fast DTs with correspondingly poor survival while mammographically diagnosed breast cancer with relatively slow DTs and good survival is no accident. It is indeed mathematically predictable.

In addition to the mathematical basis of the shape of the survival curves that reflect mortality due to metastatic disease, there is evidence that further justifies the conclusion that onset of metastatic disease occurs before

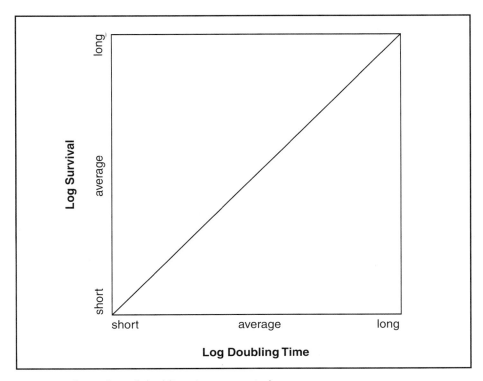

Fig. 8.6. Relationship of doubling time to survival.

clinical detection of the primary is possible. A review of the clonality of breast cancer will be helpful in this regard.

It is traditionally accepted that the metastases of primary breast cancer are clonal, based on histology. In recent years, the similar microscopic appearance of a primary and its metastases by routine pathology has been supplemented by functional characterization. Receptor analysis, estimates of ploidy and proliferative rate, tumor protein and/or oncogene analysis within technical limitations all essentially confirm the clonality of the original tumor and its secondary deposits. Only infrequently, do metastases spontaneously acquire micro-anatomical, genetic and/or molecular characteristics different from the primary that are clinically significant. With treatment selection producing suppression of sensitive clones until resistant ones emerge, changes obviously occur.

In a number of rodent tumor models, demonstration of the metastatic process very early in the life of the tumor is feasible. Observations of primary and metastatic tumor growth in such experimental systems reveal that the phenomenon closely resembles what has been observed in human pathology. Despite these findings, extrapolation of animal models to human biology as it relates to the time of metastases is not observationally definitive. Empirical plotting of tumor growth early (preclinical, microscopic) and late (clinical, macroscopic) in experimental animals is widely reported. The similarity of macroscopic growth in animals and humans is well known. Extrapolating clinical observations in humans back to microscopic, preclinical life paralleling the observations in animals is therefore reasonable.

Drawing inferences about early tumor growth, and time of metastases in humans,

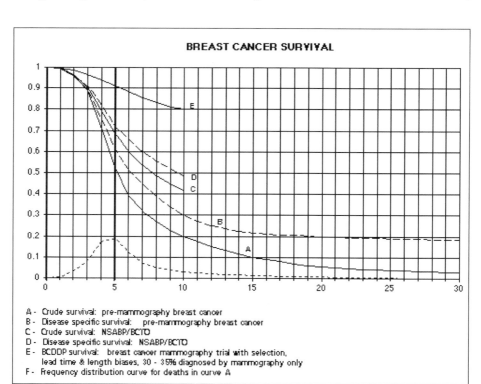

A - Crude survival: pre-mammography breast cancer
B - Disease specific survival: pre-mammography breast cancer
C - Crude survival: NSABP/BCTO
D - Disease specific survival: NSABP/BCTO
E - BCDDP survival: breast cancer mammography trial with selection,
    lead time & length biases, 30 - 35% diagnosed by mammography only
F - Frequency distribution curve for deaths in curve A

Fig. 8.7. Breast cancer survival.

with an inability to directly assess the early biological life of human cancers is a disadvantage to some casual observers, a prohibitive disadvantage. The time at which metastases are clinically detected and their size at detection, especially in relationship to the size of the primary, afford us with crucial evidence that permits a reasonable estimation of the point of origin of the metastases. This is based on the acknowledgment of a relatively predictable relationship between the duration of life of a cancer deposit and its size, whether primary or metastatic, but of necessity, unambiguously clonal. This is best seen on an arithmetic/geometric graphic (see Fig. 8.8). A straight line describes the relationship between time (a linear function) and tumor growth (an unweighted exponential function).

In order to compute the time of origin of a metastasis, certain data points have to be ascertained or at least reasonably estimated. The sizes of the primary lesion and its lymph node metastases, expressed in millimeters of diameter, are on very firm ground. If a pathologist slices through a lymph node but goes through a metastatic deposit "off center," then the size of the metastasis will be reported as smaller than it really is. Since the larger the metastasis the longer its individual biologic history and the earlier in the life of the primary was its origin. An estimated but nevertheless very important part of a calculation of onset of metastatic disease is the designation of doubling time. Although a precise DT expressed in days must be chosen for convenience in graphic representation, the number chosen need only be in a range of DTs, i.e., fast (60 days or less), medium (61-150 days), slow (151-300 days) or very slow (greater than 300 days). Variation within these groups make little difference in the final calculation of origin of metastases (see Fig. 8.9).

PERSPECTIVES

The current socio-economic scene as it impacts on medical care is bound to aggravate a system that had failings already. The time interval of 1950-1980 is usually regarded as medicine's halcyon years—certainly doctors did well financially and patients were routinely pleased. The impoverished had to obtain their medical help at charitable institutions but even in these circumstances, free or near free clinics were adequately staffed. The huge downside to this otherwise rosy picture was the double digit inflation of health care costs generating a national bill that doubled about every 5 years. The measures to combat this health hyperinflation have been severe, some say draconian. There has been progressively less reimbursement for professional services. Practicing physicians have tried to see more patients (and probably do more procedures) to make up some of the shortfall—however, more patients, more procedures, more chance for slip-ups. The other response to correcting the high cost of medical care has produced ever larger numbers of patients whose care is provided by capitated reimbursement health maintenance organizations. The irony of this is that the same (?inordinately) rapid pace of seeing patients adds greater risk to making a proper diagnosis and therefore a greater chance for real or perceived negligence. Even in the days when doctors gave patients the time the patients expected some mistakes were made that were probably overlooked by a less litigious population. Nowadays, many people have a chip on their shoulder simply because they think they have been unduly rushed in their office visits.

Many will take umbrage at my dim view of our progress in the control of breast cancer. Some will even take the cynical view that my position is dictated by a desire to deprive injured patients or their heirs from just compensation while I collect expert witness fees. Others will complain that as a physician, my failing to accept the notion that early diagnosis cures breast cancer, will lead some lay people to ignore the urging of the general medical community to participate in screening. They feel that the consequences of this will be disastrous. Others will complain that if I have no substitute for mammography why not muffle my doubts and go along. If there is only a tiny benefit from mammography, and I cannot discount this, that tiny plus is better than nothing.

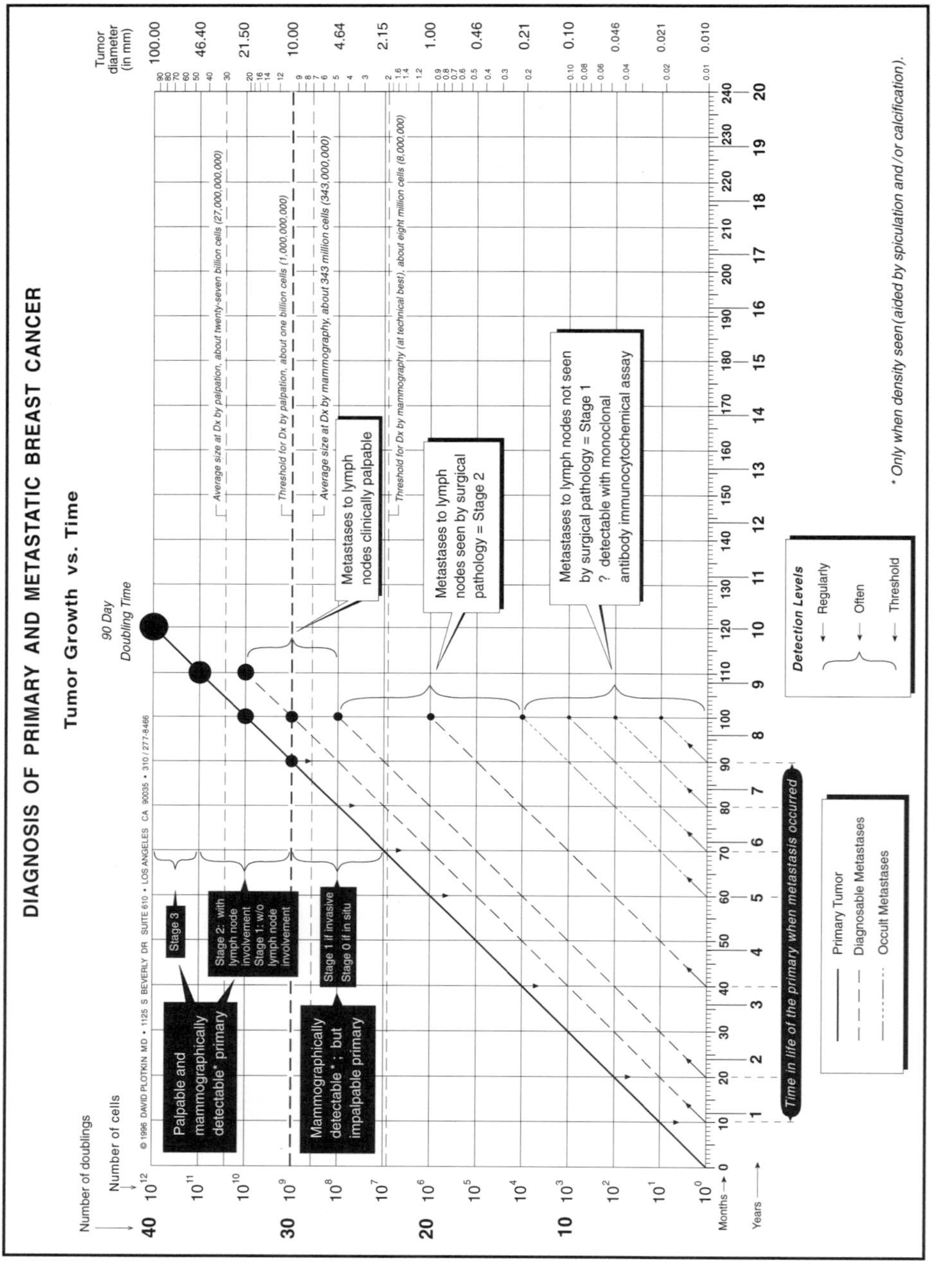

Fig. 8.8. Diagnosis of primary and metastatic breast cancer.

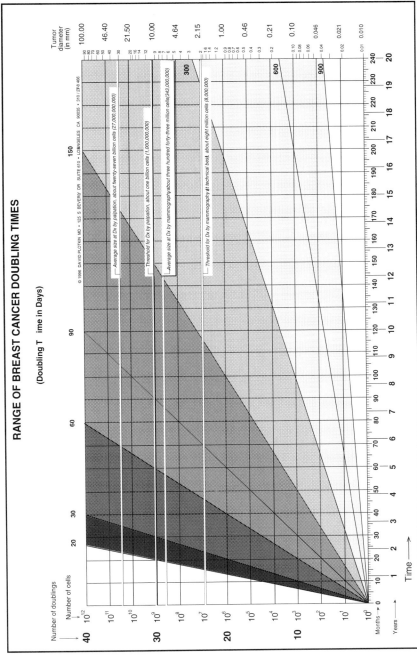

RANGE OF BREAST CANCER DOUBLING TIMES

(Doubling Time in Days)

Fig. 8.9.
Range of
breast cancer
doubling
times.

These arguments in my view are quite refutable. My role as a physician is not as important as being what I hope is an accurate interpreter and analyst of a mass of complex data. If there were truly great trust in the medical community by the public, my words of skepticism of the party line would go unheeded. In circumstances where early diagnosis clearly makes a difference, promoting screening makes total sense. Where our interventions are of dubious value, showy promotion does us great damage. When we promise a lot and deliver little, the equation produces frustration, discontent, and in our lawyer-saturated society, many inappropriate malpractice suits.

If a tiny benefit is derivable from mammography, going along with it regardless of the cost would be all right but only if we had unlimited health care resources. In an era of cost containment, prioritizing our health care efforts will be demanded of us. We all benefit by doing this responsibly.

REFERENCES

1. Feinstein AR, Sosin DM, Wells CK. Will Rogers phenomenon. Stage migration and new diagnostic techniques as a source of misleading statistics for survival in cancer. N Engl J Med 1985; 312: 1604-8.
2. Merriam Webster's Collegiate Dictionary, Tenth Edition. Merriam-Webster, Inc. Springfield, Massachusetts, 1994.
3. Cutler SJ. A description of the force of mortality associated with cancer. In Denoix P, Rouquette C, eds. Symposium of the Prognosis of Malignant Tumors of the Breast. New York: Hafner Publishing Co, 1963.
4. Berkson J, Harrington SW, Clagett OT et al. Mortality and survival in surgically treated cancer of the breast. A statistical summary of some experience of the Mayo Clinic. Proc. Staff Meet. Mayo Clinic 1957; 32:645.
5. Haybittle JL. Is breast cancer ever cured? Endocrine Related Cancer 1983; 14: 13-18.
6. Gelman R, Zelan M. Interpreting clinical data. In Harris JR, Hellman S, Henderson IC, Kinne DW, eds. Breast Diseases. Philadelphia: J.B. Lippincott, 1987:697-731.
7. Nielsen M, Thomsen JL, Primdahl S, Dyrebord U, Andersen JA. Breast cancer and atypia among young and middle aged women: a study of 110 medicolegal autopsies. Br J Cancer 1987; 56:814-9.
8. Adair F, Berg J, Joubert L, Robbins GF. Long-term follow up of breast cancer patients: the 30-year report. Cancer 1974; 33:1145-50.
9. Rutqvist LE, Wallgren A. Longterm survival of 458 young breast cancer patients. Cancer 1985; 55:658-65.
10. Mueller CB, Ames F, Anderson GD. Breast cancer in 3,558 women: age as a significant determinant in the rate of dying and causes of death. Surgery 1978; 83:123-32.
11. Rutqvist LE, Wallgren A, Nilsson BO. Is breast cancer a curable disease? A study of 14,731 women with breast cancer from the Cancer Registry of Norway. Cancer 1984; 53:1793-800.
12. Langlands AO, Pocock SJ, Kerr GR, Gore SM. Longterm survival of patients with breast cancer: a study of the curability of the disease. Br Med J 1979; 2:1247-51.
13. Spratt JA, von Fournier D, Spratt JS, Weber EE. Mammographic assessment of human breast cancer growth and duration. Cancer 1993; 71:2020-2026.
14. Harris JR, Lippman ME, Veronesi V, Willett W. Breast cancer (first of three parts). N Engl J Med 1992; 375(5): 319-328.
15. Shapiro S, Venet W, Strax P, Venet L. Selection, follow up and analysis in the Health Insurance Plan Study: A randomized trial with breast cancer screening. In Garfinkel L, Ochs O, eds. Selection, Follow up and Analysis in Prospective Studies: A Workshop. NIH Publication 85-2713; National Cancer Institute Monograph 67. Washington, D.C.: Department of Health and Human Services, Public Health Service, 1985.
16. Wright CJ. Breast cancer screening: a different look at the evidence. Surgery 1986; 100:594-598.
17. Skrabanek P. The other side of the story. BMJ 1988; 297:971-972.

18. Kusama S, Spratt JS, Donegan WL, Watson FR, Cunningham C. The gross rates of growth of human mammary carcinoma. Cancer 1972; 30:594-9.

19. Pearlman AW. Breast cancer-influence of growth rate on prognosis and treatment evaluation. Cancer 1976; 38:1826-33.

20. Spratt JS. The lognormal frequency distribution and human cancer. J Surg Res 1969; 9:151-7.

21. Lee YTN. The lognormal distribution of growth rates of soft tissue metastases of breast cancer. J Surg Oncol 1972; 4:81-8.

22. Heuser L, Spratt JS, Polk HC. Growth rates of primary breast cancers. Cancer 1979; 43:1888-94.

23. von Fournier D, Weber E. Hoeffken W, Bauer M, Kubli F, Barth M. Growth rate of 147 mammary carcinomas. Cancer 1980; 45:2198-207.

24. von Fournier D, Schiller U, Junkermann H, Legler U, Bauer M. Natural growth rate in 300 primary breast carcinomas and correlation to hormone factors. Ann NY Acad Sci 1986; 464:563-5.

25. Galante E, Gallus G, Guzzon A, Bona A, Bandieramonte G, Di Pietro S. Growth rate of primary breast cancer and prognosis: observations on a 3 to 7 year follow up in 180 breast cancers. Br J Cancer 1986; 54:833-6.

CHAPTER 9

BARRIERS TO BREAST CANCER SCREENING AND STRATEGIES TO OVERCOME THEM*

Sarah A. Fox, Richard Roetzheim and Clairice T. Velt

INTRODUCTION

A variety of socioeconomic, cultural and communication barriers appear to underlie the use of breast cancer screening. Barriers discussed in this chapter are categorized into five areas: (1) demographic characteristics such as insufficient income and urban versus rural living that might act as major barriers in the ability of some women to access screening services; (2) physician-patient communication patterns that might act as a barrier in affecting adherence with screening recommendations; (3) knowledge gaps about the importance of early detection for controlling breast cancer that might play a primary role in some women's decisions to seek breast cancer screening; (4) physicians' or patients' attitudes about some aspects of breast cancer screening such as its safety or efficacy that might negatively affect physician recommendations to seek breast cancer screening or patient adherence with screening recommendations and (5) insufficient individual or community-based activities to assist providers in educating and reminding women about the importance of having regular screening for breast cancer. A woman might experience any one or all of these barrier types.

The interpretation of differences in utilization rates of cancer screening services, like that for acute care services, is complex because there is no clear consensus on the appropriate utilization rates. For example, there is wide agreement in the medical community that screening for lung cancer with chest radiographs is not an effective means for improving health.[1] However, even for procedures for which there is a broad consensus such as mammography for breast cancer, there exists variation in the details (primarily in the recommended screening frequency for women of different ages) of screening recommendations across sets of recommendations issued by various organizations.[1,2] This variation is important to use as a guideline in interpreting utilization rates by particular groups because under-utilization of screening services should imply a lower rate than that recommended in the most conservative guidelines.

*Revised with permission from Fox SA et al, Barriers to cancer screening in the older person; Clin Geriatr Med (February), © 1997 W.B. Saunders Company.

Understanding barriers to breast cancer screening utilization is the precursor to developing and improving strategies for their reduction, thereby bring utilization rates closer to the goals set for the year 2000. Strategies to disseminate important breast cancer screening information, increase patient adherence with screening recommendations as well as access to screening services should be multilevel and include individual-level (physician or patient), cohort-level (physician and patient), practice-level and community-level efforts. Research studies currently are underway at all levels to develop, refine and implement strategies for reducing barriers to breast cancer screening.

This chapter examines major screening barriers and suggests directions for reducing or overcoming those barriers.

DEMOGRAPHIC VARIATIONS IN THE USE OF BREAST CANCER SCREENING SERVICES

Available data from national data sets indicate that the rates of utilization of a wide range of health care services vary substantially across major demographic groups. Although most utilization analyses have focused on acute care services, there exists substantial evidence of variation in cancer screening rates in general and of breast cancer screening rates in particular.

The primary demographic factors for which we have good data on utilization rates are age, race and ethnicity, income, education and urban versus rural residence. Andersen has classified the first two of these demographic factors, age and race/ethnicity, as predisposing factors; they inherently characterize a person along dimensions that cannot be changed.[3] These factors are conceptually distinguished from barrier, or conversely, enabling, demographic factors that can be changed in theory, albeit slowly if at all in, practice.[3] An underserved woman could be a member of an underserved group in one or more of these demographic areas. In general, she is elderly, economically disadvantaged and poorly educated.

Comparing utilization rates among different groups of women within demographic categories makes it possible to characterize underserved women in more detail; reported differences in rates can guide strategies regarding secondary barriers, for example, ability to access screening services, knowledge about breast cancer and breast cancer screening, and reasons underlying nonadherence when screening has been recommended. This information is important to those designing clinical and public health interventions to promote the appropriate use of screening services.

AGE

Age differences in breast cancer screening utilization have been documented since tracking of mammography utilization began in the 1987 National Health Interview Survey (NHIS).[4] Several studies have shown age to be a predictor of breast cancer screening rates, with older women being screened less frequently than younger women in every ethnic group.[5-7] Even in populations of educated women who report interest in adherence to recommended screening usage, older women are screened less frequently than younger women.[5] When there have been analyses of differences within the over 65 population, the older members of this population are still less likely to be screened. For example, among older women in the 1992 NHIS, the percentage of women who had completed a mammogram varied significantly by age.[8] While 41% among women age 60-64 had completed a mammogram, only 28% among women age 75-79 had. Thus, despite the evidence that routine screening mammograms among women 50 years of age or older can reduce breast cancer mortality by as much as 30%, these women are less likely to receive mammograms.[9] Older women are also significantly less likely to adhere to recommendations for breast cancer screening.[10,11] Harris et al found that younger women who assessed their risk of breast cancer to be high were more likely to get screened than older women whose actual risk is higher. Perhaps this is part of the reason for the lower screening rates among older women.[12]

RACE AND ETHNICITY

Breast cancer screening utilization rates are generally lower for minority than white women. Latina and African American women have been associated with less regular use of screening mammograms than Anglo women and are less likely to have ever had a mammography.[7,13,14] Among women over the age of 75 in the 1987 NHIS, 83.5% of black women and 93.2% of Latinas had never had a mammogram, compared to 75% of white women.[15] In the 1987 National Medical Expenditure Survey (NMES), fewer Blacks and Latinas 50-69 years of age had had screening mammograms than Anglos and other ethnic groups.[16]

Among the minority groups, some studies indicate that Latinas have the lowest breast cancer screening rates. In women 35-40 years and older, Latinas have been found to have lower rates of mammography screening[17-19] than non Latina women. Data also indicate that Latinas have fewer lifetime clinical breast examinations and poorer monthly performance of self breast examinations than non Latina women.[17]

African-American women also have lower breast cancer screening rates than the general population.[20-21] This situation seems to persist despite availability of screening tests at reduced costs and educational interventions[21] and despite their greater likelihood of being diagnosed with late-stage disease and dying from breast cancer compared to other racial/ethnic groups.[20,22-24] Analysis of Medicare claims in 1986 found that the relative risk of having a mammogram for white women compared to black women was 1.76.[25]

Little is known about details of specific relative patterns of use across racial and ethnic minorities (e.g., across specific Latina or Asian subpopulations). Differences across these subpopulations may have important implications for eliminating their barriers as well as barriers for other underserved groups.

SOCIOECONOMIC STATUS

Socioeconomic status, typically measured by education and income, is an important predictor of use of medical services. Both education and income have been found to be predictive of breast cancer screening in a number of studies,[7,19-20,26] including breast self examination.[27-28] As is true with many health care procedures, women with lower incomes and less education are less likely to undergo breast cancer screening compared to higher income and more educated persons. For example, among women in the 1990 NHIS above age 40, only 24% of those from families with income less than $20,000 had a mammogram, compared to 39% among those from families with incomes greater than $20,000.[29] In this same study, 23% of women above age 40 with less than a high school education had a mammogram, compared to 41% for women with more than a high school education.[29] In the1987 NMES, those women classified as "near poor" had the lowest mammography rate.[16]

URBAN VS. RURAL LIVING

Available data suggest that women living in rural settings are less likely to undergo cancer screening. In the 1990 NHIS data, 35% of urban women over 40 years of age received a mammogram compared to 26% for rural women.[29] Analyses of data from a Canadian population found similar findings: women in rural areas were less likely to report a clinical breast examination or a mammogram.[30] There is some evidence that the urban-rural distinction may increase racial/ethnic group differences in screening frequencies. For example, the Black-White gap in breast cancer screening frequencies is reportedly greater among rural than urban women;[20] also, in an analysis of 1986 Medicare data, the relative risk among white vs. black women for undergoing mammography increases from 1.67 to 2.64 when urban and rural populations are compared.[25]

One idea underlying the notion that breast cancer screening would be less frequent in rural than in urban areas is that distances to mammography facilities are generally greater and thus affect access to those services. This idea was investigated in a Michigan rural setting for women 40 years of age and older. After statistically controlling for demographic differences, there was no effect of travel distance or travel time on mammogram frequencies.[31] Potential screening barriers such as travel distance and time are especially interesting because they have known solutions (though in practice perhaps difficult to implement). More research is needed to better understand their effects in general and any differential effects they may have for women of different ethnic groups.

ACCESS TO CARE

Access to care is a dual-sided concept that is commonly used to predict use of services on the one hand and an individual's ability to access services on the other. Perhaps the factor most frequently examined as affecting access is cost of services and ability to pay for services. In this section, we look at access to care in terms of major reasons cited by women for not obtaining breast cancer screening or not complying with screening recommendations that are associated with cost. These include cost of services, insurance status, travel distance, time, lack of transportation and child care.[16,18,32-33] Since these factors can relate to cost, they are also related in large part to income.

Data from the 1987 National Medical Expenditure Survey (NMES) provide some revealing information about the role of cost in screening utilization. Many U.S. residents, most of whom have insurance, reportedly were unable to obtain a variety of needed health care services because of costs. In this survey, more than a third of women over 17 years of age had not had a clinical breast examination in the previous[1] year and over half of the women between the ages of 50-69 had never had a mammogram, including 70% of uninsured women, 63% of those with Medicaid and 50% of those privately insured.[16]

The fact that many insured women in the NMES reported cost as the reason for not utilizing needed services suggests that even relatively small costs of screening services may hinder their use for the poor. This is supported in utilization data for women covered by the new (1992) Medicare plan that reimburses for mammograms after deductibles and copayments have been met. These elderly women, who were at greater risk for late-stage breast cancer diagnoses, still were not seeking breast cancer screening unless they had supplemental policies to cover the out-of-pocket payments.[34] Elderly women with Medicare supplement policies had significantly higher cancer screening rates than those who did not.[34-35] However, interventions that provided Medicare coverage of cancer screening tests also increased the rates of cancer screening.[36] Important to increasing screening rates among women with Medicare could be informing them that the cost of mammogram screening is covered by Medicare. Coleman et al found that only 29% of Medicare recipients in their survey knew that the costs for mammogram screening were partially covered by Medicare.[37]

Not surprisingly, there is evidence that women who lack health insurance have much lower rates of breast cancer screening than the insured[8,37-38] and are more likely to be diagnosed with cancer at an advanced stage.[39] And, access to primary care[40] and the number of provider visits[6,7,41-43] are associated with higher rates of cancer screening. Some studies have found that patients enrolled in managed care HMOs receive more cancer screening services and have earlier stages of cancer at diagnosis.[44-46] However, it is not known if this is due to a greater emphasis on prevention by HMOs or simply the result of prevention-oriented physicians self-selecting into HMOs.

While costs of services and lack of health insurance coverage are certainly important barriers for some patients, other barriers discussed in this chapter also play a role in impeding access. This is evidenced by the relative ineffectiveness of interventions directed primarily at reducing screening costs unless they are supplemented with patient education[47] and by the low screening rates among poor people in countries (e.g.,

Canada) with universal health insurance.[48] Knowledge about screening, doctor-patient communication about screening, and patient's and physician's attitudes about breast cancer and breast cancer screening probably play some role in breast cancer screening decisions. These barriers are discussed in the next three sections.

PHYSICIAN-PATIENT COMMUNICATION AND BREAST CANCER SCREENING

Physician-patient communication is a topic of considerable interest to those who investigate both barrier and enabling factors that might impact patients' adherence to screening recommendations. Some researchers believe that "better" patient-physician communication about cancer and cancer screening will increase screening usage thereby decreasing mortality and morbidity levels from this disease.[49-51]

What impact, if any, do characteristics of patient/physician communications have on physician or patient behaviors? A review of the communication literature (a recent annotated bibliography by AE Beisecker) relevant to patients and their physicians highlights the possible role communication characteristics might play in health outcomes in general. Additionally, Beisecker reviewed the different components of the doctor-patient relationship that might impact patient-physician communication and patient outcomes (for example, patient adherence to physician recommendations or physician's screening recommendation).[52] These include provider and patient characteristics, for example, gender and race; the content of the encounter, for example, the type or amount of information communicated; the patient's or physician's communication style, for example, patient's assertiveness; physician's enthusiasm; and the context in which the communication takes place that could be defined along a number of screening barrier dimensions, such as the reason for the visit, or the presence of a patient's companion.

PATIENT/PHYSICIAN CHARACTERISTICS AND COMMUNICATION

There is some evidence that points to the influence of a patient's age and a physician's age, race or gender on physician's breast cancer screening recommendations. Weinberger et al found that physicians were significantly more likely to include mammography in their screening recommendations when women were under 65 years old and limit screening recommendations to clinical breast examination for women 75 years or older.[53] These physicians cited co-morbidities and an expected shortened life expectancy as reasons for their limited screening recommendations in this older age group.[53]

It seems reasonable to suppose that patient comorbidities influence patient/physician communication about screening that in turn could lead to fewer physician screening recommendations.[54] Certainly communication difficulties are inevitable and complicated when patients have cognitive deficits or hearing impairments.[54] These difficulties are seen more often in the elderly but could characterize a person of any age. Greene found evidence of communication problems between physicians and elderly patients who exhibited a confusion about what occurred during the office visits.[55] There was significantly less concordance for the older (over 65 years of age) patient-physician dyadic interactions than for the younger dyads, especially in relation to what was discussed in general and discussed medically.[55]

There have been other studies that have also found differences in screening recommendations based on physician gender. Kreuter et al found that female physicians screened younger patients (ages 35-39) for mammograms at a much higher rate than male physicians, with screening rates becoming more equal for older patients;[56] another study found that Anglo physicians and younger physicians were more likely than other physicians to report screening elderly women.[57] Finally, Fox et al found that a physician's discussion of mammography was a stronger predictor of patient adherence in the 65 years and over age group than in younger patients; it was the strongest predictor for mammography screening for women over age 50, regardless of age.

COMMUNICATION CONTENT

The notion of content in patient/physician communication carries with it characteristics of type, amount and the absence as well as the presence of certain types of information in patient/physicians encounters. At present, there seems to be a paucity of a content literature in general and with respect to breast cancer screening.

It is clear from the present literature, however, that the most salient content factor associated with breast cancer screening rates is the physician's recommendation or discussion of breast cancer screening.[43,51,58-62] But, it is possible that the positive impact of a physician's recommendation on mammography screening rates decreases with age,[62] although this finding might have occurred because older women are more easily influenced by their physician than are younger women, and physicians neglect to talk about or recommend mammography screening to their older patients.[53] There is also evidence that women believe their physician would tell them if they needed a mammogram,[42] that is, the belief that this information would be part of the regular content of the patient/physician interaction if mammograms were important to get.

There is some evidence that important information might be missing from patient/physician communications. For example, some older patients report that their problems were not addressed at their office visit and that over half of these patients had at least one important medical problem and one psychological problem of concern.[63] Adelman et al also found that older patients had difficulty getting their concerns acknowledged and that about two-thirds of the topics discussed in physician/patient interactions were ones raised by physicians rather than patients.[64] Even though these studies did not relate to cancer screening, there is

an implication here that screening topics and recommendations might be neglected if they are not on the physician's agenda.

The extent to which the patient is encouraged to participate in patient/physician interactions increases the patient's input to the interactions, thereby changing the content of the discussion. Beisecker and Beisecker (1990) found that information-seeking comments of patients were influenced by the patient's diagnosis, reason for the office visit, presence of a patient's companion, length of the doctor/patient interaction and whether the visit was an initial or repeat visit.[65] This study did not focus on breast cancer screening but explorations of these variables in a potential setting that calls for breast cancer screening discussions might yield some interesting insights into subsequent physician and patient behaviors.

Wolf et al listed categories of screening information that they recommend physicians communicate to their patients that include information on mammography and clinical breast exams.[66] Providing this information to the patient is likely to increase the quality of the patient/physician communication about cancer screening and to promote the shared decision-making environment about cancer screening that they believe to be a "central tenet of the physician-patient relationship."

COMMUNICATION STYLE

There is some evidence that the content of the physician/patient communication can be influenced by the patient's communication style and that the patient's communication style can influence physicians' behavior as well as the reverse, i.e., that the physicians' communication style can influence the patient's behavior.

Adelman and others found that audiotapes of primary care follow up appointments showed that physicians reacted differently to patients under 45 compared to those over 65 years of age.[67-68] Younger patients were perceived as asking better questions and providing better information to physicians than older patients. Physicians reacted by providing more information on physician-initiated issues and more support for patient-initiated issues; physicians were also reportedly "nicer" to younger patients.[67-68] Conversely, older patients appeared to limit amounts and kinds of information contained in the patient/physician interaction by being more passive and giving more decision-making authority to the physicians.[68-71]

There has been little exploration of physician or patient communication style on either physician or patient breast-cancer screening behavior. In one study, Fox et al found that patient's reported the enthusiasm with which her physician discussed screening mammography to be the strongest predictor of the patient's screening behavior.[51] Women who reported their physicians to have at least some enthusiasm for mammography were more than four and a half times more likely to have had a mammogram within the previous year than women who reported their physicians as having no or little enthusiasm for mammography.[51] The level of enthusiasm women reported their physicians to have for mammography screening decreased with increasing patient age and dropped markedly for women over 75 years of age. This may be a contributing factor to the lower screening rates in this group of women.[51]

COMMUNICATION CONTEXT

Context is a multifaceted construct. For example, demographics of the patient or physician, their communication styles and attitudes, and the knowledge they bring to the encounter all, by definition, change the context in which the communication takes place. These contextual variables could directly affect patient behaviors (e.g., adherence, recall) or physician behaviors (e.g., screening recommendations), or could affect an intermediary variable such as the content of the communication encounter that in turn impacts behavior.

An interesting contextual variable that has been explored is the presence of a third party accompanying the patient to the office visit. Labrecque, Blanchard et al (1991) found that physicians tended to provide more support to the less sick cancer patients when they came alone for their office visit.[72] However, physicians spent more time interacting with the sicker patients. They discussed future treatment more often when family members were present but only when the patient was sicker.

Beisecker examined audiotapes of 21 patient-doctor visits for patients aged 60-85. In nine of these visits, the patient was alone; a family member was included in 12 of the visits.[73] The presence of the family member did not appear to affect the length of the patient/doctor encounter, but rather, served to decrease the patient/doctor interaction time.[73] Coe found that, although the presence of a third party affected communication, e.g., physicians adjusted to include the presence of a third party; it was not clear whether the effect was positive or negative for the patient.[74] Both authors agreed that more research is needed on the effects that third parties bring to the patient-physician interaction and subsequent screening rate recommendations and patient adherence.

KNOWLEDGE-BASED BARRIERS TO SCREENING

It seems reasonable to believe that women and their health-care providers need a minimal knowledge base which should include breast cancer risk factors, awareness of cancer screening procedures, the importance of early detection for controlling breast cancer and the current guidelines for frequency of screening, if there is to be patient adherence regarding utilization. Lack of such knowledge can serve as a barrier to appropriate breast cancer screening recommendations on the physician's side and adherence on the patient's side.*

The literature regarding the impact of knowledge on breast cancer screening

*Knowledge of "recommended" utilization of screening mammography can understandably differ for different patients and providers given the different recommendations by different institutions and the changes in these recommendations over short periods of time.[53]

referrals by physicians and adherence by their patients is not as extensive as one might hope; additionally, it is often coupled with studies which document other barriers to screening, such as attitudes. And, the studies that do explore knowledge have focused on patient knowledge instead of provider knowledge of risk factors or screening recommendations. Studies indicate that a woman's knowledge about breast cancer, cancer detection, breast cancer screening and her risk for getting breast cancer are associated with her screening behavior and intentions.[42,43,61,74-81]

Mandelblatt et al found that older, black, low income women who reported low levels of knowledge about breast cancer also demonstrated low levels of screening utilization.[75] In other studies, less adherent patients were found to have lower levels of knowledge about breast cancer and detection issues;[76-77] women who intended to participate in regular breast cancer screening were more knowledgeable about breast cancer,[78,60] and women who actually participated in screening tests were more likely to be more informed about breast cancer and screening than those who had not had a mammogram.[42,43,79-81] Gardiner found that higher scores on a knowledge and awareness test predicted mammography screening rates, and that educational level was the most significant predictor of these scores.[79]

A woman's knowledge about her risk for getting breast cancer also appears to be a factor in her screening behavior. Mah and Bryant found that, although over half of their sample in their Canadian study had had a mammogram, the proportion decreased with age after age 60.[82] Knowledge of breast cancer risk factors was generally low as was knowledge of guidelines; both decreased with age.[82] Rimer et al demonstrated that educating women about their actual risk for breast cancer increased screening adherence.[47] They offered a health education program to retirement home residents that included teaching the older women about risk factors as well as detection techniques.[47] These women were more likely to subsequently get screened than women who were offered subsidized mammograms.[47]

Differences in knowledge levels by race/ethnicity have been found. Perez-Stable found that misconceptions about cancer were more prevalent among Latinas than Anglos.[83] However, if Latinas, especially the elderly, had acquired English and were acculturated, they were more likely to know more about cancer and to have been screened.[84-85] Flores and Mata found that Latinos in general lacked specific knowledge about screening—the procedures or recommended frequency of screening examinations[86]—which might account for Latinas' comparatively lower screening rates.

Many researchers believe that educating women about breast cancer and breast cancer screening is the means for achieving increases in breast-cancer screening rates thereby lowering morbidity and mortality rates due to this disease.[42,57,87-89] And there is some evidence for this. Friedman found that the recency of participating in an educational component of a screening program was predictive of both adherence with mammography in the past 12 months and intentions to obtain CBE in the next year.[90] Kernohan found that South Asian women who initially had the lowest levels of knowledge about screening showed the most improvement through educational interventions in terms of increases in mammograms;[87] other studies found increases in mammography screening rates after an educational intervention.[78,91]

ATTITUDINAL BARRIERS TO SCREENING

PATIENT ATTITUDES AND BELIEFS

Health beliefs and attitudes are important components of several theoretical models of patients' health behavior that have been examined in the context of cancer screening. Models such as the Theory of Reasoned Action and the Health Belief Model have been found to have reasonably good predictive value for adherence to cancer screening, suggesting that patient attitudes are important determinants of screening behavior.[92-95] Studies also have found correlations between general health attitudes and cancer screening.[96] Patient's attitudes and beliefs that have been associated with breast cancer screening rates are:

- belief in the curability[19] or incurability[7] of breast cancer;
- low perceived risk of getting breast cancer;[7,80,94,97-102]
- belief that symptoms are necessary before screening;[61,83,100-101,103-105]
- disinterest;[106]
- fear that radiation is harmful;[106]
- embarrassment and discomfort;[18,32,87,107-108]
- fear of a positive diagnosis;[32]
- perceived inefficacy of screening;[109]
- patient's poor health status: sicker patients are less likely to be screened;[99,103,105]
- belief that physician will tell the patient if a screen is necessary.[43]

Breast cancer screening rates were found to be lower when patients believed there to be a low prospect of curing breast cancer[7,19] and higher in the absence of negative attitudes (e.g., mammograms are unnecessary)[61] and when patients' believed themselves to be at a higher personal risk for breast cancer.*[97]

Latinas have cited embarrassment and fear of a positive diagnosis as reasons for not obtaining breast cancer screening.[18,32] From the perceptions of health care providers, barriers to screening for Latinas have been their fear of a positive diagnosis, a belief that the test is unnecessary, a belief that it is uncomfortable[32] and a feeling of embarrassment.[31] Latinas have also reported a belief in being susceptible to breast cancer but perceive breast cancer to be incurable;[18] those who reportedly held strong traditional Mexican family attitudes were more likely to participate in mammography screening.[85]

Latinas have reported the belief that surgery causes cancer to spread, a belief that

might not effect breast cancer screening decisions but could well be a deterrent to getting treatment.[81] Both Latinas[13,81] and African-Americans[110] believe that a blow or trauma to the breast is an important cancer risk. Powe reports that these kinds of "misinformed beliefs" are reported less frequently by Anglos than by Latinas. However, they are reported with rather high frequency by the elderly.[101,103,105] Focus groups, for instance, included discussions by older women who viewed cancer in a worst case scenario—associated with radical and painful treatments, usually fatal, and accompanied by a greatly feared dependency on others.[111] There was very little distinction made between early and late-stage disease. Cancer cures were instead attributed more often to luck or personal character traits rather than early detection with screening.[111] The association of these "fatalistic" beliefs to breast cancer screening rates is unclear. It is known, however, that both elderly and Latina women have low breast cancer screening rates compared with other age and race groups.

Attitudes may play a more important role in screening behavior for the elderly than in younger women.[109] Studies have documented a number of negative attitudes about cancer screening that are held more frequently by the elderly. These include greater worries about radiation/safety of mammography,[98,109] a greater reliance on symptoms to detect cancer rather than asymptomatic detection with screening,[83,100,101,103,104] lower perceived efficacy of screening,[109] less concern about early detection than about current medical problems,[99,103] greater embarrassment with screening[89,107-108] and, despite the striking age-related increase in cancer incidence, many paradoxically perceive less susceptibility to cancer, a belief that has been associated with lower levels of screening.[82,94,98,102] The elderly's perception that they are less susceptible to breast cancer may be a result of the failure to target screening educational programs to the elderly. Until recently, for instance, most breast cancer media promotions typically featured younger women

---

Smith found that patients greatly overestimated their personal lifetime risk and 10-year risk of breast cancer.

undergoing screening, leaving the impression that they were most vulnerable.[112]

However, it is encouraging to think that women's negative attitudes and beliefs about breast cancer screening can be altered. Burnett et al reported that the women's significant other can influence her attitudes and beliefs.[113] Others have found that social support limits the negative effects of fear/anxiety on cancer screening decisions.[114-115] A number of researchers believe that positive attitudes, beliefs and firm recommendations of the health-care professionals for breast cancer screening can positively influence their patients' attitudes.[51,61,113,116] And we have seen from the previous section that educating women about the importance of breast cancer screening can increase their mammography screening.

PHYSICIAN ATTITUDES AND BELIEFS

It appears that primary care physicians have some very positive attitudes about cancer screening in general. They overwhelmingly know and support American Cancer Society guidelines, often in preference to less aggressive guidelines like the US Preventive Services Task Force.[117-120] They also believe cancer screening is effective[121-122] and express strong interest in cancer screening education.[123] Although the yield of cancer screening is generally low in a typical primary care practice, its emotional impact can be substantial. During focus groups, physicians reported being affected greatly by the diagnosis of an early cancer by screening and also being quite affected by caring for cancer patients with terminal disease. Diagnosing cancer is likely a critical event for physicians.

Cancer screening attitudes are not uniform among primary care physicians, however. Some studies, for instance, have shown less favorable attitudes about cancer screening among older physicians. It is unclear if this is the result of a cohort effect reflecting training differences of younger and older physicians. It is also possible that attitudes about the value of breast cancer screening change as physicians age or assume care for an older patient population.

The literature strongly suggests that primary care physicians are in a crucial position to increase mammography screening rates.[14,26,43,51,58-62] Lost opportunities may result when physicians underestimate the importance of their role or overestimate the patient's resistance.[26,124] Other barriers suggested by the literature are:

- patient's attitudes and beliefs;[105]
- underestimation of the life expectancy of elderly women;[53]
- patient's current poor health status;
- uncertainty of screening guidelines (especially for elderly women);
- physician's age;[125]
- concerns about radiation and safety of elderly patients;[98,109]
- screening not emphasized.[126]

Physicians' screening recommendations are likely influenced by their perceptions of their patients' attitudes and beliefs. During focus group discussions they reported that their patients found many screening tests unpleasant or embarrassing;[122] this agrees with independent reports from patients.[89,107-108] For their elderly patients, physicians reported them to be less interested in breast cancer screening than in caring for their acute and chronic medical problems[105] and therefore more likely to refuse cancer screening recommendations.[121]

Women 65 years of age or older are at higher risk for breast cancer than younger women but they have lower screening rates across all ethnic groups. Physician attitudes and beliefs about breast cancer screening for the elderly and what affects their quality of life may in part be responsible for this lower screening rate. Physicians (and others) generally underestimate the life expectancy of older Americans.[53] For example, the average life expectancy of a 65 year old woman in reasonable health is 18 years, for a 75 year old woman 12 years, and for an 85 year old woman 7 years.[127] Physicians have no simple methods to assess life expectancy and functional life expectancy to assist in screening decisions.[128] If physicians perceive a limited life expectancy with poor quality of life for their elderly patients they might have less enthusiasm for prescribing them mammograms.

Another complication to adequate mammogram screening for older women might be the negative attitudes toward the elderly in general held by some physicians. Greene and her colleagues found that physicians were condescending, abrupt, and indifferent with older patients and showed less tendency to include them in decision-making activities when compared to younger patients.[129]

However, physicians may intend to prescribe more mammograms than they actually do. A study by Roetzheim et al suggested that mammography screening rates would significantly increase for women over 65 years of age if physicians' screening recommendation rates increased to match their stated agreements on who should be screened.[130] Gaps between physicians' intentions and behaviors may exist for other patient age groups as well.

COMMUNITY-BASED BARRIERS TO SCREENING

OFFICE INTERVENTIONS

Even physicians with a very strong commitment to screening must overcome a number of barriers, including remembering to offer screening, finding adequate time during patient encounters and the many logistical problems of screening. A fairly substantial gap between physicians intentions to screen and actual screening rates are usually reported.[130] A large number of interventions have been conducted to improve cancer screening in the primary care setting. Interventions have been directed at primary care physicians, their patients and their staff.

Physician-directed interventions have included health promotion checklists, flow sheets and chart tags that serve as reminders for screening.[131-136] These reminder systems increase screening rates by attempting to focus attention to selected cancer screening tests. In general such reminders are effective especially when directed at a small number of screening tests. They are less ef-

fective when directed at multiple screening tests with some studies finding that non-targeted screening tests may actually decrease. Clearly physicians can not focus their attention on all screening interventions.

Chart audit of screening adherence with feedback of screening rates to individual physicians has also been successfully used.[137,138] Finally computer-generated reminders have been studied extensively.[138-145] These interventions have generally shown greater increases in screening rates than chart reminders and when directed at multiple screening tests have produced more uniform effects. Computer reminders were more cost-effective than audit with feedback.[146] Patient interventions that have been found to be effective include mailed reminder postcards/letters,[136,138,147,148] history/risk factor questionnaires[144] and patient-held minirecords.[145,150] Telephone calls have not been found to be particularly effective.[141,147] Interventions targeted at both physicians and patients (physician computer reminders and patient letter or postcard)[14] have also been effective and have generally shown additive effects.[149-152] Several interventions have been directed at office nursing staff and have been effective at increasing rates of breast and colorectal screening.[153-156]

Although all of the above interventions have been successful to some extent, the long-term durability of their effects is not known. One would expect effects to wane over time as the novelty of reminder systems wears off.[157]

COMMUNITY INTERVENTIONS

A number of community-based interventions to promote cancer screening have been conducted.[158-171] Most have studied breast and cervical cancer screening. Strategies to promote screening have generally been multifaceted including efforts to educate and persuade primary care physicians to increase screening (CME, newsletters), efforts to educate/motivate women (posters, brochures, direct mailings, mass media, church/worksite programs, use of celebrities and volunteers) and efforts to overcome logistic/access barriers (mobile vans, on-site nurse practitioners, reminder systems, office staff training, subsidizing screening costs). The details of NCI-funded community interventions have recently been summarized.[172]

Several conclusions can be drawn from these trials. First multistrategy interventions have generally been more successful than more limited interventions. It is also clear that eliminating the costs of screening without addressing other barriers has not proven successful.[46] Finally, well structured community interventions have increased screening rates in an impressive variety of patient care settings, including HMO's, public hospital clinics, community health centers and private physicians' offices, and for patients of varied ethnicities, and socioeconomic status.

Several questions regarding community interventions remain unanswered. The cost-effectiveness of community interventions in general has not been established nor have individual strategies been compared with respect to their cost-effectiveness. Although community interventions have proven their effectiveness in research settings, it is also not always clear how they can be implemented in settings where resources are more limited, and specialized personnel are lacking.

STRATEGIES TO OVERCOME BARRIERS

Following are practice-based suggestions to reduce barriers to breast cancer screening.

DEMOGRAPHIC BARRIERS AND SUGGESTIONS FOR IMPROVEMENT:

The following patient groups need special encouragement by clinicians if there is to be more equity in screening rates: older persons, especially over age 74; non Anglo patients, especially those who are non English speaking; and poverty-level and lower-education persons.

In addition:

• Opposite gender (to physicians) patients should be treated with age-ap-

propriate screening practices, in spite of any clinician embarrassment.

• The number of quality years of life expectancy that older, still healthy, patients can expect is often under-estimated; health status, instead of chronological age, should be the best indicator of whether to refer patients for screening services.

• Older people are not homogeneous. Not only do they differ in personalities, they also differ by age groups. All 65 and over people are often viewed as similar when in fact 65-year-olds are quite different in comorbidities and other problems from 85-year-olds.

COMMUNICATION BARRIERS AND SUGGESTIONS FOR IMPROVEMENT:

• Taking more initiative and asking patients about their concerns at the beginning of the visit will facilitate patients getting their needs met. Likewise, patients should learn to be more verbally assertive about the reasons for the visit at its beginning.

• Adherence with screening guidelines is likely to suffer if their mention is not easily recalled by patients or reinforced with printed matter provided by the physician's office.

• Physicians would be more effective if patient fears about cancer were directly addressed by their physicians.

• Physicians have enormous influence over their patient's behaviors, even their screening behaviors; cancer screening adherence rates can be increased significantly through a more direct physician communication of their wants for their patients, e.g., that they want their patients to get screened for cancer.

• The way in which clinicians encourage patient behavior makes a difference in whether patients respond; physicians can enjoy an increased level of screening by their patients if physicians recommend screening with enthusiasm.

KNOWLEDGE BARRIERS AND
SUGGESTIONS FOR IMPROVEMENT:
- Knowledge levels of risk factors, awareness of screening procedures and knowledge of screening guidelines are all predictors of higher levels of screening adherence. These issues should be reviewed with all patients. Ideally, patients should leave each visit with printed matter that reinforces verbal instructions.

ATTITUDINAL BARRIERS AND SUGGESTIONS FOR IMPROVEMENT:
- Physician's enthusiasm for screening can be very effective in overcoming patient's pessimism regarding survival from a cancer diagnosis and accompanying pessimism regarding cancer screening.
- Survey research and focus groups suggest that older persons are generally very receptive to getting regular screening. Thus, providers should not assume that older patients will resist screening recommendations.

COMMUNITY BARRIERS AND
SUGGESTIONS FOR IMPROVEMENTS:
- Physician and patient reminders regarding screening tests improve adherence.
- Multiple barriers, e.g., reduction of screening costs and anxiety about a finding, etc., to screening need attention in order to increase patient adherence with screening.

ACKNOLWEDGMENTS

This investigation was supported in part by the National Cancer Institute (NCI#5RO1CA65879 and NCI #RO1CA65880) to S.A.F., and the Health Resources Services Administration (#2T32PE19001) to R.G.R.. The authors acknowledge the assistance of Sarah Connor in the preparation of this manuscript.

REFERENCES
1. Hayward RSA, Steinberg EP, Ford DE; Roizen MF et al. Preventive care guidelines. Ann Intern Med 1991; 114(9): 758-783.
2. Sox HC. Preventive health services in adults. N Eng J Med 1994; 330(22): 1589-1595.
3. Andersen R, Newman JF. Societal and individual determinants of medical care utilization in the United States. Milbank Memorial Fund Q 1973; 51(1):95-124.
4. US Dept of Health and Human Services. Provisional Estimates from the National Health Interview Survey Supplement on Cancer Control—United States, January-March 1987. Morbidity and Mortality Weekly Report 1988; 37(27):417-425.
5. Fried TR, Rosenberg RR, Lipsitz LA. Older community-dwelling adults' attitudes toward and practices of health promotion and advance planning activities. J Amer Geriatrics Soc 1995; 43(6):645-9.
6. Bastani R, Kaplan CP, Maxwell AE et al. Initial and repeat mammography screening in a low income multi-ethnic population in Los Angeles. Cancer Epidemiology 1995; 4(2):161-7
7. Lee JR, Vogel VG. Who uses screening mammography regularly? Cancer Epidemiology, Biomarkers and Prevention 1995; 4(8):901-6.
8. Breen N, Kessler L. Trends in Cancer Screening—United States, 1987 and 1992. Mortality and Morbidity Weekly Report. 1996; 45(3):57-61
9. Use of mammography services by women 65 or older enrolled in Medicare—US, 1991-1993. Morbidity and Mortality Weekly Report 1995; 44(41):777-81.
10. Hayward RA, Shapiro MF, Freeman HE et al. Who gets screened for cervical and breast cancer. Results from a New National Survey. Arch Intern Med 1988; 148:1177-1181.
11. Makuc DM; Fried VM, Kleinman JC. National trends in the use of preventive health care by women. Am J Public Health 1989; 79(1):21-26.
12. Harris RP, Fletcher SW, Gonzalez JJ et al. Mammography and age: are we targeting the wrong women? A community

survey of women and physicians. Cancer 1991; 67(7):2010-4.

13. Hubbell FA, Chavez LR, Mishra SI et al. From ethnography to intervention: developing a breast cancer control program for Latinas. J Natl Cancer Inst Monogr 1995; (18):109-115.

14. Fox SA, and Stein JA. Effect of physician-patient communication on mammography utilization by different ethnic groups. Med Care 1991; 29:1065-82.

15. Caplan LS; Wells BL, Haynes S. Breast cancer screening among older racial/ethnic minorities and whites barriers to early detection. J Gerontolo 1992; 47 (Special Issue):101-110.

16. Himmelstein DU, Woolhandler S. Care denied: US residents who are unable to obtain needed medical services. Amer J of Public Health1995; 85(3):341-4.

17. Tortolero-Luna G, Glober GA, Villarreal R, Palos G, Linares A. Screening practices and knowledge, attitudes, and beliefs about cancer among Hispanic and Non-Hispanic white women 35 years old or older in Nueces County, Texas. J Natl Cancer Inst Monogr, 1995; (18):49-56.

18. Perez-Stable EJ, Sabogal F, Otero-Sabogal R. Use of cancer-screening tests in the San Francisco bay area: comparison of Latinos and Anglos. J Natl Cancer Inst Monogr 1995; (18):147-153.

19. Fulton JP, Rakowski W, Jones AC. Determinants of breast cancer screening among inner-city Hispanic women in comparison with other inner-city women. Public Health Reports 1995; 110(4):476-82.

20. Earp JA, Altpeter M, Mayne L et al. The North Carolina Breast Cancer Screening Program: foundations and design of a model for reaching older, minority, rural women. Breast Cancer Research and Treatment 1995; 35(1):7-22.

21. Powe BD. Cancer fatalism among African-Americans: a review of the literature. Nursing Outlook 1996; 44(1):18-21.

22. Walker B, Figgs LW, Zahm SH. Differences in cancer incidence, mortality, and survival between African Americans and whites. Environmental Health Perspectives 1995; 103 Suppl 8:275-81.

23. Moormeier J. Breast cancer in black women. Annals of Int. Med 1996; 124 (10):897-905.

24. Mandelblatt J, Andrews H, Kao R et al. Impact of access and social context on breast cancer stage at diagnosis. J Health Care for the Poor and Underserved 1995; 6(3):342-51

25. Escarce JJ, Epstein KR, Colby DC et al. Racial differences in the elderly's use of medical procedures and diagnostic tests. Am J Public Health 1993; 83(7):948-954.

26. The NCI Breast Cancer Screening Consortium. Mammography—a missed clinical opportunity? Results of the NCI Breast Cancer Screening Consortium and National Health Interview Survey Studies. JAMA 1990; 264:54-58.

27. Phillips JM. Adherence to breast cancer screening guidelines among African-American women of differeing employment status. Cancer Nursing 1995; 18(4):258-69.

28. Morrison C. Determining crucial correlates of breast self-examination in older women with low incomes. Oncology Nursing Forum 1996; 23(1):83-93.

29. Breen N, Kessler L. Changes in the use of screening mammography: Evidence from the 1987 and 1990 National Health Interview Surveys. Am J Public Health 1994; 84:62-67.

30. Bryant H, Mah Z. Breast cancer screening attitudes and behaviors of rural and urban women. Prev Med 1992; 21:405-418.

31. Kreher NE, Hickner JM, Ruffin MT et al. Effect of distance and travel time on rural women's compliance with screening mammography: an UPRNet study. Upper Peninsula Research Network J of Family Practice 1995; 40(2):143-7.

32. Bakemeier RF, Krebs LU, Murphy JR et al. Attitudes of Colorado health professionals toward breast and cervical cancer screening in Hispanic women. J Natl Cancer Inst Monogr 1995; (19):95-100.

33. Beaulieu MD, Beland F, Roy D, Falardeau et al. Factors determining compliance with screening mammography. Canadian Med Assoc J 1996; 154(9):1335-43.

34. Blustein J. Medicare coverage, supplemental insurance, and the use of mam-

mography by older women. N Engl J Med 1995; 332:1138-43.

35. McCarthy BD, Yood MU, MacWilliam CH et al. Screening mammography use: the importance of a population perspective. Amer J of Prev Med 1996; 12(2): 91-95.

36. Morrissey J, Harris R, Kincaide-Norburn J et al. Medicare reimbursement for preventive care: Changes in performance of services, quality of life, and health care costs. Med Care 1995; 33:315-31.

37. Coleman EA, Feuer EJ, The NCI Breast Cancer Screening Consortium. Breast cancer screening among women 65-74 years of age in 1987-88 and 1991. Ann Intern Med 1992; 117:961-966.

38. Woolhandler S, Himmelstein D. Reverse targeting of preventive care due to lack of health insurance. JAMA 1988; 259: 2872-2874.

39. Ayanian J, Kohler B, Abe T et al. The relation between health insurance coverage and clinical outcomes among women with breast cancer. N Engl J Med 1993; 329:326-331.

40. Kirkman-Liff B, Kronenfeld J. Access to cancer screening services for women. Am J Public Health 1992; 82:733-735.

41. McCarthy BD, Yood MU, Janz NK et al. Evaluation of factors potentiallly associated with inadequate follow up of mammographic abnormalities. Cancer, 1996, 77(10):20700-6.

42. Navarro AM, Senn KL, Kaplan RM et al. Por La Vida intervention model for cancer prevention in Latinas. J Natl Cancer Inst Monogr 1995(18):137-45.

43. Mastroberti M, Stein JE. Barriers to timely mammography. HMO Practice 1996; 10(3):104-7.

44. Bernstein A, Thompson G, Harlan L. Differences in rates of cancer screening by usual source of medical care. Med Care 1991; 29:196-209.

45. Zapka J, Hosmer D, Costanza M et al. Changes in mammography use: Economic, need, and service factors. Am J Public Health 1992; 82:1345-1351.

46. Riley G, Potosky A, Lubitz J et al. Stage of cancer at diagnosis of Medicare, HMO and fee-for-service enrollees. Am J Public Health 1994; 84:1598-1604.

47. Rimer BK, Resch N, King E et al. Multi-strategy health education program to increase mammography use among women ages 65 and older. Pub Health Reports 1992; 107(4):369-80.

48. Katz S, Hofer T. Socioeconomic disparities in preventive care persist despite universal coverage: Breast and cervical cancer screening in Ontario and the United States. JAMA 1994; 272:530-4.

49. Wolf AM, Becker DM. Cancer screening and informed patient discussions. Truth and consequences. Archives of Internal Medicine 1996; 156(10): 1069-72.

50. Fox SA, Sui AL, Stein JA. The importance of physician communication on breast cancer screening of older women. Arch Intern Med 1994; 154:2058-68.

51. Fox SA, Siu AL, Stein JA. The importance of physician communication on breast cancer screening of older women. Arch Intern Med 1994; 154:2058-2068.

52. Beisecker AE. Older persons' medical encounters and their outcomes. Res on Aging 1996; 18(1):9-31.

53. Weinberger M, Saunders AF, Samsa GP et al. Breast cancer screening in older women: Practices and barriers reported by primary care physicians. J Am Geriatr Soc 1991; 39:22-29.

54. Erber NP. Communicating with elders: Effects of amplification. J Gerontolo Nursing 1994; 20:6-10.

55. Greene MG, Adelman RD, Charon R et al. Concordance between physicians and their older and younger patients in the primary care medical encounter. Gerontolo Soc Am 1989; 29:808-813.

56. Kreuter MW, Strecher VJ, Harris R et al. Are patients of women physicians screened more aggressively? A prospective study of physician gender and screening. J of General Int Medicine 1995; 10(3):119-25.

57. Roetzheim RG, Fox SA, Leake B. Physician-reported determinants of screening mammography in older women: The impact of physician and practice characteristics. J of the Amer. Geriatrics Soc 1995; 43(12):1398-402.

58. Friedman LC, Woodruff A, Lane M et al. Breast Cancer Screening Behaviors and intentions among asymptomatic women

50 years of age and older. Amer J of Prev Med 1995; 11(4):218-23.

59. Johnson MM, Hislop TG, Kan L et al. Compliance with the screening mammography program of British Columia: will she return? Canadian J of Public Health. (Revue Canadienne de Sante Publique) 1996; 87(3):176-180.

60. Sparks BT, Ragheb NE, Given BA et al. Breast cancer screening in rural populations: a pilot study. J of Rural Health 1996; 12(2) 120-9.

61. O'Connor AM, Perrault DJ. Importance of physician's role highlighted in survey of women's breast screening practices. Canadian J of Public Health 1995; 86 (1):42-5.

62. Dolan NC, Reifler DR, McDermott MM et al. Adherence to screening mammography recommendations in a university general medicine clinic. J of General Int. Med 1995; 10(6):299-306.

63. Rost K, Frankel R. The introduction of the older patient's problems in the medical visit. J Health and Aging 1993.

64. Adelman RD, Greene MG, Charon R et al. The content of physician and elderly patient interaction in the medical primary care encounter. Comm Res 1992; 19:370-380.

65. Beisecker AE, Beisecker TD. Patient information-seeking behaviors when communicating with doctors. Med Care 1990; 28:19-28

66. Wolf AM, Becker DM. Cancer screening and informed patient discussions. Truth and Consequences. Arch Int Med 1996; 156(10):1069-72

67. Adelman RD, Greene MG, Charon R. Issues in the physician-elderly patient interaction. Aging and Society 1991; 2:127-148.

68. Street RL. Information-giving in medical consultations: The influence of patients' communicative styles and personal characteristics. Soc Sci Med 1991; 32: 541-548.

69. Beisecker AE. Aging and the desire for information and input in medical decisions: Patient consumerism in medical encounters. The Gerontologist 1988; 28:330-335.

70. Kreps GL. A systematic analysis of health communication with the aged. In: Giles H, Coupland N, Wuemann JM, eds. Communication, Health and the Elderly. London: Manchester University Press, 1990:135-154.

71. Waitzkin H. Information giving in medical care. J Health Soc Behavior 1985; 26:81-101.

72. Labrecque MS, Blanchard CG, Ruckdeschel JC et al. The impact of family presence on the physician-cancer patient interaction. Soc Sci Med 1991; 33:1253-61.

73. Beisecker AE. The influence of a companion on the doctor-elderly patient interaction. Health Comm 1989; 1:55-70.

74. Coe RM, Communication and medical care outcomes: Analysis of conversations between doctors and elderly patients. In: Ward RA, Tobin SS eds. Health in Aging. New York: Springer, 1987.

75. Mandelblatt J, Traxler M, Lakin P et al. Mammography and Papanicolaou smear use by elderly poor black women. The Harlem Study Team. J Am Geriatri Soc 1992; 40(10):1001-7.

76. Champion VL. Compliance with guidelines for mammography screening. Cancer Detection and Prevention 1992; 16(4):253-8.

77. Fox SA, Klos DS, Tsou CV et al. Breast cancer screening recommendations: Current status of women's knowledge. Fam Comm Health 1987; 10(3):39-50.

78. Richardson A. Factors likely to affect participation in mammographic screening. New Zealand Med J 1990; 103(887): 155-6.

79. Gardiner JC, Mullan PB, Rosenman KD et al. Mammography usage and knowledge about breast cancer in a Michigan farm population before and after an educational intervention. J Cancer Educ 1995; 10(3):155-62.

80. Phillips JM. Adherence to breast cancer screening guidelines among African-American women of differeing employment status. Cancer Nursing 1995; 18(4): 258-69.

81. Morgan C, Park E, Cortes DE. Beliefs, knowledge, and behavior about cancer among urban Hispanic women. J Natl Cancer Inst Monogr 1995; (18):57-63.

82. Mah Z, Bryant H. Age as a factor in breast cancer knowledge, attitudes and screening behavior. Can Med Assoc J 1992; 146(12):2167-74.

83. Perez-Stable EJ, Sabogal F, Otero-Sabogal R et al. Misconceptions about cancer among Latinos and Anglos. JAMA 1992; 268(22):3219-23.

84. Ruiz MS, Marks G, Richardson JL. Language acculturation and screening practices of elderly Hispanic women. The role of exposure to health-related information from the media. J Aging and Health 1992; 4(2):268-81.

85. Suarez L, Pulley L. Comparing acculturation scales and their relationship to cancer screening among older Mexican-American women. J Natl Cancer Inst Monogr 1995(18):41-7.

86. Flores ET, Mata AG. Latino male attitudes and behaviors on their spouses' and partners' cancer-screening behavior: focus group findings. J Natl Cancer Inst Monogr 1995(18):87-93.

87. Kernohan EE. Evaluation of a pilot study for breast and cervical cancer screening with Bradford's minority ethnic women; a community development approach, 1991-93. Br J Cancer 1996; 74(29):s42-6.

88. Lieberman DA. Cost-effectiveness model for colon cancer screening. Gastroenterology 1995; 109(6):1781-90.

89. Morisky D, Fox SA, Murata P et al. The role of needs assessment in designing a community-based mammography education program for urban women. Health Educ Res 1989; 4:469-478.

90. Friedman LC, Woodruff A, Lane M et al. Breast cancer screening behaviors and intentions among asymptomatic women 50 years or age and older. Am J Prev Med 1995; 11(4):218-23.

91. Herman CJ, Speroff T, Cebul RD. Improving compliance with breast cancer screening in older women. Results from a randomized controlled trial. Arch Int Med 1995; 155(7):717-22.

92. Montano D, Taplin S. A test of an expanded theory of reasoned action predict mammography participation. Soc Sci Med 1991; 32:733-741.

93. Stein J, Fox S, Murata P et al. Mammography usage and the health belief model.

Health Educ Q 1992; 19:1-16.

94. Aiken L, West S, Woodward C et al. Health beliefs and compliance with mammography-screening recommendations in asymptomatic women. Health Psychol 1994; 12:122-9.

95. Hyman R, Baker S, Ephraim R et al. Health belief model variables as predictors of screening mammography utilization. J Beh Med 1994; 17:391-406.

96. O'Connor A, Perrault D. Importance of physician's role highlighted in survey of women's breast screening practices. Can J Public Health 1995; 86:42-5.

97. Wardle J. Women at risk of ovarian cancer. J Natl Cancer Inst Monogr 1995; 17:81-5.

98. Vernon S, Vogel V, Halabi S et al. Breast cancer screening behaviors and attitudes in three racial/ethnic groups. Cancer 1992; 69:165-74.

99. Burg M, Lane D, Polednak A. Age group differences in the use of breast cancer screening tests. J Aging Health 1990; 2:514-30.

100. Constanza M, Stoddard A, Gaw V et al. The risk factors of age and family history and their relationship to screening mammography utilization. J Am Geriatr Soc 1992; 40:774-778.

101. King E, Resch N, Rimer B et al. Breast cancer screening practices among retirement community women. Prev Med 1993; 22:1-19.

102. Lerman C, Rimer B, Trock B et al. Factors associated with repeat adherence to breast cancer screening. Prev Med 1990; 19:279-290.

103. Sutton S, Eisner E, Burklow J. Health communications to older Americans as a special population: The National Cancer Institute's consumer-based approach. Cancer 1994; 74:2194-9.

104. Rimer B, Keintz M, Kessler H et al. Why women resist screening mammography: Patient related barriers. Radiology 1989; 172:243-246.

105. Zapka J, Berkowitz E. A qualitative study about breast cancer screening in older women: Implications for research. J Gerontolo 1992; 47(Supplement):93-100.

106. Lidbrink E, Frisell J, Brandberg Y et al. Nonattendance in the Stockholm mam-

mography screening trial: relative mortality and reasons for nonattendance. Breast Cancer Research and Treatment 1995; 35(3):267-75.

107. Burack R, Liang J. The acceptance and completion of mammography by older black women. Am J Public Health 1989; 4:721-726.

108. Richardson J, Marks G, Solis J et al. Frequency and adequacy of breast cancer screening among elderly Hispanic women. Prev Med 1987; 16:761-774.

109. Taplin S, Montano D. Attitudes, age, and participation in mammographic screening: A prospective analysis. J Am Board Fam Pract 1993; 6:612-23.

110. Wardlow H, Curry RH. "Sympathy for my body": breast cancer and mammography at two Atlanta clinics. Med Anthropol 1996; 16(4):319-40.

111. Sutton S, Eisner E, Burklow J. Health communications to older Americans as a special population: The National Cancer Institute's consumer-based approach. Cancer 1995; 74:2194-9.

112. Roetzheim R, Van DD, Brownlee H et al. Reverse targeting in a media-promoted breast cancer screening project. Cancer 1992; 70:1152-1158.

113. Burnett CB, Steakley CS, Tefft, MC. Barriers to breast and cervical cancer screening in underserved women of the District of Columbia. Oncology Nursing Forum 1995; 22(10):1551-7.

114. Suarez L, Lloyd L, Weiss N et al. Effect of social networks on cancer-screening behavior of older Mexican-American women. J Natl Cancer Inst 1994; 86: 775-9.

115. Kang S, Bloom J: Social support and cancer screening among older black Americans. J Natl Cancer Inst 1993; 85: 737-742.

116. Slenker S, Grant M. Attitudes, beliefs and knowledge about mammography among women over forty years of age. J Cancer Educ 1989; 4:61-65.

117. Czaja R, McFall S, Warnecke R et al. Preferences of community physicians for cancer screening guidelines. Ann Intern Med 1994; 120:602-8.

118. Weinberger M, Saunders A, Bearon L et al. Physician-related barriers to breast cancer screening in older women. J Gerontol 1992; 47:111-117.

119. Stange K, Kelly R, Chao J et al. Physician agreement with US Preventive Services Task Force recommendations. J Fam Pract 1992; 34:409-16.

120. US Preventive Services Task Force. Guide to Clinical Preventive Services, 2nd ed. Baltimore: Williams and Wilkins, 1996.

121. Clasen C, Vernon S, Mullen P et al. A survey of physician belief and self-reported practices concerning screening for early detection of cancer. Soc Sci Med 1994; 39:841-9.

122. Montano D, Manders D, Phillips W. Family physician beliefs about cancer screening: Development of a survey instrument. J Fam Pract 1990; 30:313-9.

123. Warner S, Worden J, Solomon L et al. Physician interest in breast cancer screening education. J Fam Pract 1989; 29:281-285.

124. Lemkau JP, Grady K, Carlson S. Maximizing the referral of older women for screen mammography, 1996. Arch Fam Medicine, 1996, 5(3):174-78.

125. Lichtman SM. Physiological aspects of aging. Impl for tmnt of cancer, Drugs and Aging, 1995, 7(3):212-225.

126. Williams P, Williams M. Barriers and incentives for primary care physicians in cancer prevention and detection. Cancer 1988; 61:2382-2390.

127. Costanza M. The extent of breast cancer screening in older women. Cancer 1994; 74(Suppl):2046-50.

128. Cohen H. Breast cancer screening in older women: The geriatrician/internist perspective. J Gerontol 1992; 47:134-6.

129. Greene M; Adelman R; Charon R et al. Ageism in the medical encounter: An exploratory study of the doctor-elderly patient relationship. Lang Commun 1986; 6:113-124.

130. Roetzheim R, Fox S, Leake B. Physician-reported determinants of screening mammography in older women: The impact of physician and practice characteristics. J Am Geriatr Soc 1995; 43:1-5.

131. Cohen D, Littenberg B, Wetzel C et al. Improving physician compliance with preventive medicine guidelines. Med Care 1982; 20:1040-5.

132. Prislin M, Vandenbark M, Clarkson Q. The impact of health screening flow sheet on the performance and documentation of health screening procedures. Fam Med 1986; 18:290-2.

133. Cheney C, Ramsdell J. Effect of medical records' checklists on implementation of periodic health measures. Am J Med 1987; 83:129-36.

134. Schreiner D, Petrusa E, Rettie C et al. Improving compliance with preventive medicine procedures in a housestaff training program. South Med J 1988; 81:1553-7.

135. Robie P. Improving and sustaining outpatient cancer screening by medicine residents. South Med J 1988; 81:902-5.

136. Pierce M, Lundy S, Palanisamy A et al. Prospective randomized controlled trials of methods of call and recall for cervical cytology screening. Br Med J 1989; 299: 160-2.

137. Winickoff R, Coltin K, Morgan M et al. Improving physician performance through peer comparison feedback. Med Care 1984; 22:527-34.

138. McPhee S, Bird J, Jenkins C et al. Promoting cancer screening. A randomized, controlled trials of three interventions. Arch Intern Med 1989; 149:1866-1872.

139. McDonald C, Hui S, Smith D et al. Reminders to physicians from an introspective computer medical record a two-year randomized trial. Ann Intern Med 1984; 100:130-8.

140. Tierney W, Hui S, McDonald C. Delayed feedback of physician performance vs. immediate reminders to perform preventive care. Med Care 1986; 24:659-66.

141. McDowell I, Newell C, Rosser N. Computerized reminders to encourage cervical screening in family practice. J Fam Pract 1989; 28:420-4.

142. Chambers C, Balaban D, Carlson B et al. Microcomputer-generated reminders: Improving the compliance of primary care physicians with mammography screening guidelines. J Fam Pract 1989; 29:273-280.

143. Chodroff C. Cancer screening and immunization quality assurance using personal computer. QRB Qual Rev Bull 1990; 16:279-87.

144. Turner B, Day S, Borenstein B. A controlled trial to improve delivery of preventive care: Physician or patient reminders? J Gen Intern Med 1989; 4: 403-9.

145. Burack RC, Gimotty PA, George J et al. Promoting screening mammography in inner-city settings: a randomized controlled trial of computerized reminders as a component of a program to facilitate mammorgraphy. Med Care, 1994, Jun;32(60:609-24.

146. Bird J, McPhee S, Jenkins C et al. Three strategies to promote cancer screening: How feasible is wide-scale implementation? Med Care 1990; 28:1005-1012.

147. Petravage J, Swedberg J. Patient response to sigmoidoscopy recommendations via mailed reminders. J Fam Pract 1988; 27:387-9.

148. Wolosin R. Effect of appointment scheduling and reminder postcards on adherence to mammography recommendations. J Fam Pract 1990; 30:542-7.

149. Nattinger A, Panzer R, Janus J. Improving the utilization of screening mammography in primary care practices. Arch Intern Med 1989; 149:2087-2092.

150. McPhee S, Bird J, Fordham D et al. Promoting cancer prevention activities by primary care physicians. JAMA 1991; 266:538-544.

151. Kiefe CI, McKay SV, Halevy A et al. Is cost a barrier to screening mammography for low-income women receiving Medicare benefits? A randomized trial. Arch Int Med 1994, June 13; 154(11): 1217-24.

152. Becker D, Gomez E, Kaiser D et al. Improving preventive care at a medical clinic: How can the patient help? Am J Prev Med 1989; 5:353-9.

153. Davidson R, Fletcher S, Retchin S et al. A nurse-initiated reminder system for the periodic health examination: Implementation and evaluation. Arch Intern Med 1984; 144:2167-70.

154. Thompson R, Michnich M, Gray J et al. Maximizing compliance with Hemoccult screening for colon cancer in clinical practice. Med Care 1986; 24:904-14.

155. Belcher D. Implementing preventive services: Success and failure in an outpa-

tient trial. Arch Intern Med 1990; 150: 2533-41.

156. Foley E, D'Amico F, Merenstein J. Improving mammography recommendation: A nurse-initiated intervention. J Am Board Fam Pract 1990; 3:87-92.

157. Dietrich A, Sox C, Tosteson T, Woodruff C. Durability of improved physician early detection of cancer after conclusion of intervention support. Cancer Epidemiol Biomarkers Prev 1994; 3:335-40.

158. Suarez L, Nichols D, Brady C. Use of peer role models to increase Pap smear and mammogram screening in Mexican-American and black women. Am J Prev Med 1993; 9:290-6.

159. Herman C, Speroff T, Cebul R. Improving compliance with breast cancer screening in older women: Results of a randomized controlled trial. Arch Intern Med 1995; 155:717-22.

160. Lantz P, Stencil D, Lippert M et al. Breast and cervical cancer screening in a low-income managed care sample: The efficacy of physician letters and phone calls. Am J Public Health 1995; 85:834-6.

161. Costanza M, Zapka J, Harris D et al. Impact of a physician intervention program to increase breast cancer screening. Cancer Epidemiol Biomarkers Prev 1992; 1:581-589.

152. Trock B, Rimer B, King E et al. Impact of an HMO-based intervention to increase mammography utilization. Cancer Epidemiol Biomark Prev 1993; 2:151-6.

163. Zapka J, Harris D, Hosmer D et al. Effect of a community health center intervention on breast cancer screening among Hispanic American women. Health Serv Res 1993; 28:223-235.

164. Lane D, Polednak A, Burg M. Effect of continuing medical education and cost reduction on physician compliance with mammography screening guidelines. J Fam Pract 1991; 33:359-368.

165. Mandelblatt J, Traxler M, Lakin P et al. A nurse practitioner intervention to increase breast and cervical cancer screening for poor, elderly, black women. The Harlem Study Team. J Gen Intern Med 1993; 8:173-8.

166. Fletcher S, Harris R, Gonzalez J et al. Increasing mammography utilization: A controlled study. J Natl Cancer Inst 1993; 85:112-120.

167. Forsyth M, Fulton D, Lane D et al. Changes in knowledge, attitudes and behavior of women participating in a community outreach education program on breast cancer screening. Patient Educ Couns 1992; 19:241-50.

168. Zapka J, Costanza M, Harris D et al. Impact of a breast cancer screening community intervention. Prev Med 1993; 22:34-53.

169. Bastani R, Marcus A, Maxwell A et al. Evaluation of an intervention to increase mammography screening in Los Angeles. Prev Med 1994; 23:83-90.

170. Lane D, Burg M. Strategies to increase mammography utilization among community health center visitors: Improving awareness, accessibility, and affordability. Med Care 1993; 31:175-81.

171. Yancey AK, Tanjasiri SP, Klein M et al. Increased cancer screening behavior in women of color by culturally sensitive video exposure. Prev Med 1995; Mar, 24(2):142-8

172. Haynes S, Mara J. The picture of health: How to increase breast cancer screening in your community. National Cancer Institute; 1993; No. 94-3604.

CHAPTER 10

GENETIC TESTING FOR BREAST CANCER PREDISPOSITION

Jeffrey N. Weitzel

B reast and ovarian cancers are common, often lethal malignancies in women. Improved survival may result from early detection programs. Inheritance plays a role in the development of all human cancers to varying degrees. It is estimated that 5-10% of breast cancer and ovarian cancer cases occur as part of heritable syndromes due to mutations in highly penetrant genes. The cumulative risk for developing breast cancer in hereditary breast ovarian cancer (HBOC) families is estimated at 51% by age 50 years and 85% by age 70 years. The cloning of the *BRCA1* gene on chromosome 17, and of a second high-risk locus on chromosome 13 (*BRCA2*), has provided the opportunity to examine the role of specific BRCA genotypes in cancer predisposition. Genetic and allelic heterogeneity make screening for mutations in complex genes, such as *BRCA1* or *BRCA2*, relatively difficult, so general population analysis is not feasible or appropriate at this time. However, laboratory testing to detect genetic cancer predisposition has the potential to provide clinically useful information for populations targeted because of high-risk features or among whom only specific mutations are prevalent. Biotechnology companies have scrambled to market susceptibility testing for breast cancer risk based on these findings. Still, a perceived lack of effective therapeutic interventions and potential adverse effects on cost of premiums and eligibility for insurance are significant barriers to widespread application of this new technology. This chapter will provide an overview of cancer genetics and characteristics of hereditary breast cancer syndromes. The current status, benefits and limitations of genetic susceptibility testing for breast and ovarian cancer will be discussed.

BACKGROUND

CLINICAL FEATURES OF HEREDITARY CANCER AND THE ROLE OF TUMOR SUPPRESSOR GENES

As a group, specific familial cancer syndromes make up only about 5% of all cancers. However, lessons learned from identifying the underlying genetic abnormalities in some of these disorders have been instrumental in understanding normal cell cycle controls and the genetic basis of common sporadic cancers. The existence of tumor suppressor genes was postulated by Alfred Knudson in 1971, based on statistical observations of the distinguishing clinical features of familial retinoblastoma compared to the sporadic form of the disease (primarily earlier onset and multifocal disease in the familial cases).[1] Knudson suggested that patients with the hereditary form of the disease already have a germline mutation in all cells and that the likelihood of acquiring a second mutation or "hit" in the remaining functional copy of the critical gene in any given cell was consequently greater. Thus, multifocal tumors may occur at an earlier age. This "two-hit hypothesis" is one of the fundamental tenets of the molecular basis of hereditary predisposition to cancer. The gene responsible for retinoblastoma susceptibility (Rb1) was localized to chromosome 13 and cloned in 1987.[2] Molecular genetic and functional analysis of Rb1 confirmed the mechanism of inheritance and its role as a tumor suppressor gene.[3,4] The retinoblastoma trait may be passed on by a single mutated allele in the germline, hence the pattern of inheritance is autosomal dominant with a 50% risk of passing the abnormal allele on to each offspring. However, the genetic mechanism in an individual cancer cell is recessive, requiring the loss of function of the remaining wild type (normal) copy of the gene. With few exceptions, the Mendelian (single gene trait) cancer predisposition disorders are autosomal dominant and are caused by germline mutations in putative tumor suppressor genes.[5]

Hallmarks of hereditary cancer susceptibility are outlined in Table 10.1 (below).[6-8] Most of the single gene disorders that may predispose patients to cancer are rare. However, hereditary breast ovarian cancer

(HBOC) and hereditary nonpolyposis colorectal cancer (HNPCC) are exceptions to this rule.

MODELS USED FOR PREDICTING BREAST CANCER RISK IN THE GENERAL POPULATION

Improvements in screening techniques have made significant contributions to the early detection of breast cancer. Improved survival may result from early detection. Physicians thus face the task of identifying their patients at increased risk, such as women with a family history of breast or ovarian cancer, and providing appropriate tumor surveillance for them. There are a variety of factors that may influence a woman's risk for breast and/or ovarian cancer, which share several epidemiologic, genetic and hormonal features. Factors associated with increased risk include: prolonged exposure to sex hormones, early menarche, late menopause, and nulliparity. Having a close relative with breast or ovarian cancer confers an increased risk of breast cancer (two- to three-fold in the general population). Epidemiologic data indicates that 6-19% of women with breast cancer have a relative with breast or ovarian cancer.[9] Empiric risk estimates may be derived from this type of data and several investigators have constructed working models to predict an individual's risk. Gail et al developed a method to estimate the chance that a woman with given age and risk factors will develop breast cancer over a specified interval.[10] The risk factors used were age at menarche, age at first live birth, number of previous breast biopsies and number of first degree relatives with breast cancer. The formula has only been validated for Anglo women

---

Table 10.1. Hallmarks of hereditary cancer

- Cancer at an unusually young age (or in the less usually affected sex)
- Vertical transmission of cancer within a family
- Multifocal or bilateral disease in paired organs
- Multiple primary cancers in an individual
- Clustering of unusual or rare cancers

undergoing regular mammographic screening, and really only applies for women whose families do not otherwise fit the profile of hereditary breast ovarian cancer syndrome (HBOC, see below).[11] Although the model is being used clinically in some centers, and in the research setting (risk estimated by the model is used as part of the entrance criteria for the tamoxifen breast cancer prevention research trial), it has yet to gain widespread acceptance.

An often underutilized risk assessment tool is the family history. Claus et al determined useful age-specific risk estimates, based on the number and age of first and second degree relatives with breast cancer, from analysis of epidemiologic data from the Cancer and Steroid Hormone (CASH) study.[12] These tables can be used for the purpose of counseling women at a higher risk of breast cancer development. One can use both of these clinical tools to help fit women into broad risk categories; low (baseline population risk), moderate and high risk (possibly fitting the phenotype of highly penetrant hereditary breast cancer syndromes).[13] Counseling and surveillance recommendations may then be tailored to each risk category.

INHERITED BREAST CANCER SUSCEPTIBILITY

An estimated 5-10% of breast cancer and ovarian cancer cases occur as part of heritable syndromes due to mutations in highly penetrant genes.[12] Several separate syndromes are thought to exist. Hereditary breast ovarian cancer (HBOC) syndrome is discussed at length below. Breast cancer predisposition is seen in the rare Li-Fraumeni syndrome (associated with germline p53 mutations), in women with a mutation in one copy of the ataxia telangiectasia (ATM) gene and in association with Cowden disease (a genodermatosis with variable susceptibility to breast cancer, as well as fibroproliferative breast disease and ovarian cysts). Table 10.2 lists genes implicated in breast cancer susceptibility thus far. Increased risk for ovarian cancer and endometrial cancer may be seen in hereditary nonpolyposis colon cancer (HNPCC) families, though breast cancer does not appear to be increased in this disorder.[14] Clinical features of hereditary breast cancers include earlier age of occurrence than is usual for that neoplasm and more frequent occurrence of bilateral disease. Genetic segregation studies of breast cancer have demonstrated that, among women with breast cancer diagnosed before age 30, approximately one-third may have their disease because of an inherited susceptibility.[12]

Hereditary breast ovarian cancer syndrome and *BRCA1*

The HBOC syndrome is characterized by inherited susceptibility to carcinomas of the breast and of the ovary, with breast tumors generally being more common. A highly penetrant disease, the cumulative risk of developing breast or ovarian cancer in the disorder approaches 90% over a woman's lifetime.[15] This is in striking contrast to the

---

Table 10.2. Hereditary breast cancer genes

- *BRCA1*
- *BRCA2*
- *BRCA3...?*
  - Estrogen receptor locus (2 families linked)
  - Chromosome 8p12-22 (8 families, LOD score 2.5)
- Cowdens disease locus (chromosome 10q22)
- *p53*
- *ATM* (Ataxia telangiectasia mutated)
- Rare *HRAS*1-variable number of tandem repeat (VNTR) Alleles

lifetime risk of 11% for sporadic occurrence of breast cancer in the general population. Most impressive is the earlier age at onset typical of the inherited form of this disease, with 51% of women developing breast cancer by age 50 years, compared to 2% for the general population. Analysis of segregation data suggested the existence of a rare autosomal dominant gene trait to account for a subset of families at extraordinary risk.[16,17] Mary-Claire King and associates provided the first convincing evidence for localization of a gene (BReast CAncer gene 1), responsible for a proportion of HBOC, to the long arm (q-arm) of chromosome 17.[18] Based on this landmark study, an international consortium of breast cancer researchers collaborated in the linkage analysis of 214 breast cancer families.[15] Linkage was strongest for families that included ovarian cancer. Studies of tumor-specific deletions of chromosome 17q, and of informative recombinations of genetic markers within BRCA1-linked families, focused the search on a relatively small segment of the chromosome.[19-22] After what seemed like a long wait (two genes associated with hereditary nonpolyposis colon cancer were discovered in the interim),[23,24] the cloning of a candidate BRCA1 gene was finally announced in 1994.[25] The coding region of BRCA1 contains 5,592 base pairs split into 22 exons and is distributed over a 100,000 base pair segment of chromosome 17. Identification of families linked to a second locus on chromosome 13q (BRCA2)[26] has provided the opportunity to examine the role of specific BRCA genotypes in HBOC kindreds. Germline mutations in BRCA1 account for cancer susceptibility in 40%-50% of female breast cancer families and >80% of breast-ovarian cancer families.[27] More than 100 different mutations in BRCA1 have been reported, most of them "private" (unique to a given family).[28-31] The majority of observed BRCA1 mutations result in a truncated (nonfunctional) protein.[28] The Breast Cancer Information Core (BIC) database was created to compile mutations in both BRCA1 and BRCA2 (see below). Figure 10.1 depicts the genetic organization of BRCA1

and BRCA2, along with the position, frequency and type of mutations that have been reported to the database as of 1996.

A second gene involved in HBOC: BRCA2

At about the same time that the cloning of BRCA1 was finally announced, Wooster and colleagues localized the second major gene associated with hereditary breast cancer, BRCA2, to chromosome 13q.[26] The locus was distinct from the nearby retinoblastoma gene and appeared to be responsible for almost half of site-specific breast cancer families and the majority of male breast cancer families. A portion of the gene was cloned and the first mutations reported by the same group shortly thereafter.[32] The complete sequence was subsequently obtained and reveals a large gene with over 11,000 nucleotides in 27 coding exons, spread out over 70,000 bases of genomic DNA.[33] The gene encodes a 3,418 amino acid protein of as yet unknown function. Similar to BRCA1, numerous distinct mutations have been identified, the majority of which are predicted to interrupt the BRCA2 coding sequence leading to a truncated protein product. BRCA2 mutations were found in 8 of 49 site-specific breast cancer families in a recent study using single strand conformation analysis (SSCA) followed by direct sequencing.[34] Mutations were found in all four families that included male breast cancer. Other factors which predicted the presence of a BRCA2 mutation included a case of breast cancer diagnosed at age 35 or below (P = 0.01) and a family history of pancreatic cancer (P = 0.03).[34] BRCA2 mutations were found in the germline of 14% (7/50) of men with breast cancer in a series not selected on the basis of family history. Still, six of the seven gene-positive cases were found to have a family history of breast cancer.[35] Although early-onset breast cancer is a feature of most HBOC families characterized to date, families with later-onset breast cancer have also been identified in studies of specific BRCA2 mutations.[36]

Overall, mutations in BRCA1 or BRCA2 account for the vast majority of families with

HBOC.[37] The cumulative age-specific penetrance risks for breast and ovarian cancer have been estimated from the *BRCA1*-linked family data.[38] These studies also revealed an increased risk of prostate cancer (three-fold or 8% risk by age 70 years) in men with a *BRCA1* mutation and a four-fold increased risk of colon cancer in both men and women carriers (6% by age 70, compared with 1-2% in noncarriers). The cumulative risk for developing breast cancer in HBOC families is 51% by age 50 years and 85% by age 70 years.[27,38] The specific risk for ovarian cancer among these families is extremely variable, ranging from 20-60% by age 70 years. The greatest likelihood for linkage to *BRCA1* (>80%) was found among the families that included at least one case of ovarian cancer. Families with two or more cases of early-onset breast cancer and two or more cases of ovarian cancer have a 92% probability of being linked to *BRCA1*.[39] Since all of the earlier studies were affected by ascertainment bias (favoring families with multiple breast cancers of early onset), the risk associated with *BRCA1* mutations in families without a prominent cancer history is unclear. The frequency of highly penetrant *BRCA1* mutations in the general population has been estimated at 1:300 to 1:800, based on epidemiologic modeling. The frequency of less penetrant mutations is not yet known because general population-based screening for *BRCA1* and *BRCA2* mutations is technically difficult and prohibitively expensive at present.

Special considerations for defined populations

Although the majority of *BRCA1* mutations are unique to a given family, several mutations have been observed repeatedly, and haplotype analyses suggested the possibility of founder mutations in some cases.[40] Founder effects may be seen in any genetically and/or geographically isolated population. Nine mutations in *BRCA1* were found in 15 of 47 (32%) HBOC families in Southern Sweden. Haplotype analysis of the four recurrent mutations suggested the existence of founder effects.[41] Similarly, a high prevalence of the *BRCA2* 999del5 mutation in Icelandic breast and ovarian cancer patients associated with a common haplotype suggested a founder effect.[42,43] Nearly half of all male breast cancer in Iceland is attributable to this single mutation.[42] Historically, some ethnic groups may be at particular risk. A team of investigators at the National Center for Human Genome Research found that the 185delAG mutation of *BRCA1* (the deletion of two nucleotides, AG, at position 185 in the gene) was detected in approximately 1% of Jews of Eastern European descent (Ashkenazim) in a population not selected for cancer.[44] The investigators estimated that the 185delAG mutation might account for 16% of breast cancers and 39% of ovarian cancers occurring in Ashkenazi women before age 50 years. Other genetic disorders such as Tay Sachs disease have also been observed predominantly within the Jewish Ashkenazi population or at a significantly higher level than in the general population. Epidemiological studies of one such disorder, idiopathic torsion dystonia (ITD), suggest that a small founder population from the "Jewish Pale of Settlement" (historically the western part of Lithuania, Poland and Belarus) may have given rise to the existing Ashkenazi Jewish population.[45] Moreover, haplotype analyses of *BRCA1* mutations in 61 HBOC families indicated that the 185delAG mutation is estimated to have arisen approximately 38 generations or 760 years ago, around 1235 A.D., overlapping with the estimate for the appearance of the ITD gene.[46] This data along with events in European Jewish history support the concept of a founder effect in Ashkenazim.[47] Additional studies have detected the 185delAG mutation in 8 of 39 Jewish women (21%) with breast cancer at or before the age of 40.[48] None of these women had a family history of breast cancer definitive for HBOC, although seven of the eight had at least one affected first- or second-degree relative. One can calculate attributable risks using the prevalence figure of 1 in 107 for the 185delAG mutation in Jewish women and the age-dependent penetrance curves for the observed risk of breast

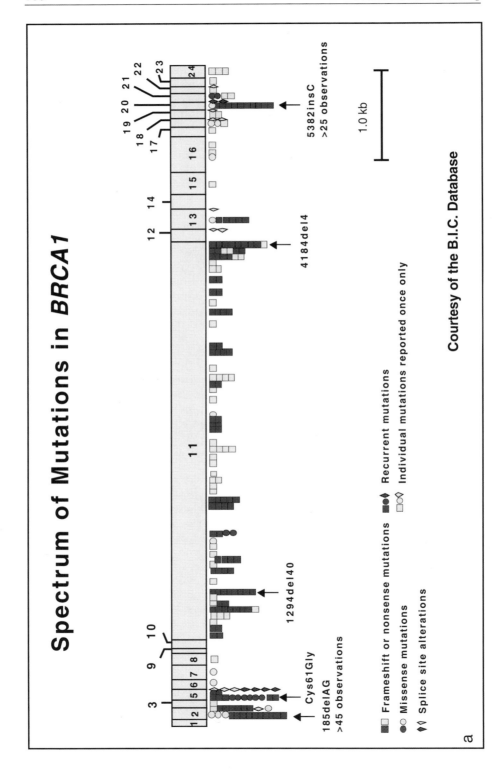

Spectrum of Mutations in *BRCA1*

Courtesy of the B.I.C. Database

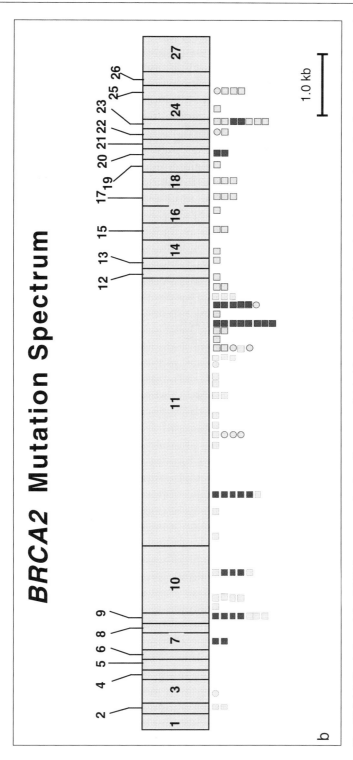

Fig. 10.1 (a) Depiction of the *BRCA1* gene organization. Exons are divided by vertical lines and numbered on or above the diagram. The type of mutation (frameshift or nonsense, missense, or splice site), location and recurrent or individual status is indicated. The 185delAG and 5382insC mutations are prevalent in persons of Ashkenazi Jewish decent and/or Baltic decent, respectively. Three other relatively common mutations are also indicated.

(b) *BRCA2* gene organization is depicted, along with the same mutation information as described for *BRCA1*. Both diagrams are courtesy of the Breast Cancer Information Core (BIC) database and are available through the world wide web.

cancer in families with *BRCA1* mutations. For Jewish women under 40 with breast cancer, 27% would be expected to have germline *BRCA1* mutations.[31] Unfortunately, the frequent occurrence of this mutation in Ashkenazim does not exclude the possibility of other *BRCA1* mutations within the same population. Families with the 5382insC mutation in *BRCA1* also share an ancestral chromosome.[30,40] A recent report suggested that the 6174delT (the deletion of a thymidine nucleotide, T, at position 6174 in the gene) frame shift mutation in the *BRCA2* gene was also relatively common among Jewish women with breast cancer (8% of those diagnosed before age 42 years).[49] Thus, either the *BRCA1* 185delAG or the *BRCA2* 6174delT mutation were detected in 29% of Jewish women who developed breast cancer before the age of 42. Table 10.3 summarizes several population-based surveys that were performed among persons of Jewish decent to approximate the frequency of these specific *BRCA* mutations in cohorts not selected for cancer history.[44,50,51] Remarkably, 1 in 40 are predicted to be carriers of one of these mutations. Approximately 2-3% of the North American population, or about six million people, are of Jewish decent. The frequency of three recurrent *BRCA1* mutations and one recurrent *BRCA2* mutation was assessed for 220 North American Ashkenazi Jewish breast cancer

families (selected on the basis of having a minimum of two women affected by breast cancer, at least one of which occurred before age 50).[52] Although the 188del11 mutation in *BRCA1* was seen in four Ashkenazi Jewish women in a previous report,[53] none were found in this cohort of 220 families. These studies resulted in important observations about the prevalence of specific mutations in a defined population, the incidence of cancers other than breast or ovarian and a crude estimate of genotype-specific penetrance.

Given the high prevalence of these specific *BRCA* mutations in the Jewish population, it is not unexpected that homozygotes (inheriting the same mutation from each parent) or double heterozygotes (bearing mutation in both *BRCA1* and *BRCA2*) may be found. A recent report documented the co-inheritance of both the *BRCA1* 185delAG and the *BRCA2* 6174delT mutations in an individual.[54] Interestingly, this patient developed both breast and ovarian cancer, but neither occurred when she was young. Because of the possibility of independent *BRCA* mutations segregating on both the paternal and maternal sides of a family of Ashkenazi Jewish decent, it would be prudent to test for the presence of all three common mutations in each family member, even when one of these mutations has already been identified.

Table 10.3. Frequency of specific BRCA1 and BRCA2 mutations in the Jewish population and in Jewish breast cancer families

| | Mutation | | | |
	185delAG	5382insC	6174delT	Total
Population Frequency	1.05%	0.11%	1.36%	2.52%
Site-specific Breast Cancer	20.3%	5.1%	3.6%	29%
Breast Ovarian Cancer Syndrome	52.4%	15.9%	4.9%	73.2%

Data compiled from refs. 44, 50, 51, 52.

In a series of ovarian cancer patients ascertained without regard to family history, 6 of 31 (19.4%) Jewish patients were carriers of the *BRCA1* 185 delAG mutation compared to 0 of 23 Jewish controls.[55] None of the 6 patients with the mutation had a family history consistent with hereditary breast ovarian cancer syndrome. The same mutation was detected in 38.9% of ovarian cancer patients with a positive family history, and 13.3% of family history negative ovarian cancer cases in an Israeli series.[56]

Genotype—Phenotype correlations

Prior studies have failed to demonstrate a significant difference in the histology of breast cancers occurring in women bearing *BRCA1* mutations and that in sporadic disease, although there was a trend toward higher grade in the *BRCA1*-associated tumors.[57] There are no conclusive studies of the influence, if any, of *BRCA1* genotype on prognosis for age–stage-matched breast tumors. However, a recent report suggested the possibility of a less penetrant mutation in *BRCA2* (6174 delT).[52] Tonin et al observed that this mutation was seen in only 4% of 220 North American Jewish breast cancer families (each with two or more breast cancer cases), in spite of the fact that the 6174delT allele is ten times more frequent in the Jewish population than the *BRCA1* 5382insC mutation seen in 22% of breast cancer families in this study. Lifetime risk for breast cancer was estimated to be < 25%, compared to > 85% for *BRCA1* mutations. Prospective studies designed to assess penetrance of the 6174delT mutation in a population-based survey will be necessary to confirm the true risk for women bearing this mutation in the germline.

Ovarian cancer risk is particularly variable among HBOC kindreds. Early reports suggested that ovarian cancer was more likely to be associated with *BRCA1* than *BRCA2*.[37] It has been suggested that there is a modest correlation between ovarian cancer occurrence and inactivating mutations in the 5' two-thirds of *BRCA1* versus mutations in the 3' end of the gene.[58] Although exceptions to this generalization are numer-ous for *BRCA1*, recent analysis of the mutation distribution along the length of the *BRCA2* gene indicated a significant genotype-phenotype correlation for breast and ovarian cancer risk. The highest risk for ovarian cancer relative to breast cancer was associated with a cluster of mutations in a small region of exon 11 (between nucleotides 3035 and 6629).[59] Observations such as this may be important in counseling women at risk for cancer due to *BRCA2*. In addition, better survival was reported for *BRCA1*-associated advanced stage ovarian cancer cases compared to age- and stage-matched controls (77 months vs. 29 months).[60] Interestingly, there is precedent for a less aggressive phenotype being associated with hereditary cases for colon cancer associated with HNPCC.[61,62]

Finally, the spectrum of tumors that may be associated with mutations in *BRCA1* and *BRCA2* continues to grow as more families are characterized. As noted above, patients bearing mutations in *BRCA1* are at modestly increased risk for prostate cancer and colon cancer. In addition, cancers of the fallopian tube (4 of 4 families) and pancreatic cancers (14 of 19 families) were seen significantly more frequently among *BRCA1* and *BRCA2* carriers than would have normally been expected.[52]

BRCA1 biology

The human *BRCA1* gene encodes an 1,863 amino acid (aa) protein of unknown function, though somatic deletion (loss of heterozygosity, LOH) studies imply that BRCA1 functions as a tumor suppressor. Subsequent analysis indicates the presence of a RING domain near the N-terminus.[25] RING domains are cysteine-rich zinc-binding motifs found in a variety of regulatory proteins. Transfection studies of *BRCA1* provided direct evidence for tumor suppressive activity.[63] Wild-type *BRCA1* gene specifically inhibits growth in vitro of several breast and ovarian cancer cell lines, but not fibroblasts or cancer cells from other tumor types. Moreover, a retroviral vector expressing wild-type BRCA1 significantly inhibits tumor growth and resulted in increased survival among mice with established MCF-7 tumors. Studies of the developmental pattern of murine *BRCA1* gene expression imply that *BRCA1* is involved in proliferation and differentiation in multiple tissues, notably in the mammary gland, in response to ovarian hormones.[64] Other studies indicated that steroid hormones may affect BRCA1 expression indirectly by altering the proliferative status of the cells.[65] Together these results suggest that BRCA1 may be a hormone-induced growth regulator. BRCA1 appears to be critical for normal development in mice. Analysis of the effects of BRCA1 deficiency in mice homozygous for mutant *BRCA1* alleles revealed early embryonic lethality, with evidence for significant neuroepithelial abnormalities.[66] Interestingly, a natural human "knockout" has been reported, wherein the affected individual inherited identical inactivating *BRCA1* mutations from each parent. Although the patient developed breast cancer at age 32, she reportedly had no obvious developmental abnormalities and the cancer phenotype was indistinguishable from her affected family members who inherited a single mutated allele.[67]

In contrast to APC (responsible for the colon cancer-associated syndrome familial adenomatous polyposis coli), which is altered somatically in most sporadic colorectal tumors,[68] initial surveys of sporadic breast and ovarian cancers revealed very few tumors with somatic alterations of *BRCA1* sequences.[69] In fact, the specific *BRCA1* mutations discovered by screening the tumors was also present in the germline in all four breast cancer cases. However, exclusively somatic *BRCA1* mutations have been detected in up to 5% of unselected ovarian cancers.[70] The fact that overall patterns of LOH are similar for both sporadic and HBOC-related breast cancer indicates that multiple steps are required for the acquisition of the full tumorigenic phenotype in both cases, though the initiating events may differ.[71] A rapid decline in the relative risk for breast cancer in gene carriers over the age range 30-70 years old suggests that there

may be mechanistic differences between cancers caused by *BRCA1* and sporadic breast cancers.[72]

Aberrant subcellular localization of the BRCA1 protein in most breast and ovarian cancers was recently demonstrated.[69,73] This suggests that abnormalities in BRCA1 are fundamental to the initiation or progression of most breast and ovarian cancers, sporadic as well as familial. Discovering the molecules responsible for the transport of BRCA1 from its site of synthesis to its normal site of action in the nucleus is the focus of intense research, as mutations in these molecules may represent alternative ways to inactivate the crucial function of BRCA1. Recently, a novel BRCA1-associated RING domain protein (BARD1) was identified.[74] Missense mutations that segregate with breast cancer susceptibility disrupt the interaction between BRCA1 and BARD1. Thus, BARD1 may mediate tumor suppression by BRCA1.

BREAST CANCER OCCURRING IN OTHER CONDITIONS WHERE THE GENETIC BASIS IS KNOWN OR SUSPECTED

Cowden disease (CD, multiple hamartoma syndrome) is a cancer-associated autosomal dominant genodermatosis with characteristic mucocutaneous findings including multiple smooth facial papules (cutaneous tricholemmomas), acral keratosis and multiple oral papillomas. Central nervous system manifestations of CD may include megalencephaly, epilepsy and dysplastic gangliocytomas of the cerebellum (Lhermitte Duclos disease).[75] Other associated lesions include benign and malignant disease of the thyroid, intestinal polyps and genitourinary abnormalities. Expression of the disease is variable and penetrance of the dermatological lesions is thought to be complete by age 20. Early diagnosis is important since females with CD have a high frequency of mammary carcinoma in early middle age.[76] The incidence of breast cancer in affected females ranges from 22-50%.[76-78] Recent observations of early onset breast cancer among women with only subtle cutaneous manifestations of the disease raises concern that the syndrome may be unrecognized in many cases. The gene for Cowden disease was recently localized to chromosome 10q22-23 by linkage analysis.[79] Although presently a research tool, DNA-based predictive testing may soon be possible for informative families undergoing linkage analysis.

ATM, a gene that is mutated in the autosomal recessive disorder ataxia telangiectasia (AT), was identified on chromosome 11q22-23.[80] Homozygous AT is characterized by cerebellar degeneration, immunodeficiency, chromosomal instability, cancer predisposition, radiation sensitivity and cell cycle abnormalities. Heterozygotes for AT (estimated to be as frequent as 1% of the population) mildly manifest two of the disease characteristics: cancer predisposition and radiation sensitivity. Cancer predisposition in this group has been estimated to be about three- to four-fold that of the general population, with a relative risk for breast cancer in women carriers five-fold that of women with two normal copies of the ATM gene.[81,82] Genotypic studies of ATM in women with breast cancer are ongoing. Testing for germline mutations is restricted to the research setting at present.

Li-Fraumeni Syndrome family members are at significant risk for the development of several tumor types, particularly sarcomas, breast cancer, brain tumors, leukemias and adrenocorticocarcinomas. Germline *p53* gene mutations are implicated in this highly penetrant disorder (50% cancer incidence by age 30).[83] Testing for germline mutations has been undertaken in these rare families, modeled after the experience with genetic testing for Huntington's disease (HD).[84] Lessons from the HD experience served as an example upon which subsequent protocols for testing in other cancer predisposition syndromes have been developed.[85] Genetic testing for detection of germline *p53* mutations in these rare families is carried out in some research-based programs as well as through commercial testing programs. Increased surveillance for breast cancer is generally recommended for

women in LFS families. However, the efficacy of surveillance programs for the other diverse malignancies seen in LFS is uncertain.

Moderate risk loci and modifier genes

Rare variable number of tandem repeat (VNTR) alleles of the *HRAS1* gene confer a modest risk of breast cancer alone (two- to four-fold).[86] However, since these cancer-associated VNTR alleles are relatively prevalent in the population (3-6%), the attributable breast cancer burden may be as high as 9%. The value of knowing the allelotype at loci such as this is uncertain as an independent risk factor for individuals. An important question researchers are studying is whether interactions between moderate-risk loci such as *HRAS1* help explain the greater than 90% of breast cancer classified as sporadic disease. Another important question is whether these loci act as *modifier genes.* Thus far, differences in cancer penetrance and expressivity of breast and ovarian cancer among families with specific *BRCA1* mutations is not explained. However, one recent study indicated that the *HRAS1* locus may influence the penetrance of ovarian cancer among *BRCA1* mutation carriers.[87] A modifier locus (modifier of MIN, or MOM) was identified for the mouse model of hereditary polyposis (mouse intestinal neoplasia, MIN).[88] MOM influences the expression of polyps and neoplasia in animals with germline mutation of the murine homolog of the human *FAP* gene (mAPC).

Though not discussed here, there are also genetically determined differences in individual susceptibility to mutagens that could play a role in breast cancer risk. For example, cigarette smoking was recently implicated as a breast cancer risk factor for a subset of women with particular N-acetyl-transferase 2 isoenzymes that have a slower acetylation rate.[89]

CLINICAL APPLICATION OF CANCER GENETICS KNOWLEDGE

The opportunity to use emerging technologies based on our current understanding of the molecular genetic basis for some forms of inherited breast and ovarian cancer is exciting indeed. The most appropriate application of these new tools is not yet clearly defined. The basic elements of a genetic cancer risk assessment service are outlined in Table 10.4. To begin with, one must appreciate that a high-risk subset exists. The most important step is using family history as a clinical tool. In our own clinic we obtain at least a three generation pedigree, as well as additional information about reproductive history, diet and possible environmental exposures.[8] The pedigree is analyzed to determine if the pattern of cancers in the family is consistent with a genetic disorder. In many cases, family structure limits the amount of useful information available. This is compounded by the fact that sporadic cases of breast cancer are common. Therefore, identifying clinical features suggestive of hereditary disease, such as early-onset and/or multifocal cancer, is an important part of the analysis. Selection criteria for patients who may benefit from assessment and counseling are outlined below. In addition, information on ancestry can influence recommendations for genetic testing.

LABORATORY METHODS

Several techniques/strategies for detecting mutations in cancer genes have been adopted by different researchers and commercial vendors. These include methods for gene scanning (e g., single strand conformation polymorphism analysis (SSCP) or conformation sensitive gel electrophoresis (CSGE)) or heteroduplex analysis, assays designed to detect only specific mutations (allele-specific oligonucleotide hybridiza-tion assays, ASO), functional assays, such as the protein truncation test (PTT), and complete sequencing of coding exons and flanking splice junction sequences in PCR-amplified genomic DNA (for review, see Weber, BL 1996).[90] In an attempt to bring the economies of scale and automation to genetic testing, silicon chip-based technologies are being developed.[91] There are limitations to all these approaches. For example, virtually all these techniques will miss deleterious mutations in the upstream regulatory sequences of genes and may miss large deletions. There are examples of HBOC families with no detectable mutation in coding sequences but strong linkage to *BRCA1*.[92] Examination of mRNA revealed mono-allelic expression in the germline and loss of expression in tumors, implying a defect in gene regulation.

In general, discovery of an inactivating or "deleterious" mutation of either *BRCA1* or *BRCA2* is indicative of a high probability of developing breast and/or ovarian cancer, especially if the mutation is detected in affected family members. One of the greatest challenges is the interpretation of missense mutations. These mutations have been documented in several HBOC kindreds.[28] They are more likely to be of significance if the mutation is located in an evolutionarily conserved or functionally critical region of the protein. However, in many cases the clinical significance of the alteration depends on prior disease association (i.e., associated with disease previously in other families) and/or documented absence of the alteration in the general population. In the absence of a clear disease association it is often difficult to exclude the possibility that a given missense alteration simply represents

---

Table 10.4. Genetic cancer risk assessment components

a. Assess family history of cancer by formal pedigree analysis
b. Obtain epidemiologic data by questionnaire
c. Provide counseling and education
c. Obtain informed consent prior to collecting blood and/or tumor tissue for genetic testing
e. Provide post-test counseling, including discussion of management options

a rare polymorphism. The same can be said for minor DNA sequence variations that would not be expected to change the amino acid specified by the codon. A testing service may designate such changes as "genetic variants of uncertain significance."

There are several important considerations in choosing a genetic testing laboratory. They should have an American Board of Medical Genetics certified Director, and the laboratory should be CLIA (Clinical Laboratory Improvement Amendments of 1988)-approved. Protocols for the clinical validation of the genetic tests should receive the approval of an institutional review board, and quality control standards are essential. The sensitivity, specificity and positive predictive value (PPV) are all important measures. The PPV of a test depends on the prevalence of the disorder in the population being tested and is also influenced by incomplete penetrance.

Currently, three vendors offer analysis of *BRCA1* coding sequences. The Genetic Diagnostic Laboratory at the University of Pennsylvania uses CSGE analysis of PCR products of genomic DNA or cDNA to screen for mutations in BRCA1 on a fee-for-service basis. The first person in the family to be screened should be affected with breast or ovarian cancer, and they should have a family history suggestive of a dominantly inherited cancer susceptibility gene. Sequencing is used to identify the basis for any shifted bands. Myriad Genetic Laboratories, of Salt Lake City, uses automated sequencers for full sequence determination from both strands of genomic DNA representing the coding sequences and adjacent intronic splice junction sequences for both *BRCA1* and *BRCA2*. PCR amplification products from 83 reactions (35 for BRCA1 and 48 for BRCA2) are directly sequenced and compared with a consensus wild-type sequence to detect genetic variants. As for all the vendors, they concede that the assay will not detect deletion of complete exons or genes, or errors in RNA transcript processing unrelated to DNA exon sequence. Together these types of abnormalities are estimated to account for 5-15% of clinically significant

defects in *BRCA1* and *BRCA2*. OncorMed, based in Gaithersburg, MD, offers a staged analysis of *BRCA1* and *BRCA2*, beginning with a directed analysis (ASO) for several of the most common mutations (including the mutations prevalent in persons of Jewish decent) for a specified price. If no mutations are found in this initial screen, stage II analysis consists of a functional gene scanning methodology (PTT) which is estimated to pick up an additional 27-37% of mutations in *BRCA1* and *BRCA2*. For additional cost, stage III analysis (only available for *BRCA1* at the time of this writing) uses direct sequencing to detect an estimated 16% of alterations not detectable by the previous two approaches. The combined sensitivity of the three assays is claimed to approach 90%, with an inability to detect the same types of mutations missed by the other listed testing services. OncorMed, along with other vendors, also offers a directed assay called a "Heritage Panel" to screen for the three specific mutations that are prevalent in the Ashkenazi Jewish population. Since a directed assay is technically much easier to perform reliably, the cost is significantly less than that for complete gene screening.

Most protocols emphasize the importance of initially focusing genetic testing on family members with cancer, because of the limitations inherent in current mutation detection technologies. Even if one is convinced that a family has HBOC based on clinical criteria, there is only a 50% chance that an offspring or sibling of an affected patient will have inherited the deleterious allele. Therefore, only a positive test (detection of a known or likely deleterious mutation) is truly informative. Until the "familial mutation" is known, a negative test result could mean either of two things: the unaffected person being tested did not inherit the cancer susceptibility mutation or they inherited the disease associated gene but the mutation was not detectable by the methods used. However, in many cases there are no affected family members available for testing. In that case one may proceed, but only in the context of thorough counseling regarding the risks, benefits and *limitations* of genetic testing.

The rapid pace of research on the molecular genetics of cancer has garnered much attention from the media and consequently the lay public, resulting in many "worried well" individuals due to misinterpretation of scientific information. Unless there is suggestive family history, cancer susceptibility testing is not considered appropriate for screening unaffected individuals in the general population. However, an exception is testing unaffected persons in ethnic groups where specific ancestral mutations are prevalent.

Individuals who may benefit from genetic cancer risk assessment

Most patients will have family histories that do not suggest inheritance of an increased risk for cancer. Cancer screening for these patients should be based on current clinical practice guidelines and recommendations of national organizations such as the American Cancer Society. However, all patients should be asked about their extended family history because family structure may limit the usefulness of immediate family history or generations may be "skipped" if the cancer expression is sex-limited. Furthermore, the ethnic origin of a patient's ancestors could play a role in determining cancer risk. The following steps, designed to ascertain the contribution of family history to cancer risk, serve as an initial screen for patients that could benefit from genetic cancer risk assessment. This approach is not limited to breast cancer families.

STEP 1. Obtain accurate family history and construct a pedigree. Collect information on cancer(s) in the patient, their offspring, siblings, parents, aunts, uncles and grandparents.

For gender specific cancers such as breast, ovarian and prostate, one may need to collect cancer histories on more distant relatives. A family history of breast cancer on a patient's father's side could be missed in an initial family history.

STEP 2. Determine the number of relatives with cancer, biological relationship to the patient and the types of cancer in the family.

Is there a first degree relative (parent, sibling or offspring) with cancer? Are there two or more second degree relatives (aunts, uncles, grandparents) with cancer? Are there two or more relatives with the same type of cancer?

STEP 3. For affected relatives determine the age at cancer diagnosis and the occurrence of synchronous or metachronous tumors.

Is the age of onset unusually early? For example, breast cancer less than age 45 or colon cancer less than age 50.

Does one of the relatives have multiple primary malignancies?

STEP 4. Consider referral for comprehensive risk assessment for any two positive responses in step 2 or one positive response in both steps 2 and 3.

The American Society of Clinical Oncology (ASCO) recommends that cancer predisposition testing be offered only when: (1) the person has a strong family history of cancer or very early age of onset of disease; (2) the test can be adequately interpreted; (3) the results will influence the medical management of the patient or family member.[93]

Patients with only a single close relative affected, but exceptionally high levels of anxiety about cancer risk in spite of limited counseling, may benefit from more comprehensive counseling by a cancer genetics professional. In general, a reasonable threshold for offering genetic testing would be a prior probability of ≥ 20% that the disease occurring in the family or individual has a hereditary basis. The other setting where testing unaffected individuals with limited family history may be appropriate is if specific mutations are prevalent in a genetically homogenous population, such as persons of Ashkenazi Jewish decent.

Individual risk estimates for women undergoing genetic testing for cancer susceptibility

Attributable risk estimates for the development of breast cancer among women bearing BRCA gene mutations were largely derived from analysis of markedly affected families ascertained for linkage analysis. This was necessary in order to select for the most clearly identifiable phenotype, especially given that breast cancer is a relatively common disease in the general population. Several apparently sporadic cases have been documented in nonmutation carriers within families bearing *BRCA1* mutations.[37] Now that the genes responsible for the majority of families with HBOC are known, it is expected that less penetrant mutations will be discovered in people with less formidable pedigrees. Of concern is the fact that current technology misses 10-15% of pathologic alterations in *BRCA1* and *BRCA2*. Therefore, the meaning of a "negative" test will carry little weight in the setting of a strong family history. Conversely, the meaning of a positive test in the absence of a strong family history of cancer is unclear at present. These problems highlight the importance of encouraging anyone undergoing genetic testing for breast cancer susceptibility to participate in research studies designed to capture and correlate genotypic data with observations of clinical phenotype. In addition, studies of risk management strategies and outcome data are critical to define the optimal interventions.

Clinical management options in the face of inherited susceptibility to cancer

General guidelines for evaluation and management of genetic cancer risk may be drawn from clinical expertise, review of the literature, professional society position statements and from working group recommendations (for example; materials being developed by the Cancer Studies Consortium (ELSI Branch) Task Force on Preventive Recommendations. An example of how genetic testing can help members of a family with HBOC choose appropriate interventions is illustrated in Figure 10.2. The consultand (indicated by an arrow) was 47 years old and unaffected at the time of consultation, though she was certain she would develop cancer. She was contemplating both prophylactic mastectomy and oophorectomy because her mother and two of her sisters died of breast or ovarian cancer. She was also concerned about her own daughters' risk. A mutation in *BRCA1* (4184del4) had been found in her sister just prior to her death from breast cancer at age 50. After extensive counseling, the consultand decided to pursue genetic testing for the familial mutation. Fortunately, testing revealed that she did not carry the mutation. She canceled the surgical procedures after being told that her risk for breast or ovarian cancer was no more than that of the general population (11% and 1.6%, respectively). Moreover, she was relieved to learn that her daughters were not at increased risk either, since she had not inherited the familial mutation and thus could not pass it on to them. Other family members also came forward for testing. Her 45-year-old sister was found to carry the familial mutation (indicated by • in Fig. 10.2). Prior to counseling and testing she was so anxious about her cancer risk that she was unable to examine her own breasts. However, in spite of "bad news" about her carrier status, she was empowered to pursue appropriate interventions from the surveillance and preventive surgery options presented. Genetic testing had a real impact on health care decisions in this carefully counseled high-risk family and presumably reassured some individuals and spared them from unnecessary procedures.

The goal of increased surveillance is the detection of cancer at its most curable stage. Current recommendations for cancer screening, among women who are carriers of deleterious mutations in *BRCA1* or *BRCA2*, are outlined in Table 10.4. The relative merits and methods of screening for breast cancer in the general population are discussed at length in other chapters of this volume, so they will not be commented on

HEREDITARY BREAST AND OVARIAN CANCER

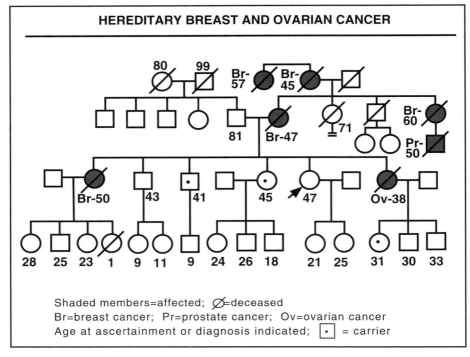

Shaded members=affected; ⌀=deceased
Br=breast cancer; Pr=prostate cancer; Ov=ovarian cancer
Age at ascertainment or diagnosis indicated; ⟨•⟩ = carrier

Fig. 10.2. Pedigree of a Hereditary Breast and Ovarian Cancer Family. Shaded members = affected; ⌀ = deceased; Br = breast cancer; Pr = prostate cancer; Ov = ovarian cancer. Age at ascertainment or diagnosis indicated; ⟨•⟩ = carrier; □ = male, ○ = female.

further here. Familial cancer patients present a special challenge. Increased density of breast tissue in premenopausal women may prevent adequate visualization by mammography. There are no controlled trials of mammography or prophylactic mastectomy that relate to women in the high-risk subset. Therefore, the options presented represent the state of knowledge and the best tools available at the present time. Anecdotal experience suggests that prophylactic or preventive surgery significantly decreases, but does not eliminate, the risk of developing breast cancer. The surgical technique for breast cancer risk reduction is simple mastectomy. Any skin-sparing techniques should involve the removal of all mammary tissue, including the nipple and areola.

There are currently no proven methods of screening for ovarian cancer. Although

of uncertain benefit, the techniques listed in Table 10.5 for early detection have been suggested for women at increased risk.

Although elevated CA125 levels are seen in 80% of advanced stage epithelial ovarian cancer cases, they are detectable in only 50% of stage I ovarian cancers. Moreover, false-positive elevations can be seen in benign disorders, such as endometriosis, uterine fibroids, pelvic inflammatory disease, biliary disease and in some nonovarian cancers. Ultrasound examination can often detect subtle alterations in ovarian architecture. The use of a transvaginal ultrasound probe is generally more sensitive than the transabdominal approach. However, false-positive scans are problematic, especially for premenopausal women where the detection of functional ovarian cysts may necessitate a period of heightened surveillance with follow up scans at a short interval. This can

Table 10.5. Risk management options for BRCA mutation carriers*

Recommended for breast cancer detection or prevention
- Monthly self-examination of the breasts beginning in late teen years

Beginning at age 25-35 (or at least 10 years before the earliest-onset cancer in the kindred):
- Clinician breast exam every 6 months
- Annual mammography

Discussed as options:
- Prophylactic bilateral simple mastectomy (± reconstruction)
- Participation in clinical trials for chemo-prevention (i.e., the BCPT)

Recommended for ovarian cancer detection or prevention
- Pelvic examination and PAP smear annually
- Serum CA125 annually
- Transvaginal ultrasound (TVUS) annually

Discussed as options:
- Prophylactic oophorectomy upon completion of childbearing
- Oral contraceptive use
- Reproductive counseling (?earlier childbearing)

*Also offered to women at increased risk because of their position in HBOC families, but for whom genotypic information is not available.

lead to increased anxiety in the individual. Furthermore, surgery (laparotomy or laparoscopy) is often necessary to evaluate unresolved abnormalities detected by ultrasound or CA125 testing. Most cases are revealed to be nonmalignant conditions.[94,95] Oral contraceptive use has been associated with a 40% reduction in risk of ovarian cancer in the general population,[96] but has never been studied in the setting of familial cancer. Men who are *BRCA* mutation carriers should be counseled about their increased risk (albeit modest) of developing prostate cancer. Options for prostate cancer screening generally conform to the American Cancer Society (ACS) guidelines: rectal examination and prostate specific antigen (PSA) level, annually, beginning at age 50. Similarly, because of the four-fold increased risk of colon cancer in both men and women carriers of *BRCA1* mutations, adherence to the relevant ACS colorectal cancer screening guidelines for the general public is recommended at a minimum. The guidelines call for flexible sigmoidoscopy every 3-5 years, beginning at age 50, as well as annual

testing of the stool for occult blood. Of course, women with normal *BRCA* genes still have at least the general population risk for breast cancer. Therefore, self-examination technique and ACS guidelines for breast cancer screening should be reviewed with all women.

How knowledge of genetic cancer risk could influence management of patients who already have breast cancer

The data from the Breast Cancer Linkage Consortium suggests that the cumulative risk of developing a second primary breast cancer is 65% by age 70 among *BRCA1* mutation carriers who have already had a breast cancer. Thus, knowledge of genetic status for a woman affected with breast cancer might influence the initial surgical approach (e.g., bilateral mastectomy instead of a more conservative procedure). Moreover, since ovarian cancer risk may be markedly increased in women with *BRCA1* mutations additional measures such as surveillance for presymptomatic detection of early-stage tumors or consideration of oophorectomy may be warranted. It is important to appreciate that elevated risk for ovarian cancer can be present in families who have not previously had anyone affected with ovarian cancer.

Potential benefits/potential harm from genetic testing

Genetic counseling for cancer risk assessment, based on advances in the molecular genetics knowledge base, has begun in earnest in many cancer centers. The ability to identify individuals at highest risk for cancer holds the promise of improved prevention and early detection of cancers. It is natural that consumers seek "testing" or clarification from their primary care physicians, who may not be prepared to address the complex issues surrounding genetic testing for cancer risk assessment. Most physicians have not had adequate genetics training in medical school. Further, increasing pressures for productivity in the context of managed care leaves little time for counseling patients. This problem is compounded by the rush of biotechnology concerns to market cancer susceptibility testing. There are potential medical, psychological and other personal risks that must be addressed in the context of informed consent for genetic testing. However, several barriers to identification and counseling of patients and families at risk abound. Chief among these barriers is the lack of access to competent counseling and education services that are equipped to handle the rapidly evolving medical, technological and ethical issues. Further, lack of understanding or even "disinformation" in the lay public, fears, adverse publicity and appropriate concerns about insurability or discrimination probably contribute to underutilization of existing services. Genetics professionals are rightly concerned that biotechnology companies may end up encouraging unproven clinical practices if educational measures and inclusive well-designed research protocols are not forthcoming.

Several professional associations and patient advocacy groups have issued policy statements in an effort to frame the issues and help shape clinical practice guidelines.

- National Advisory Council for Human Genome Research. Statement on the use of DNA testing for presymptomatic identification of cancer risk. JAMA 271:785, 1994
- National Breast Cancer Coalition. Presymptomatic genetic testing for heritable breast cancer risk. July, 1994
- Statement of the American Society of Human Genetics on genetic testing for breast and ovarian cancer patients. AJHG 55:i-iv, 1994
- Genetic discrimination and health insurance: an urgent need for reform. Policy forum: Recommendations. Science 270:391-393, 1995
- Statement of the American Society of Clinical Oncology: Genetic testing for cancer susceptibility. JCO 1996; 14:1730-1736.

Most of these groups acknowledge that assessment of inherited mutations of cancer predisposition genes will have a significant impact on the practice of clinical and preventive oncology. Given the daunting task of identifying and counseling the 5-10% of persons destined to develop breast cancer because of relatively penetrant genetic susceptibility traits, there are currently inadequate numbers of health care providers with cancer genetic counseling ability and experience. The problems associated with the evaluation and management of incompletely penetrant adult onset autosomal dominant disorders are many. Examples can be drawn from the experience with molecular diagnosis for Huntington's disease (HD), which is viewed as the paradigm for testing of late-onset disorders.[85] It is clear that there are many issues in common with genetic testing for cancer susceptibility, particularly the psychosocial consequences (increased anxiety, survivor guilt, etc.) and medico-legal issues (insurability, job discrimination). There is the often cited problem of the Tiresias complex: The blind sear Tiresias confronted Oedipus with the dilemma: 'It is but sorrow to be wise when wisdom profits not' (from Oedipus the King by Sophocles).[85] Some consumer advocates debate whether or not obtaining the knowledge of higher cancer risk alone is empowerment. However, in contrast to HD, cancer susceptibility conditions are generally incompletely penetrant, and surveillance methodologies exist which have presumed but unproven efficacy for early detection. In addition, preventive measures such as prophylactic surgery in selected cases, chemo-prevention (e.g., tamoxifen) or nutritional and lifestyle interventions may have a role in management of hereditary cancer risk. Therefore, cancer susceptibility testing is unique in the ability to potentially "offer something" to the consultand. Certainly there is a great need for clinical research to evaluate these options. Just as new chemotherapy regimens need to be applied first in the research setting, with informed consent of participants, before being incorporated into the practice of clinical oncology, so too do the new genetic risk assessment technologies.

The legal and privacy issues surrounding genetic testing are as complex as the testing technologies. Although several state laws regarding the privacy of medical information, genetic testing and insurance and employment discrimination have been passed, they vary widely. California, Colorado, Georgia, Minnesota, New Hampshire, New Jersey, Ohio, Oregon and Wisconsin have laws which prohibit insurers from requiring or requesting genetic tests and from using tests to determine premiums and benefits; similar legislation was recently pending in other states. Alabama, California, Florida, New York and North Carolina have laws in place which offer some protection to persons with specific genetic conditions such as the sickle-cell trait or Tay-Sachs disease. Maryland prohibits discrimination in insurance rates based on any trait unless there is actuarial justification. "The Health Insurance Portability and Accountability Act of 1996," US public law 104-191, stipulates that genetic information may not be treated as a preexisting condition in the absence of a diagnosis of the condition related to such information. Further, it prohibits group medical plans from basing rules for eligibility or costs for coverage on genetic information. However, the law does not address genetic privacy issues. Federal legislation is now pending that would govern ERISA as well as all other insurance plans. I would refer the reader to world wide web sites for government, the National Center for Human Genome Research (NCGR) and to breast cancer information services for updates.

SUMMARY

Genetic cancer risk assessment technologies have made the transition from the bench to the bedside. Hereditary forms of breast cancer constitute only approximately 7% of breast cancer cases overall.[97] However, the magnitude of the probability that a woman will develop cancer if she inherits a highly penetrant cancer gene mutation justifies the intense interest in predictive testing. Several genes can contribute to inherited susceptibility to breast cancer. Testing for *BRCA1* and *BRCA2* mutations, responsible for the majority of HBOC families, is now available commercially. There is clearly a potential to benefit carefully selected and counseled families who choose to undergo genetic testing. Numerous barriers to the application of this emerging technology exist. Identification of the correct syndrome is important (caveat: different genes can cause the same phenotype). Efficacy of the testing for a given gene (sensitivity, specificity and predictive value) influences the quality and surety of the advice one can offer. Psychologic, financial (insurability and cost) and social barriers exist that may preclude genetic testing in some cases. Legislation regarding insurance discrimination and privacy of genetic information is being crafted and debated at both the State and Federal level. Still, these exciting new technologies promise to change the face of preventive medicine. Education and adequately trained health care professionals are key elements to the successful integration of genetic cancer risk assessment into clinical practice. Studies of genotype-phenotype correlations and efficacious genetic testing techniques, along with the development of effective clinical screening modalities and preventive measures, are critical needs as we move into the 21st century.

ACKNOWLEDGMENTS

JNW is supported in part by Clinical Investigator Award #1 KO8 CA1574 from the NIH/NCI, and by a Breast Cancer Research Award from the Massachusetts Department of Public Health. I would like to thank Deborah MacDonald, R.N., M.S., and Pauli Morin for helpful comments on the manuscript.

REFERENCES

1. Knudson AG. Mutation and cancer: statistical study of retinoblastoma. Proc Natl Acad Sci USA 1971; 68:820-823.
2. Lee WH, Bookstein R, Hong F, Young LJ, Shew JY, Lee EY-HP. Human retinoblastoma susceptibility gene: cloning, identification, and sequence. Science 1987; 235:1394-1399.
3. Weinberg RA. The Rb gene and the negative regulation of cell growth. Blood 1989; 74:529-532.
4. Fung Y-KT, Murphree AL, T'Ang A, Qian J, Hinrichs SH, Benedict WF. Structural evidence for the authenticity of the human retinoblastoma gene. Science 1987; 236:1657-1661.
5. Weitzel JN. Cancer genetics. In: Diamond MPaD, A H ed. Infertility and Reproductive Medicine Clinics of North America. Philadelphia: Saunders, 1994: 121-142.
6. Albano WA, Lynch HT, Recabaren JA et al. Familial cancer in an oncology clinic. Cancer 1981; 47(May 1, 1981):2113-2118.
7. Parry DM, Berg K, Mulvihill JJ, Carter CL, Miller RW. Strategies for controlling cancer through genetics: Report of a workshop. Amer J Human Genetics 1987; 41:63-69.
8. Weitzel JN. Genetic counseling for familial cancer risk. Hospital Practice 1996; 31(2):57-69.
9. Slattery ML, Kerber RA. A comprehensive evaluation of family history and breast cancer risk: the Utah population database. JAMA 1993; 270:1563-1568.
10. Gail MH, Brinton LA, Byar DP et al. Projecting individualized probabilities of developing breast cancer for white females who are being examined annually. J Natl Cancer Inst 1989; 81:1879-1886.
11. McGuigan KA, Ganz PA, Breant C. Agreement between breast cancer risk estimation methods. J Natl Cancer Inst 1996; 88(18, Sept):1315-1317.
12. Claus EB, Risch N, Thompson WD. Autosomal dominant inheritance of early-onset breast cancer; implications for risk prediction. Cancer 1994; 73:643-651.
13. Hoskins KF, Stopfer JE, Calzone KA et al. Assessment and counseling for women with a family history fo breast cancer—a guide for clinicians. JAMA 1995; 273 (No.7):577-585.
14. Lynch HT, Smyrk TC, Watson P et al. Genetics, natural history, tumor spectrum, and pathology of hereditary nonpolyposis colorectal cancer: an updated review. Gastroenterology 1993; 104: 1535-1549.
15. Easton DF, Bishop DT, Ford D, Crockford GP, Consortium BCL. Genetic linkage analysis in familial breast and ovarian cancer: Results from 214 families. Amer J Human Genetics 1993; 52:678-701.
16. Claus EB, Risch N, Thompson WD, Carter D. Relationship between breast histopathology and family history of breast cancer. Cancer 1993; 71(1): 147-153.
17. Claus EB, Risch N, Thompson WD. Genetic analysis of breast cancer in the cancer and steroid hormone study. Amer J Human Genetics 1991; 48:232-242.
18. Hall JM, Lee MK, Newman B et al. Linkage of early-onset familial breast cancer to chromosome 17q21. Science 1990; 250:1684-1689.
19. Bowcock AM, Anderson LA, Friedman LS et al. THRA1 and D17S183 flank an interval of <4 cM for the breast-ovarian cancer gene (BRCA1) on chromosome 17q21. Amer J Human Genetics 1993; 52:718-722.
20. Chamberlain JS, Boehnke M, Frank TS et al. BRCA1 maps proximal to D17S579 on chromosome 17q21 by genetic analy-

sis. Amer J Human Genetics 1993; 52: 792-798.

21. Neuhausen SL, Marshall CJ. Loss of heterozygosity in familial tumors from three *BRCA1*-linked kindreds. Cancer Res 1994; 54:6069-6072.

22. Simard J, Feunteun J, Lenoir G et al. Genetic mapping of the breast-ovarian cancer syndrome to a small interval on chromosome 17q12-21: exclusion of candidate genes EDH17B2 and RARA. Human Molecular Genetics 1993; 2:1193-1199.

23. Bronner CE, Baker SM, Morrison PT et al. Mutation in the DNA mismatch repair gene homologue *hMLH 1* is associated with hereditary non-polyposis colon cancer. Nature 1994; 368:258-261.

24. Fishel R, Lescoe MK, Rao MRS et al. The human mutator gene homolog *MSH2* and its association with hereditary non-polyposis colon cancer. Cell 1993; 75: 1027-1038.

25. Miki Y, Swensen J, Shattuck-Eidens D et al. A strong candidate for the breast and ovarian cancer susceptibility gene *BRCA1*. Science 1994; 266:66-71.

26. Wooster R, Neuhausen SL, Mangion J et al. Localization of a breast cancer susceptibility gene, *BRCA2*, to chromosome 13q12-13. Science 1994; 265:2088-2090.

27. Easton DF, Narod SA, Ford D, Steel M. and the Breast Cancer Linkage Consortium. The genetic epidemiology of *BRCA1*. Lancet 1994; 344:761.

28. Shattuck-Eidens D, McClure M, Simard J et al. A collaborative survey of 80 mutations in the BRCA1 breast and ovarian cancer susceptibility gene: implications for presymptomatic testing and screening. JAMA 1995; 273:535-541.

29. Hogervorst FBL, Cornelis RS, Bout M et al. Rapid detection of *BRCA1* mutations by the protein truncation test. Nature Genetics 1995; 10:208-212.

30. Friedman LS, Szabo Cl, Ostermeyer EA et al. Novel inherited mutations and variable expressivity of BRCA1 alleles, including the founder mutation 185delAG in Ashkenazi Jewish families. Amer J Human Genetics 1995; 57:1284-1297.

31. Collins FS. *BRCA1*— Lots of mutations, lots of dilemmas. New Eng J Med 1996; 334:186-188.

32. Wooster R, Bignell G, Swift S et al. Identification of the breast cancer susceptibility gene *BRCA2*. Nature 1995; 378: 789-792.

33. Tavtigian SV, Simard J, Rommens J et al. The complete *BRCA2* gene and mutations in chromosome 13q-linked kindreds. Nature Genetics 1996; 12:333-337.

34. Phelan CM, Lancaster JM, Tonin P et al. Mutation analysis of the *BRCA2* gene in 49 site specific breast cancer families. Nature Genetics 1996; 13:120-122.

35. Couch FJ, Farid LM, DeShano ML et al. *BRCA2* germline mutations in male breast cancer cases and breast cancer families. Nature Genetics 1996; 13: 123-125.

36. Berman DB, Costalas J, Schultz DC, Grana G, Daly M, Godwin AK. A common mutation in BRCA2 that predisposes to a variety of cancers is found in both Jewish Ashkenazi and Non-Jewish individuals. Cancer Res 1996; 56(Aug): 3409-3414.

37. Narod SA, Ford D, Devilee P et al. Genetic heterogeneity of breast-ovarian cancer revisited. Amer J Human Genetics 1995; 57:957-958.

38. Ford D, Easton DF, Bishop DT, Narod SA, Goldgar DE, Consortium TBCL. Risks of cancer in *BRCA1*-mutation carriers. Lancet 1994; 343:692-695.

39. Narod SA, Ford D, Devilee P et al. An evaluation of genetic heterogeneity in 145 breast-ovarian cancer families. Amer J Human Genetics 1995; 56:254-264.

40. Simard J, Tonin P, Durocherl F et al. Common origins of *BRCA1* mutations in Canadian breast and ovarian cancer families. Nature Genetics 1994; 8: 392-398.

41. Johannsson O, Ostermeyer EA, Hakansson S et al. Founding *BRCA1* mutations in hereditary breast and ovarian cancer in Southern Sweden. Amer J Human Genetics 1996; 58:441-450.

42. Thorlacius S, Olafsdottir G, Tryggvadottir L, Neuhausen S, Jonasson J, Tavtigian S. A single BRCA2 mutation in male and female breast cancer families from Iceland with varied cancer phenotypes. Nature Genetics 1996; 13: 117-119.

43. Johannesdottir G, Gudmundsson J,

Bergthorsson J et al. High prevalence of the 999del5 mutation in Icelandic breast and ovarian cancer patients. Cancer Res 1996; 56:3663-3665.

44. Struewing JP, Abeliovich D, Peretz T et al. The carrier frequency of the *BRCA1* 185delAG mutation is approximately 1 percent in Ashkenazi Jewish individuals. Nature Genetics 1995; 11:198-200.

45. Risch N, de Leon D, Ozelius L et al. Genetic analysis of idiopathic torsion dystonia in Ashkenazi Jews and their recent descent fro ma small founder population. Nature Genetics 1995; 9(Feb): 152-159.

46. Neuhausen SL, Mazoyer S, Friedman L et al. Haplotype and phenotype analysis of six recurrent BRCA1 mutations in 61 families: results of an international study. Amer J Human Genetics 1996; 58: 271-280.

47. Motulsky AG. Jewish diseases and origins. Nature Genetics 1995; 9(Feb): 99-101.

48. Fitzgerald MG, MacDonald DJ, Krainer M et al. Germline *BRCA1* mutations in Jewish and non-Jewish women with early-onset breast cancer. New Eng J Med 1996; 334:143-149.

49. Neuhausen S, Gilewski T, Norton L et al. Recurrent *BRCA2* 6174delT mutations in Ashkenazi Jewish women affected by breast cancer. Nature Genetics 1996; 13:126-128.

50. Roa BB, Boyd AA, Volcik K, Richards CS. Ashkenazi Jewish population frequencies for common mutations in *BRCA1* and *BRCA2*. Nature Genetics 1996; 14:185-187.

51. Oddoux C, Struewing JP, Clayton CM et al. The carrier frequency of the *BRCA2* 6174delT mutation among Ashkenazi Jewish individuals is approximately 1%. Nature Genetics 1996; 14:188-190.

52. Tonin P, Weber B, Offit K et al. Frequency of recurrent BRCA1 and BRCA2 mutations in Ashkenazi Jewish breast cancer families. Nature Medicine 1996; 2:1179-1183.

53. Berman DB, Wagner-Costalas J, Schultz DC, Lynch HT, Daly M, Godwin AK. Two distinct origins of a common *brca1* mutation in breast-ovarian cancer families: a genetic study of 15 185delAG-mutation kindreds. Amer J Human Genetics 1996; 58:1166-1176.

54. Ramus SJ, S. FL, Gayther SA, Ponder BAJ. A breast/ovarian cancer patient with germline mutations in both *BRCA1* and *BRCA2*. Nature Genetics 1996; 15:14-15.

55. Muto MG, Cramer DW, Tangir J, Berkowitz R, Mok S. Frequency of the *BRCA1 185delAG* mutation among Jewish women with ovarian cancer and matched population controls. Cancer Res 1996; 56:1250-1252.

56. Modan B, Gak E, Sade-Bruchim RB et al. High frequency of *BRCA1* 185delAG mutation inovarian cancer in Israel. JAMA 1996; 276:1823-1825.

57. Eisinger L, Stoppa-Lyonnet D, Longy M et al. Germline mutation at BRCA1 affects the histoprognostic grade in hereditary breast cancer. Cancer Res 1996; 56:471-474.

58. Gayther SA, Warren W, Mazoyer S et al. Germline mutations of the BRCA1 gene in breast and ovarian cancer families provide evidence for a genotype-phenotype correlation. Nature Genetics 1995; 11:428-433.

59. Gayther SA, Mangion J, Russell P et al. Variation of risks of breast and ovarian cancer associated with different germline mutations of the *BRCA2* gene. Nature Genetics 1996; 15:103-105.

60. Rubin SC, Ivor B, Kian B et al. Clinical and pathological features of ovarian cancer in women with germline mutations of BRCA1. New Eng J Med 1996; 335:1413-1416.

61. Lynch PM. Hereditary nonpolyposis colorectal carcinoma (HNPCC): clinical application of molecular diagnostic testing. Annals of Medicine 1994; 26: 221-228.

62. Sankila R, Altonen LA, Jarvinen HJ, Mecklin J-P. Better survival rates in patients with MLH1-associated hereditary associated colorectal cancer. Gastroenterology 1996; 110:682-687.

63. Holt JT, Thompson ME, Szabo C et al. Growth retardation and tumor inhibition by *BRCA1*. Nature Genetics 1996; 12: 298-302.

64. Marquis ST, Rajan JV, Wynshaw-Boris A

et al. The developmental pattern of *Brca1* expression implies a role in differentiation of the breast and other tissues. Nature Genetics 1995; 11:17-26.

65. Gudas JM, Nguyen H, Li T, Cowan KH. Hormone-dependent regulation of BRCA1 in human breast cancer cells. Cancer Res 1995; 55:4561-4565.

66. Gowen LC, Johnson BL, Latour AM, Sulik KK, Koller BH. BRCA1 deficiency results in early embryonic lethality characterized by neuroepithelial abnormalities. Nature Genetics 1996; 12:191-194.

67. Boyd M, Harris F, McFarlane R, Davidson HR, Black DM. A human *BRCA1* gene knockout. Nature 1995; 375:541-542.

68. Ichii S, Takeda S, Horii A et al. Detailed analysis of genetic alterations in colorectal tumors from patients with and without familial adenomatous polyposis (FAP). Oncogene 1993; 8:2399-2405.

69. Futreal PA, Liu Q, Shattuck-Eidens D et al. *BRCA1* mutations in primary breast and ovarian carcinomas. Science 1994; 266:120-122.

70. Takahashi H, Behbakht K, McGovern PE et al. Mutation analysis of the BRCA1 gene in ovarian cancers. Cancer Res 1995; 55:2998-3002.

71. Lindblom A, Skoog L, Rotstein S, Werelius B, Larsson C, Nordenskjold M. Loss of heterozygosity in familial breast carcinomas. Cancer Res 1993; 53:4356-4361.

72. Easton DF, Ford D, Bishop DT, Corsortium* BCL. Breast and ovarian cancer incidence in BRCA1-mutation carriers. Amer J Human Genetics 1995; 56:265-271.

73. Chen Y, Chen C-F, Riley DJ et al. Aberrant subcellular localization of BRCA1 in breast cancer. Science 1995; 270:789-791.

74. Wu LC, Wang ZW, Tsan JT et al. Identification of a RING protein that can interact in vivo with the BRCA1 gene product. Nature Genetics 1996; 14:430-440.

75. Albrecht S, Haber RM, Goodman JC, Duvic M. Cowden syndrome and Lhermitte-Duclos disease. Cancer 1992; 70:869-876.

76. Brownstein MH, Wolf M, Bikowski JB. Cowden's disease: A cutaneous marker of breast cancer. Cancer 1978; 41:2393-2398.

77. Starink TM, Veen JPWVD, Arwert F et al. The Cowden syndrome: a clinical and genetic study in 21 patients. Clinical Genetics 1986; 29:222-233.

78. Walton BJ, Morain WD, Baughman RD, Jordan A, Crichlow RW. Cowden's disease: A further indication for prophylactic mastectomy. Surgery 1986; 99:82-86.

79. Nelen MR, Padberg GW, Peeters EAJ et al. Localization of the gene for Cowden disease to chromosome 1Oq22-23. Nature Genetics 1996; 13:114-116.

80. Savitsky K, Bar-Shira A, Gilad S et al. A single ataxia telangiectasia gene with a product similar to PI-3 kinase. Science 1995; 268:1749-1753.

81. Swift M, Reitnauer PJ, Morrell D, Chase CL. Breast and other cancers in families with ataxia-telangiectasia. New Eng J Med 1987; 316:1289-1294.

82. Swift M, Morrell D, Massey RB, Chase CL. Incidence of cancer in 161 families affected by ataxia-telangiectasia. New Eng J Med 1991; 325:1831-1836.

83. Malkin D, Li FP, Strong LC et al. Germline p53 mutations in a familial syndrome of breast cancer, sarcomas, and other neoplasms. Science 1990; 250:1233-1237.

84. Li FP, Garber JE, Friend SH et al. Recommendations on predictive testing for germline p53 mutations among cancer-prone individuals. J Natl Cancer Inst 1992; 84:1156-1160.

85. Wexler NS. The Tiresias complex: Huntington's disease as a paradigm of testing late-onset disorders. FASEB J. 1992; 6:2820-2825.

86. Krontiris TG, Devlin B, Karp DD, Robert NJ, Risch N. An association between the risk of cancer and mutations in the *HRAS1* minisatellite locus. The New Eng J Med 1993; 329:517-523.

87. Phelan CM, Rebbeck TR, Weber BL et al. Ovarian cancer risk in *BRCA1* carriers is modified by the *HRAS1* variable number of tandem repeat (VNTR) locus. Nature Genetics 1996; 12:309-311.

88. MacPhee M, Chepenik KP, Liddell RA, Nelson KK, Siracusa LD, Buchberg AM.

The secretory phospholipase A2 gene is a candidate for the *Mom1* locus, a major modifier of Apc^Min-induced intestinal neoplasia. Cell 1995; 81:957-966.

89. Ambrosome CB, Freudenheim JL, Graham S et al. Cigarette smoking, N-Acetyltransferase 2 genetic polymorphisms, and breast cancer risk. JAMA 1996; 276(No. 18):1494-1501.

90. Weber BL. Genetic testing for breast cancer. Scientific American Science & Medicine 1996; (Jan/Feb):12-21.

91. Hacia JG, Brody LC, Chee MS, Fodor SPA, Collins FS. Detection of heterozygous mutations in BRCA1 using high density oligonucleotide arrays and two-colour fluorescence analysis. Nature Genetics 1996; 14(Dec):441-447.

92. Serova O, Montagna M, Torchard D et al. A high incidence of BRCA1 mutations in 20 breast-ovarian cancer families. Amer J Human Genetics 1996; 58:42-51.

93. ASCO. Statement of the American Society of Clinical Oncology: genetic testing for cancer susceptibility. Journal of Clinical Oncology 1996; 14:1730-1736.

94. Muto MG, Cramer DW, Brown DL et al. Screening for ovarian cancer: The preliminary experience of a familial ovarian cancer center. Gynecologic Oncology 1993; 51:12-20.

95. Bourne TH, Whitehead MI, Campbell S, Roysto P, Bhan V, Collins WP. Ultrasound screening for familial ovarian cancer. Gynecologic Oncology 1991; 43:92-97.

96. Cash, Development TCaSHSotCfDCatNIoCHaH. The reduction in risk of ovarian cancer associated with oral-contraceptive use. New Eng J Med 1987; 316:650-655.

97. Claus E, Schildkraut J, Thompson W, Risch N. The genetic attributable risk of breast and ovarian cancer. Cancer 1996; 77:2318-2324.

CHAPTER 11

MANAGEMENT GUIDELINES FOR THE WOMAN AT INCREASED RISK FOR BREAST CANCER

S. Eva Singletary

INTRODUCTION

Deciding how to manage the woman at increased risk for breast cancer is an emotional and intellectual challenge for both the patient and the physician.[1-3] This chapter will outline the current approach to mammographic screening, elective (prophylactic) mastectomy and primary prevention strategies for the woman at increased risk.

MAMMOGRAPHIC SCREENING

Although annual mammographic screening in women 50 years of age or older has been shown to reduce breast cancer mortality by 25-30%, continued debate exists about the magnitude of benefit that mammographic screening provides for women younger than 50 years of age.[4-7] For young women who are known to be at increased risk for breast cancer, the prevalence of disease is increased and may approach the breast cancer prevalence seen in older populations.[8] The ability to image breast cancers in young women appears to be similar to that in older women even though the denseness of the breast tissue in young women can create problems with visualization.[9]

Early detection of small breast cancers by mammographic screening may lead to less radical surgery and possibly to a decrease in breast cancer mortality of a yet-undetermined degree, especially in women younger than 40 years of age. The disadvantages of mammographic screening in this young age group are the additional tests and biopsies for benign lesions, the possibility of overtreating a premalignant or low-grade in situ carcinoma that may be clinically insignificant, false reassurance from a negative mammogram or psychological distress from a false-positive mammogram, the possible lack of insurance coverage for screening mammography and potential cumulative radiation risk.[10-13] Although there are no current public health recommendations regarding mammographic screening in women who are heterozygotes for the ataxia telangiectasia (AT) gene, female AT heterozygotes are

---

Breast Cancer Screening, edited by Ismail Jatoi. © 1997 Landes Biosience.

estimated to have a six-fold increased risk of developing breast cancer after exposure to ionizing radiation compared with non-exposed controls.[14] Owing to the recent cloning of the AT gene,[15] identification of AT heterozygotes, who compose about 1% of the general population, may soon be feasible.

The first step in determining when to initiate and how often to perform mammographic screening is to obtain a valid estimate of a woman's lifetime probability of developing breast cancer. Many young women who are at increased risk for breast cancer overestimate their true risk by as much as 20 times.[13] The next step is to determine if the patient is attempting to become pregnant, is pregnant, or is lactating. Although minimal, any radiation dose to a fetus from screening mammography should be avoided. Imaging of lactating breasts often generates false-positive readings.

Annual mammographic screening beginning at age 30 may be considered in the following circumstances in asymptomatic women who are not pregnant or lactating but who are at high risk for breast cancer: (1) strong evidence of genetic predisposition or familial clustering, particularly with a family history of premenopausal breast cancer; (2) family history of breast cancer and a breast biopsy showing either lobular carcinoma in situ or proliferative disease with atypia; and (3) a Gail model risk score of five or greater.[16] In all other cases, routine mammographic screening should begin at age 40. Annual mammography should be sufficient unless an indeterminate low-risk mammographic abnormality is identified, in which case, an initial 6 month follow up study should be performed.

In addition to regular mammographic screening, all women should have regular thorough physical examination of the breasts and regional nodal basins by an experienced health-care provider. Although controversial, breast self-examination performed by the patient may be useful if the technique is properly taught to the motivated individual who prefers to take an active role in her health care.

Ultrasonography is not recommended for routine screening but should be performed if a mass lesion is detected on screening mammography. The imaging roles of magnetic resonance scans[17] and sestamibi scintigraphy[18] are still being explored.

ELECTIVE MASTECTOMY AND BREAST RECONSTRUCTION

Genetic testing to identify women who may carry genes such as *BRCA1, BRCA2, p53* or *ataxia telangiectasia* that substantially increase the risk of breast cancer has brought considerable attention to the role of elective (prophylactic) mastectomy. This procedure is controversial because it does not guarantee freedom from breast cancer. Experimental studies of elective mastectomy in rats given chemical carcinogens showed that tumors still occurred in residual breast tissue despite mastectomy.[19] Even in mice not exposed to mammary carcinogens, prophylactic mastectomies did not prevent the development of spontaneous breast malignancies.[20] Although a total mastectomy is defined as the complete removal of breast tissue, some breast tissue may still actually remain after mastectomy. Temple et al demonstrated that with careful pathologic examination of the chest wall and axilla in women who had undergone mastectomy for breast cancer, breast tissue could still be detected in the axilla and pectoralis fascia.[21] With less extensive subcutaneous mastectomies, subsequent invasive carcinomas have been reported in at least 1% of cases.[22-24] Thus, the term "prophylactic mastectomy" is misleading and should be replaced with "elective mastectomy."

The relative indications for elective mastectomy are given in Table 11.1. The first question to be addressed when elective mastectomy is being considered is whether the patient has an existing breast cancer. A careful history and physical examination with bilateral diagnostic (not screening) mammograms is essential.

If the diagnostic work up is negative, the next question is whether the patient understands her true risk for the development of breast cancer. Most patients overestimate

Table 11.1. Relative indications for elective mastectomy

1. Genetic carriers of *BRCA1, BRCA2, p53, ataxia telangiectasia,* or other predisposing genes
2. Family history consistent with a genetic pattern: family history of bilateral, premenopausal breast cancer in one or more first-degree relatives or multiple affected relatives in several generations
3. Family history of breast cancer in first-degree relative(s) plus a breast biopsy showing atypical hyperplasia
4. Past or current history of lobular carcinoma in situ
5. Difficult-to-examine breasts: significant scarring from repeated breast biopsies or multiple nodular densities and/or diffuse microcalcifications on mammograms
6. Asymmetry of the contralateral breast in patients who desire immediate or delayed breast reconstruction after mastectomy
7. Psychological disability due to extreme fear of breast cancer

their risk or fail to put their relative risk in proper perspective with other competing causes of health problems. The patient should be made aware that removal of both breasts will not necessarily prevent breast cancer. As elective mastectomy is an irreversible surgical procedure, the clinician must aid the patient in sorting out her emotional needs.[25] If the patient has any doubt about proceeding with elective mastectomy, she is not a candidate for this procedure. If unwarranted cancer phobia is present, psychological counseling is necessary to determine the appropriateness of the patient's level of anxiety about her cancer risk.

The third question that needs to be explored with the patient is whether she is interested in immediate breast reconstruction. If the answer is yes, the different types of reconstruction that are now available should be discussed. The two basic methods currently used for recreating a breast mound are saline- or silicone-filled implants and autogenous-tissue flaps.

The advantage of implants for immediate reconstruction is that they can be inserted at the time of mastectomy with minimal operative time and morbidity. The disadvantage of implants is the continual risk of implant failure in the form of infection, rupture, extrusion or capsular contracture. In a series of 300 breast recon-structions performed using tissue expanders and implants, the incidence of complications was as follows: significant capsular contracture, 5.8%; implant exposure, 5.1%; implant loss, 4.6%; deflation, 4.5%; and infection, 2.5%.[26] Another consideration with the use of implant reconstruction is the need to stretch the soft-tissue mastectomy skin flaps over 4-6 months to achieve enough skin laxity so that the implant has the correct cosmetic ptosis. This stretching process requires the patient to make numerous office visits for inflation of the tissue expander. Finally, the issue of whether implants contribute to or induce autoimmune disorders has created a great deal of patient anxiety, although no evidence thus far has confirmed a link between silicone implants and autoimmune diseases.[27-29] It should be remembered that even the saline-filled implants and tissue expanders have a silicone envelope so their long-term safety is also still controversial.

With the recent advances in autogenous-tissue reconstructions, more plastic surgeons and their patients are choosing this method of reconstruction. One of the most commonly used autogenous-tissue flaps is the transverse rectus abdominis myocutaneous (TRAM) flap.[30] In the conventional pedicled TRAM flap, the flap is transferred with the muscle pedicle based superiorly with the blood supply derived from perforating blood vessels of the underlying rectus abdominis muscle. Disadvantages of the pedicled TRAM flap technique include the sacrifice of most of the rectus muscle, which may result in abdominal wall weakness; possible flap ischemia since the major blood supply to the lower abdominal skin is from the inferior epigastric system rather than the superior epigastric vessels; and the bulge in the inframammary region from tunneling the flap to the chest wall area.

An alternative to the pedicled TRAM flap is to transfer the TRAM flap to the mastectomy site using a microvascular anastomosis of the inferior epigastric vessels to the thoracodorsal vessels in the axilla (free TRAM flap). This free-flap technique has the advantages of a more reliable blood supply, minimal rectus abdominis muscle resection and the elimination of the tunneling bulge (Fig. 11.1). The disadvantage is the risk of losing the entire flap if thrombosis of the microvascular anastomosis occurs. In the initial experience at The University of Texas M. D. Anderson Cancer Center, flap loss occurred in only 3 of 211 flaps in 163 patients (48 patients had bilateral reconstructions), for a 99% success rate.[31] No flap loss happened in the subsequent 162 flaps.[31] Fat necrosis (defined as persistent induration beyond 2 months after surgery) or partial flap loss from ischemia occurred in 7% of patients. This ischemia correlated with a history of cigarette smoking as 12 (12%) of 99 smokers had fat necrosis, compared with 3 (3%) of 112 nonsmokers.

Other tissue sources available for autogenous-tissue breast reconstruction include the extended latissimus dorsi flap,[32] the gluteal free flap[33] and the recently described "Ruben's fat pad" flap, which uses fatty tissue in the flank overlying the iliac crest.[34] The disadvantages of these flaps are possible donor site deformity and, in the case of the latter two flaps, technical difficulty.

Nipple reconstruction is performed after the edema of the reconstructed breast has resolved. The projection of the nipple can be recreated by the use of small local flaps elevated from the reconstructed breast

mound.[35] The areola is simulated with micropigmentation using a medical-grade tattoo.

Although today's new techniques of breast reconstruction allow creation of a simulated breast mound that is judged by clinicians to be cosmetically acceptable, the patient has to be the lifetime satisfied consumer. In one series,[36] 20% of women perceived their reconstructed breasts either were too small or were in the wrong position, and 60% reported a negative change in their sexual relationships. It is important that women realize that erogenous sensitivity will be absent from the reconstructed nipple-areola complex and that the reconstructed breast mound itself may be insensate. Finally, the patient has to answer the question of whether she would have any severe regrets about choosing elective mastectomies if the reconstruction failed. If the answer is yes, the patient is probably not a good candidate for elective mastectomy. In our experience at M. D. Anderson Cancer Center, the patient who initiates the discussion of elective mastectomy and is able to persist in her argument for this surgical procedure even as the clinician presents the disadvantages of elective mastectomy is the patient most likely to be content with this surgical option.

PRIMARY PREVENTION STRATEGIES

The ideal strategy after identifying women at high risk for breast cancer would be to eradicate or reduce this risk by primary prevention before the breast cancer actually occurred. Several pharmacologic agents for primary prevention are now under investigation: tamoxifen, retinoids and gonadotropin-releasing hormone agonists. As data collection and analysis are still ongoing, these agents should not be used as a preventive for women at increased risk for breast cancer except in the context of a clinical trial.

TAMOXIFEN

Tamoxifen is an antiestrogen that binds to the estrogen receptor of the cell, resulting

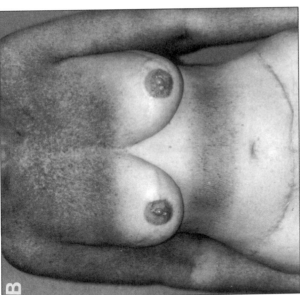

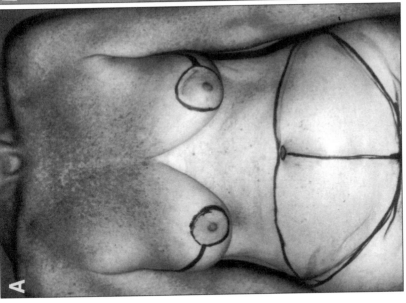

Fig. 11.1. (A) Patient with a history of lobular carcinoma in situ who elected bilateral total mastectomies with immediate reconstruction for treatment of invasive ductal carcinoma of the left breast. (B) Results of immediate breast reconstruction using a transverse rectus abdominis musculocutaneous free flap with microvascular anastomosis of the inferior epigastric vessels to the axillary thoracodorsal vessels. The nipple was reconstructed 6 weeks later using double opposing skin flaps from the breast mound area. Symmetry with the opposite nipple-areola complex was created by tattooing. Photographs reprinted with permission of Stephen S. Kroll, M.D., Department of Plastic Surgery, The University of Texas M.D. Anderson Cancer Center.

in a decrease in cell proliferation. Tamoxifen may also exert an effect on tumor cell growth by inducing transforming growth factor-beta, an inhibitor of epithelial cell growth, and by decreasing circulating insulin-like growth factor.[37] Tamoxifen has also been associated with an increase in circulating steroid hormone binding globulin that may decrease the availability of free estrogen.[37]

The growing interest in tamoxifen as a primary preventive agent for breast cancer developed from the observation that the incidence of contralateral breast cancer is reduced in patients receiving tamoxifen. In the meta-analysis of more than 18,000 women enrolled in 42 separate, randomized trials with a placebo control versus tamoxifen therapy, 184 cases (2.0%) of second primary breast cancer developed among 9,135 women treated with placebo, while 122 second primary breast cancers (1.3%) developed among 9,128 women who received 10-40 mg of tamoxifen daily for a median of 2 years.[38] This reduction in the incidence of contralateral breast cancer appeared to be related to duration of tamoxifen therapy. For women who received < 2 years of therapy, the actuarial risk of a second primary breast cancer was reduced by 26%; for women who received tamoxifen for exactly 2 years, the risk was reduced by 37%. The risk was reduced by 56% for women who received tamoxifen for > 2 years. No significant preventive benefit was detected for tamoxifen use of < 1 year.[39]

Before tamoxifen can be recommended for primary prevention of breast cancer in healthy women, the agent's long-term side effects and potential toxicity must be carefully weighed against the putative gains. Secondary advantages of tamoxifen may be its positive effect on cardiovascular disease and bone mineral density.

In the meta-analysis, the tamoxifen-treated group had a 12% reduction in nonbreast-cancer deaths and a 25% reduction in deaths due to cardiovascular events.[38] This reduction in mortality from cardiovascular disease[40,41] may be due in part to the observed decreases in low-density-lipoprotein cholesterol levels accompanied by either no change or an increase in high-density-lipoprotein cholesterol levels.[42,43] Studies have indicated that a 15-20% decrease in the low-density-lipoprotein cholesterol level may result in a 6-20% decrease in the incidence of coronary heart disease.[44,45] Unfortunately, tamoxifen's beneficial effect on a patient's lipid profile appears to reverse after cessation of tamoxifen use.[46] Another reported action of tamoxifen that may also be related to the drug's cardiovascular effect is a decrease of 16% or greater in fibrinogen levels with a 10% reduction in antithrombin III levels.[47] An inverse relationship between fibrinogen levels and myocardial infarctions and strokes has been proposed in population studies.[48,49]

The effect of tamoxifen in preserving bone mineral density in postmenopausal women is thought to be due to its estrogenic agonist effect on osteoclasts that slows bone resorption.[50,51] In vitro data demonstrated that tamoxifen can block bone resorption induced by parathyroid hormone, prostaglandin E2 and 1,25-dihydroxyvitamin D3.[52] In oophorectomized rats, tamoxifen was shown to block bone loss[53] and to increase osteoclast activity.[54] However, a troubling recent observation is that while tamoxifen increases bone mineral density in postmenopausal women by 1.8%, it may actually reduce bone mineral density in premenopausal women by 1.9%.[55]

Common side effects of tamoxifen therapy are hot flashes, nausea and vomiting.[56] Other less frequently reported adverse reactions include vaginal bleeding, vaginal discharge, weight gain, hirsutism, hair loss[57] and dry skin and skin rash.[55] In premenopausal women, tamoxifen may significantly increase estradiol levels[55] or cause amenorrhea, and rarely, ovarian cysts.[55] Other side effects that have been described include anorexia, depression, dizziness, thromboembolic events and retinal and corneal eye changes.[55]

Of most concern is whether tamoxifen may have carcinogenic properties. In animal studies, tamoxifen was shown to be a possible carcinogen for hepatocellular carcinoma.[58,59] There have also been preliminary reports of hepatic neoplasms in women receiving 40 mg of tamoxifen daily.[60] However, no increase in the incidence of hepatic neoplasms has yet been demonstrated in women receiving the standard dose of 20 mg daily. Similarly, the previously reported finding of a possible increased incidence of gastrointestinal neoplasms in women with prior exposure to tamoxifen[61] was not confirmed in the meta-analysis, which showed a reduction in the incidence of second primary malignancies except for endometrial carcinomas.

A definite association has been established between tamoxifen and an increased incidence of endometrial carcinoma. Initial data from the randomized trial from Sweden in which women received 40 mg of tamoxifen daily showed a 6.5-fold higher incidence of uterine tumors in the women who received tamoxifen than in those who received placebo. The cumulative frequency of uterine tumors (both endometrial carcinomas and uterine sarcomas) was 0.4% in the control group, 0.9% in women who received tamoxifen for 2 years and 5.5% in women who received tamoxifen for 5 years.[60,62] Initial results from the National Surgical Adjuvant Breast and Bowel Project trial B-14, which examined the benefit of adjuvant tamoxifen in women with node-negative breast cancer, also indicated a relative risk of 7.5 with the use of tamoxifen as compared to placebo.[63] The hazard rate was calculated to be 0.2 per 1,000 women in the placebo group and 1.6 per 1,000 women in the tamoxifen group. A subsequent analysis revealed more occurrences of endometrial carcinomas in the placebo group. This lowered the relative risk to approximately four.

The use of tamoxifen as a chemopreventive agent is currently being investigated in the ongoing National Surgical Adjuvant Breast and Bowel Project Prevention Trial P-01 which began in 1992.[64] In this prospective clinical trial, women at increased risk for breast cancer are randomly assigned to receive tamoxifen or a placebo for 5 years. This trial defines women at increased risk as women age 60 years or older or women between the ages of 35-59 who are at in-

creased risk as calculated by the Gail model.[16] The trial involves 16,000 women and will evaluate the effect of tamoxifen on the incidence of breast cancer, patients' lipid profile and bone mineral density, and the incidence of bone fractures. Patients without breast cancer should not be prescribed tamoxifen as a breast cancer preventive unless enrolled in a clinical study.

RETINOIDS

Retinyl acetate and the synthetic retinoid N-(4-hydroxyphenyl)-retinamide (4-HPR, fenretinide) have been shown to inhibit breast cancers that have been chemically induced in rats.[65] This tumor inhibition by 4-HPR was further potentiated when the rats were oophorectomized. Similar to tamoxifen, retinoids also induce the synthesis of transforming growth factor-beta and lower circulating levels of insulin-like growth factor-I.[66]

A phase III randomized trial was initiated in Italy in 1987 to evaluate the efficacy of 4-HPR in preventing second primary breast cancers in women with previous stage I disease.[67] Women were randomly assigned to either 4-HPR 200 mg/day for 5 years or no treatment. Accrual was completed in 1993 with 2,972 participants. An interim analysis[68] at a median follow up of 65 months suggests a treatment benefit in young, premenopausal patients. Side effects were reported in 10-20% of 4-HPR-treated women as compared to 2-5% of women in the control group. The most common toxicities noted were diminished visual adaptation to darkness, eye dryness, skin disorders and vague gastrointestinal symptoms. Whether a combination of tamoxifen and retinoids can further enhance inhibition of breast cancer development remains to be tested in clinical trials.[69]

GONADOTROPIN-RELEASING HORMONE AGONISTS

Several risk factors for breast cancer are mediated by the estrogen regulatory pathway (e.g., early age at menarche, late onset of menopause, older maternal age at first live birth). It has been proposed that continuous estrogen-related proliferation of breast epithelium without subsequent complete cellular differentiation may increase the risk of genetic errors.[70-72] A pilot trial using leuprolide acetate depot as a gonadotropin-releasing hormone agonist to suppress ovarian steroid production has produced favorable mammographic changes of decreased density of the imaged breast tissue.[71] However, low-dose replacement of conjugated estrogen and medroxyprogesterone acetate were added to ameliorate the hypoestrogenic effects of the leuprolide. An androgen was also included to protect against loss of bone density in the lumbar spine. Until more mature data are available, this approach should be used only in a closely monitored clinical trial.

CONCLUSION

Guidelines for the optimal management of women at increased risk of breast cancer are still evolving. The use of frequent and careful physical examinations and annual mammographic screening remains the current standard of care. The role of elective mastectomy is still unknown, but this procedure may be indicated in selected subgroups of women. Chemopreventive strategies should be explored in the setting of well-designed clinical trials.

REFERENCES

1. Vogel VG, Yeomans A, Higginbotham E. Clinical management of women at increased risk for breast cancer. Breast Cancer Res Treat 1993; 28:195-210.
2. Morrow M. Identification and management of women at increased risk for breast cancer development. Breast Cancer Res Treat 1994; 31:53-60.
3. Bilimoria M, Morrow M. The woman at increased risk for breast cancer: Evaluation and management strategies. CA Cancer J Clin 1995; 45:263-278.
4. Smart CR, Hendrick RE, Rutledge JH et al. Benefits of mammography screening in women ages 40 to 49 years—current evidence from randomized controlled trials. Cancer 1995; 75:1619-1626.
5. Vogel VG. Screening younger women at

risk for breast cancer. Monogr Natl Cancer Inst 1994; 16:55-60.
6. Miller AB, Baines CJ, To T et al. Canadian national breast screening study. 1. Breast cancer and death rates among women aged 40 to 49 years. Can Med Assoc J 1992; 147:1459-1476.
7. Sickles EA, Kopans DB. Deficiencies in the analysis of breast screening data. J Natl Cancer Inst 1993; 85:1621-1624.
8. Mettlin C. Breast cancer risk factors—contributions to planning breast cancer control. Cancer 1992; 69:1904-1910.
9. Meyer JE, Kopans DB, Oot R. Breast cancer visualized by mammography in patients under 35. Radiology 1983; 147:93-94.
10. Lerman C, Rimer B, Trock B et al. Psychological and behavioral implications of abnormal mammograms. Ann Intern Med 1991; 114:657-661.
11. Lerman C, Trock B, Rimer B et al. Psychological side-effects of breast cancer screening. Health Psychol 1991; 10:259-267.
12. Kash JM, Holland JC, Halper MS et al. Psychological distress and surveillance behaviors of women with a family history of breast cancer. J Natl Cancer Inst 1992; 84:24-30.
13. Blank WC, Nease RF Jr, Tostesm ANA. Perceptions of breast cancer risk and screening effectiveness in women younger than 50 years of age. J Natl Cancer Inst 1995; 87:720-731.
14. Swift M, Morrell D, Massey RB et al. Incidence of cancer in 161 families affected by ataxia telangiectasia. N Engl J Med 1991; 325:1831-1836.
15. Savitsky K, Bar-Shira A, Gilad S et al. A single ataxia telangiectasia gene with a product similar to PI-3 kinase. Science 1995; 268:1749-1753.
16. Gail MH, Bronton LA, Byar DP et al. Projecting individualized probabilities of developing breast cancer for white females who are being examined annually. J Natl Cancer Inst 1989; 81:1879-1886.
17. Lewis-Jones HG, Whitehouse GH, Leinster SJ. The role of MRI in the assessment of local recurrent breast carcinoma. Clin Radiol 1991; 43:197-204.
18. Kalkhali I. New horizons in breast im-

aging: A complementary role of technetium 99m sestamibi for the diagnosis and staging of breast carcinoma. Breast Journal 1996; 2:23-25.

19. Wong JH, Jackson CF, Swanson JS et al. Analysis of the risk reduction of prophylactic partial mastectomy in Sprague-Dawley rats with 7,12-dimethylbenzanthracene-induced breast cancer. Surgery 1986; 99:67-71.

20. Nelson H, Miller SH, Buck D et al. Effectiveness of prophylactic mastectomy in the prevention of breast tumors in C3H mice. Plast Reconstr Surg 1989; 83: 662-669.

21. Temple WJ, Lindsay RL, Magi E et al. Technical considerations for prophylactic mastectomy in patients at high risk for breast cancer. Am J Surg 1991; 161: 413-415.

22. Goodnight JE Jr, Quagliana JM, Morton DL. Failure of subcutaneous mastectomy to prevent the development of breast cancer. J Surg Oncol 1984; 26:198-201.

23. Pennisi VR, Capozzi A. Subcutaneous mastectomy data: A final statistical analysis of 1500 patients. Aesthetic Plast Surg 1989; 13:2115-2122.

24. Ziegler LD, Kroll SS. Primary breast cancer after prophylactic mastectomy. Am J Clin Oncol 1991; 14:451-454.

25. Kroll SS, Miller MJ, Schusterman MA et al. Rationale for elective contralateral mastectomy with immediate bilateral reconstruction. Ann Surg Oncol 1994; 1:457-461.

26. Gibney J: The long-term results of tissue expansion for breast reconstruction. Clin Plast Surg 1987; 14:509-518.

27. Kessler DA. The basis for the FDA's decision on breast implants. N Engl J Med 1992; 326:1713-1715.

28. Shons AR, Schubert W. Silicone breast implants and immune disease. Ann Plast Surg 1992; 28:491-501.

29. Varga J, Schumacher HR, Jimenez SA. Systemic sclerosis after augmentation mammoplasty with silicone implants. Ann Intern Med 1989; 111:377-383.

30. Hartrampf CR, Bennett GK. Autogenous tissue reconstruction in the mastectomy patient: A critical review of 300 patients. Ann Surg 1987; 205:508-518.

31. Schusterman MA, Kroll SS, Miller MJ et al. The free TRAM flap for breast reconstruction: One center's experience with 211 consecutive cases. Ann Plast Surg 1994; 32:234-241.

32. McCraw JB, Papp C, Edwards A et al. The autogenous latissimus breast reconstruction. Clin Plast Surg 1994; 21: 279-288.

33. Elliot LF, Beegle PH, Hartrampf CR Jr. The lateral transverse thigh flap, an alternative for autogenous-tissue breast reconstruction. Plast Reconstr Surg 1990; 85:169-178.

34. Hartrampf CR Jr, Noel RT, Drazan L et al. Ruben's fat pad for breast reconstruction: A peri-iliac soft-tissue free flap. Plast Reconstr Surg 1994; 93:402-407.

35. Kroll SS. Nipple and areolar reconstruction. In: Kroll SS, ed. Oncologic Plastic Surgery: Reconstructive Surgery for Cancer Patients. Philadelphia: Mosby, 1996: 314-318.

36. Wapnir IL, Rabinowitz B, Greco RS. A reappraisal of prophylactic mastectomy. Surg Gynecol Obstet 1990; 171:171-184.

37. Vogel VG. Tamoxifen for the prevention of breast cancer. In: DeVita VT Jr, Helman S, Rosenberg SA, eds. Important Advances in Oncology—1995. Philadelphia: J. B. Lippincott, 1995; 187-200.

38. Early Breast Cancer Trialists' Collaborative Group. Systemic treatment of early breast cancer by hormonal, cytotoxic, or immune therapy. 133 randomized trials involving 31,00 recurrences and 24,000 deaths among 75,000 women. Lancet 1992; 339:1-15.

39. Andersson M, Storm HH, Mouridsen HT. Carcinogenic effects of adjuvant tamoxifen treatment and radiotherapy for early breast cancer. Acta Oncol 1992; 31:259-263.

40. McDonald CC. Fatal myocardial infarction in the Scottish adjuvant tamoxifen trial. BMJ 1991; 303:435-437.

41. Rutqvist LE, Mattson A. Cardiac and thromboembolic morbidity among postmenopausal women with early-stage breast cancer in a randomized trial of adjuvant tamoxifen. J Natl Cancer Inst 1993; 85:1398-1406.

42. Bruning PF, Bonfrer JMG, Hart AAM et

al. Tamoxifen, serum lipoproteins and cardiovascular risk. Br J Cancer 1988; 58:497-499.

43. Love RR, Newcomb PA, Wiebe DA et al. Effects of tamoxifen therapy on lipid and lipoprotein levels in postmenopausal patients with node-negative breast cancer. J Natl Cancer Inst 1990; 82:1327-1332.

44. Bush T, Fried LP, Barrett-Connor E. Cholesterol, lipoprotein and coronary heart disease in women. Clin Chem 1988; 34:60-70.

45. Yusuf SA, Wittes J, Friedman L. Overview of results of randomized clinical trials in heart disease. II. Unstable angina, heart failure, primary prevention with aspirin and risk factor modification. JAMA 1988; 260:2259-2263.

46. Cuzick J, Allen D, Baum M et al. Long-term effects of tamoxifen—Biological Effects of Tamoxifen Working Party. Eur J Cancer 1993; 29:15-21.

47. Love RR, Wiebe DA, Newcomb PA et al. Effects of tamoxifen on cardiovascular risk factors in postmenopausal women. Ann Intern Med 1991; 115:860-864.

48. Kannel WB, Wolf PA, Castelli WP et al. Fibrinogen and risk of cardiovascular disease. JAMA 1987; 258:1183-1186.

49. Hoffman CJ, Miller RH, Lawson WE et al. Elevation of factor VII activity and mass in young adults at risk of ischemic heart disease. J Am Coll Cardiol 1989; 14:941-946.

50. Love RR, Mazess RB, Borden HS et al. Effects of tamoxifen on bone mineral density in postmenopausal women with breast cancer. N Engl J Med 1992; 326: 852-856.

51. Kristensen B, Ejlertsen B, Dalgaard P et al. Tamoxifen and bone metabolism in postmenopausal low-risk breast cancer patients: A randomized study. J Clin Oncol 1994; 12:992-997.

52. Stewart PJ, Stern PH. Effects of the antiestrogens tamoxifen and clomiphene on bone resorption in vitro. Endocrinology 1986; 118:125-131.

53. Jordan VC, Phelps E, Lingren JU. Effect of antiestrogens on bone in castrated and intact female rats. Breast Cancer Res Treat 1987; 10:31-35.

54. Turner RT, Wakley GK, Hannon KS et al. Tamoxifen inhibits osteoclast-mediated resorption of trabecular bone in ovarian hormone deficient rats. Endocrinology 1988; 122:1146-1150.

55. Powles TJ, Hickish TF, Kanis JA et al. Tamoxifen preserves bone mineral density in post-menopausal women but causes loss of bone density in premenopausal women. Proc Am Soc Clin Oncol 1995; 14:165.

56. Product Information: Nolvadex-ICI Pharma. In: Barnhart ER, ed. Physicians Desk Reference. Oradell, NJ: Medical Economics Company Inc., 1991:1070-1072.

57. Dukes MNG. Sex hormones: Tamoxifen. In: Dukes MNG, ed. Meyler's side effects of drugs: An encyclopedia of adverse drug reactions and interactions. New York: Elsevier, 1984; 773.

58. Hirsimaki P, Hirsimaki Y, Nieminen L et al. Tamoxifen induces hepatocellular carcinoma in rat liver: A 1-year study with two antiestrogens. Arch Toxicol 1993; 67:49-54.

59. Williams GM, Iatropoulos MJ, Djordjevic MV et al. The triphenylethylene drug tamoxifen is a strong liver carcinogen in the rat. Carcinogenesis 1993; 14:315-317.

60. Fornander T, Rutqvist LE, Cedermark B et al. Adjuvant tamoxifen in early breast cancer: Occurrence of new primary cancers. Lancet 1989; 1:117-120.

61. Rutqvist LE, Johansson H, Signomklao T et al. Adjuvant tamoxifen therapy for early stage breast cancer and second primary malignancy. J Natl Cancer Inst 1995; 87:645-651.

62. Fornander T, Hellstrom A-C, Moberger B. Descriptive clinicopathological study of 17 patients with endometrial cancer during or after adjuvant tamoxifen in early breast cancer. J Natl Cancer Inst 1993; 85:1850-1855.

63. Fisher B, Costantino JP, Redmond CK et al. Endometrial cancer in tamoxifen-treated breast cancer patients: Findings from the National Surgical Adjuvant Breast and Bowel Project (NSABP) B-14. J Natl Cancer Inst 1994; 86:527-537.

64. Nayfield SG, Karp JE, Ford LG et al. Potential role of tamoxifen in prevention of breast cancer. J Natl Cancer Inst

1991;83:1450-1459.

65. Vogel VG, Lippman SM, Boyd N. Is breast cancer preventable? Can J Oncol 1991; 1:28-37.

66. Torrisi R, Pensa F, Orengo MA et al. The synthetic retinoid fenretinide lowers plasma insulin-like growth factor I levels in breast cancer patients. Cancer Res 1993; 53:4769-4771.

67. Costa A, Formelli F, Chiesa F et al. Prospects of chemoprevention of human cancers with the synthetic retinoid fenretinide. Cancer Res 1994; 54:2032s-2037s.

68. Veronesi U, DePalo G, Costa A. Breast cancer prevention with retinoids. Ninth International Congress on Breast Disease. April 28-May 2, 1996. Houston, Texas. p. 118.

69. Ratco TA, Detrisac CJ, Dinger NM et al. Chemopreventive efficacy of combined retinoid and tamoxifen treatment following surgical excision of a primary cancer in female rats. Cancer Res 1989; 49: 4472-4476.

70. Spicer DV, Krecker EA, Pike MC. The endocrine prevention of breast cancer. Cancer Invest 1995; 13:495-504.

71. Spicer DV, Pike MC. Breast cancer prevention through modulation of endogenous hormones. Breast Cancer Res Treat 1993; 28:179-193.

72. Battersby A, Anderson TJ. Proliferative and secretory activity in the pregnant and lactating human breast. Virchows Arch 1988; 418:189-196.

INDEX

A

American Cancer Society, 11, 20, 26, 35, 53, 77, 144, 168, 171
American College of Radiology, 36
American Medical Association, 36
American Society of Clinical Oncology (ASCO), 168, 172
Ashkenazim, 159, 161-162, 167-168
Ataxia-telangiectasia (AT), 44, 165, 179-180
Autogenous-tissue reconstruction, 181

B

BARD1, 164
Biannual mammography, 60
Breast cancer
  age-adjusted incidence, 123
  biology of, 59, 111, 124
  early-onset, 158-159, 166
  later-onset, 158
  pharmacologic agents for the prevention of
    gonadotropin-releasing hormone agonists, 182
    Retinoids, 182, 185
  radiation-induced, 61
  stage creep, 118
Breast Cancer Detection Demonstration Project (BCD, 15, 43, 53-54, 57, 60, 67, 98, 100-101, 104, 121, 123-124
Breast cancer detection rate, 9, 40, 74, 100
Breast Cancer Information Core (BIC) database, 158, 161
Breast cancer mortality, 1, 10, 36-43, 46-47, 54, 56-59, 68-69, 72, 81, 86, 89, 90, 92-93, 120, 122-124, 136, 179
Breast Cancer Trialists Organization (BCTO), 124-125, 127
Breast self examination (BSE)
  component(s), 88
  technique, 88-89, 91

C

"Cancer control window", 65-66
Cigarette smoking, 165, 182
Comedo cancer(s) (low grade ductual invasive cancer), 5
Cowden disease, 157, 164, 165
Cure(s)
  actuarial, 113, 122, 125
  concept of, 113
  personal, 114, 125
  statistical, 114

D

DNA-based predictive testing, 165
DOM project, 57
Ductual carcinoma in situ (DCIS), 44-45

E

Epidemiology of screening, 5
Estrogen receptor positive tumor(s), 41
European Society of Mastology (EUSOMA), 35, 57

F

Familial adenomatous polyposis coli, 164
Familial retinoblastoma, 156
Family pedigree, 166, 168-170
Fast-growing tumors, 2
Finnish pilot screening program, 3
Forum on Breast Cancer Screening, 58

G

Gene(s)
  BRCA1, 155, 157-159, 161-167, 169, 171, 173, 180
  BRCA2, 155, 158-159, 162-163, 166-167, 169, 173, 180
Gothenburg study, 69